DPT:
A Shot in the Dark

DPT:
A SHOT
in the DARK

Harris L. Coulter
and Barbara Loe Fisher

Harcourt Brace Jovanovich, Publishers
San Diego · New York · London

Requests for permission to make copies of any part of the work
should be mailed to:
Permissions, Harcourt Brace Jovanovich, Publishers, Orlando,
Florida 32887

Most names and residences of parents interviewed for this
book have been changed.

Library of Congress Cataloging in Publication Data
Coulter, Harris L.
    DPT, a shot in the dark.
    Bibliography: p.
    1. Whooping-cough—Preventive inoculation—Complications
and sequelae.   2. DPT vaccine.   I. Fisher, Barbara Loe.
II. Title.   III. Title: D.P.T., a shot in the dark.
RA644.W6C68   1985   614.5′43   84-12933
ISBN 0-15-126481-3

Designed by Victoria Hartman
Printed in the United States of America

B C D E

The authors wish to thank the following for permission to quote from the sources listed:

From *Every Second Child* by Archie Kalokerinos, M.D., copyright © 1981 by Keats Publishing, Inc., New Canaan, CT, used with permission. Lines from "Ceremony After a Fire Raid" by Dylan Thomas, *Poems of Dylan Thomas*, copyright 1946 by New Directions Publishing Corporation, reprinted by permission of New Directions. Material reproduced from *Bulletin of World Health Organization* 59(1):9–15 (1981), C. R. Manclark. "Letter from Abroad—Campaign of Terror," *A. J. Dis. Child.* 137, September 1983, pp. 922–23. Lines from "A Prayer for My Daughter" from *The Poems* by W. B. Yeats, edited by Richard J. Finneran, copyright 1924 by Macmillan Publishing Co., Inc., renewed 1952 by Bertha Georgie Yeats. From "Division of Biologics Standards: The Boat That Never Rocked" by N. Wade, *Science*, Vol. 175, pp. 1225–30, 17 March 1972, copyright © 1972 by the American Association for the Advancement of Science. Quotations from Transcript No. 2042: "DPT Danger," MacNeil/Lehrer Newshour. Letter from Howard H. Frankel, Ph.D., excerpted by permission of *The New England Journal of Medicine* 301:3 (July 19, 1979), p. 159. Sentences from *Pediatric Red Book*, 19th edition, 1982. From the International Symposium on Combined Vaccines, 1967 (Marburg, FGR), *Symp. Series immunobiol. Standard.*, Vol. 7, pp. 21–28, George Dick, "Reactions to the Pertussis Component of Quadriple and Triple Vaccines." From "Illness After Whooping Cough Vaccination" by J. M. H. Hopper, *The Medical Officer*, October 20, 1961, pp. 241–44. From "Multiple Antigen Immunization of Infants against Poliomyelitis, Diphtheria, Pertussis, and Tetanus" by Clarence D. Barrett et al., *Pediatrics* 30 (1962), pp. 720–36, copyright © by the American Academy of Pediatrics. From "Diphtheria-Tetanus Toxoids-Pertussis Vaccination and Sudden Infant Deaths in Tennessee" commentary on Bernier, etc. by J. M. Garfunkel, p. 419, R. H. Bernier, et al., p. 421, *The Journal of Pediatrics* 101:419–421, 1982. From "Vaccine Reactions: The Challenge to Pediatricians" by Janice L. Cockrell, M.D., *Virginia Medical*, June 1982, pp. 380–81. From "Choruses from 'The Rock'" in *Collected Poems* 1909–1962 by T. S. Eliot, copyright 1936 by Harcourt Brace Jovanovich, Inc.; copyright © 1963, 1964 by T. S. Eliot, reprinted by permission of the publisher. From *Silent Spring* by Rachel Carson, copyright © 1962 by Rachel L. Carson, reprinted by permission of Houghton Mifflin Company. From *Whooping Cough: Reports from the Committee on Safety of Medicines and the Joint Committee on Vaccination and Immunization*, 1981, reproduced with permission of the Controller of Her Britannic Majesty's Stationery Office.

Julie Middlehurst-Schwartz was three years old when she died in status epilepticus in March 1984. The daughter of Jeffrey Schwartz and Donna Middlehurst, she went into her first grand mal convulsion within hours of her third DPT shot. From the day of that shot to the day of her death, she suffered with uncontrollable convulsions. But Julie, like so many vaccine-damaged children, never let the pain she did not understand break her spirit or take away her enthusiasm for life.

This book is for Julie, and for all the other children whose health has been destroyed or whose lives have been taken from them, and for their parents, who will always love them.

Contents

Acknowledgments

DPT: A Shot in the Dark was born out of a shared vision by parents, physicians, scientists, journalists, and others who recognized that public education about the pertussis vaccine would help prevent unnecessary vaccine damage. It could not have been written without the support of those who believed in the need to tell the pertussis vaccine story and also believed in us. To each of them, we owe our deepest gratitude for time freely given and encouragement provided during the years we wrote this book.

Most especially, we thank Paul McCluskey, our editor, without whose understanding and personal commitment this book would not have been published; Kathleen Bursley, for her professional expertise and the very special attention she gave to the manuscript; Claudia Menza, who recognized the importance of this book and carefully guided us through the publishing process; Kevin Geraghty, M.D., for his tireless dedication and hours spent reviewing the manuscript, and the excellent advice he offered; and Lea Thompson and the staff of WRC-TV in Washington, D.C., for having led the way with their landmark 1982 documentary, "DPT: Vaccine Roulette," which alerted American parents to the risks of pertussis vaccine.

We also want to acknowledge Justus Ström, M.D., Gordon Stewart, M.D., and Wolfgang Ehrengut, M.D., for their pioneering research; Anne Lambright, Monty Preiser, Andrew Dodd, Sid McMath, William Schroeder, Robert Kaufman, and Allen McDowell for their work on behalf of vaccine-damaged children; John Chriss Hoffman, J. Anthony Morris, Dan and Mary Resciniti, and Mary Alleshouse Koppel for their help at the beginning of our search for information; Senator Paula Hawkins for her concern for the health of children that led to congressional hearings on childhood vaccinations; as well as all those individuals who have tried for years to inform the public about vaccine risks and who have endured so much in their lonely struggle.

Separately, we would like to thank our personal friends and members of our family who contributed immeasurably to our well-being and made it possible for us to continue working under sometimes difficult circumstances. Barbara Loe Fisher thanks Gerrie, Janet, Wendy, Maryl, Kathi, and Susan for their steadfast friendship and words of encouragement. But most of all, she thanks her parents, Robert and Adah Loe, for always being there when she needed them and for providing love and care for her children during the writing of this book; her husband, Ken, for his moral support and endless patience; and her children, Christian and Ryan, who she hopes will forgive her for being so preoccupied during the past three years. Harris L. Coulter thanks his wife and children for listening patiently to an inordinate number of monologues on the pertussis vaccine while this book was being written.

Finally, the authors owe special gratitude to the more than one hundred mothers and fathers who selflessly shared their experiences with us so that fewer parents need suffer the pain of watching their once-healthy children die or become permanently brain damaged after a routine DPT vaccination. We will always be grateful to them and all the others who provided information to us during the research and writing of this book.

Note to Parents

This book is a compilation of information about a very controversial subject: the mass, mandatory use of the pertussis vaccine in the United States. It is not intended as medical advice. As with any medical procedure involving a child, parents should gather all available information and discuss the decision of whether or not to vaccinate with one or more doctors and in consideration of the laws of the state in which they reside. There is no substitute for informed medical opinion.

1

A Shot in the Dark?

Truth in all its kinds is most difficult to win and truth in
medicine is the most difficult of all.

Peter Mere Latham

T oday, nearly all our children get the DPT shot—D for diphtheria,
P for pertussis, or whooping cough, and T for tetanus. These three
different vaccines are combined into one shot to combat three dreaded
diseases that have, in past centuries, caused children to die or become
permanently handicapped.

We have been taught to believe in the wisdom of vaccination. But
how much do parents, or even scientists and doctors, really know about
the crippling side effects of vaccines? Particularly in the case of the
pertussis vaccine, which is supposed to protect against whooping cough,
are we giving our children a shot in the dark?

In the history of immunization, no vaccine has been as controversial
as the one for pertussis. It was designed to wipe out the ravaging
whooping cough epidemics that invaded turn-of-the century homes and
sometimes claimed the lives of every child in the household. Since its
development in the mid-1930s and its widespread use in the late 1950s,
the pertussis vaccine has been denounced and praised with equal zeal by
scientists and doctors in both America and Europe.

For the past half century, there have been repeated reports by parents and medical researchers that children were being permanently injured by the whooping cough vaccine and left with medication-resistant
convulsions, mental retardation, and physical handicaps. There have
been indications, although most government health authorities and
members of the medical establishment hotly deny them, that one cause

1

of the feared and unexplained Sudden Infant Death Syndrome (SIDS) is the pertussis vaccine administered to our newborns at two, four, and six months of age. Other researchers have theorized that the more subtle forms of damage caused by the vaccine may include varying degrees of learning disabilities and hyperactivity, although these suggestions also have been vehemently denied by most physicians.

At present, however, few doctors or government health officials deny that the pertussis vaccine can cause the following serious reactions: high fever (over 103 degrees Fahrenheit); convulsions (with or without a fever); unusual high-pitched screaming; persistent crying for many hours during which the child cannot be comforted; excessive somnolence (a deep sleep from which the child can only be awakened with great difficulty); collapse (a sudden loss of consciousness); encephalopathy (brain damage); and death.

All these serious reactions are documented in the scientific literature and most are mentioned in guidelines produced for doctors by the American Medical Association (AMA), American Academy of Pediatrics (AAP), the Centers for Disease Control (CDC), and vaccine manufacturers. But how many American parents are aware that their child can die or become brain damaged after a serious reaction to a DPT shot? How many parents have been told to watch their child carefully after a DPT shot for evidence of these serious reactions? How many know that a child who suffers any one of these reactions should never again receive the P, or pertussis, portion and should only be given the DT (diphtheria and tetanus) shot thereafter?

The pertussis vaccine story is a dramatic one that reveals a puzzling half century of silence on the part of the physicians, scientists, drug manufacturers, and government health agencies responsible for developing, testing, and setting vaccine policy. They have essentially kept the facts about the pertussis vaccine from the American public. Very few Americans know that some Western European countries have stopped recommending mass immunization with the pertussis vaccine because they have decided the risk of vaccine damage is greater than the risk of catching the milder form of whooping cough prevalent in developed nations today.

This is an alarming story of ignorance, and in some cases negligence, on the part of American physicians who give the pertussis vaccine to our children. This reality is made painfully clear when parents tell how their children were injured by repeated injections of pertussis vaccine even after severe reactions to previous DPT shots.

It is a frustrating story of the curious failure by American scientists to produce a safer pertussis vaccine even though Japan has developed and used a safer vaccine for several years. It is a disturbing story of big-name drug manufacturers treating the vaccine as merely another commercial product while failing to adequately monitor adverse reactions. Yet the costs of producing the pertussis vaccine are rising steeply as parents seek financial compensation for their vaccine-damaged children and, in June 1984, a leading DPT manufacturer abruptly withdrew from the pertussis vaccine market.

It is a frightening story of our federal health agencies aggressively promoting a vaccine they know to be highly reactive but failing to organize a credible national adverse reaction reporting system to assess the true incidence of permanent vaccine damage; failing to conduct large-scale clinical tests for safety; failing to improve the laboratory tests for vaccine potency and toxicity; and ignoring information about vaccine reactions.

It is a thought-provoking story of how our state governments, whose constitutions are founded on individual rights, have passed laws requiring every American child to be injected with a vaccine of unknown toxicity before attending school, thereby abolishing a parent's right to freely choose whether or not a child should be vaccinated. How many Americans know that the countries in Eastern Europe have mandatory pertussis vaccination laws while most countries in Western Europe do not?

And finally, this is a profoundly moving story of the true victims of this medical scandal: the unknown numbers of vaccine-damaged children and their parents who, like soldiers in a terrible war, have given their lives for a society that refuses to accept any responsibility for the sacrifice it has required them to make.

In the following pages, parents explain what happened to their once-healthy children after being given one of the five DPT shots routinely administered to nearly 96 percent of American children. This is their story and they share it in the hope that other children will be saved from death and handicap because those who read it, parents and doctors alike, will come away better informed and with an understanding that this kind of tragedy must not happen again.

2

Profile:
Forgive Us Your Death

> Forgive
> Us forgive
> Us your death that myselves the believers
> May hold it in a great flood
> Till the blood shall spurt,
> And the dust shall sing like a bird
> As the grains blow, as your death grows,
>   through our heart.
>   *Dylan Thomas*

"It was January 12, 1983, and I was getting ready to take my two-month-old son, Richie, to the pediatrician for his checkup," Janet recalled. "My sister-in-law called and asked me if I had watched the *Phil Donahue Show* on the side effects of vaccines that morning. I told her I hadn't had time to watch it, but that I'd call her later to learn more."

In two months, Richie's weight had climbed to eleven pounds, nine ounces from his six-pound, six-ounce, birth weight. He frequently had loose stools the first eight days after he came home from the hospital until his formula was changed to plain Similac without iron and the loose stools stopped. He was a good eater and very even-tempered, despite a nagging problem with gas that had prompted Janet's pediatrician to put him on the antiflatulent Mylicon. An alert and active baby, he was awake more than most newborns during the day and wanted to eat several times a night.

4

"Well, I can't find anything wrong with this baby," Janet's pediatrician said, after checking Richie over. He proceeded to give Richie his first DPT shot and oral polio vaccine and told Janet to "give him half a baby aspirin or children's Tylenol in four hours."

"I knew the DPT shots produced a lot of discomfort," Janet admitted, "because my five-year-old son, Ryan, had terrible problems with all his DPT shots. After Ryan's first DPT shot, his leg got red and hot and swollen from the hip to the knee. It was so swollen, I was worried about the circulation in his leg. His temperature always zoomed to over 103 degrees and he screamed uncontrollably. Nothing could stop his screaming. He also had diarrhea and vomiting. All this lasted for about forty-eight hours after each shot. When I phoned my pediatrician to report on Ryan's condition and asked what I should do, he always told me it was a normal reaction to the DPT shot and not to worry."

A licensed practical nurse, Janet works on the orthopedic-neurology floor of a community hospital. While she has received an education in nursing and has practiced for five years, she says she was never informed about adverse reactions or contraindications to vaccines in nursing school.

"We were never taught about reactions to vaccines, and I have asked my friends who are RN's if they were taught about vaccine reactions or which children should not receive the vaccines, and they have all said no. Some of them have advanced degrees. From what I know now about the pertussis vaccine, my pediatrician should have reviewed our family history, which includes epilepsy, deafness, and blindness caused by unexplained neurologic damage, Bell's Palsy, rheumatic heart disease, diabetes, and allergies including milk intolerance, and migraine headaches before he gave either of my sons the pertussis vaccine. He never discussed it with me."

Janet trusted her pediatrician when he said that Ryan's violent reactions to his DPT shots were normal. She had no reason to suspect they were not.

Janet remembers taking Richie home, hoping his reaction to his first DPT shot would not be as bad as his older brother's had been. By that evening, however, Richie's hip had started to swell just like Ryan's had after his shots. But Richie's hip then turned from red to dark purple, and later, the purple started to spread out from the site of the injection in round patches. Richie did not have a fever and drank from his bottle, but he cried if Janet touched his leg.

"He woke up about one-thirty in the middle of the night crying," Janet said. "After a couple of sucks on the bottle he went back to sleep until six that morning. When he woke up, he started screaming off and on. He sounded like a cat in pain. His scream was high and forceful, and then he would fall asleep. I put a soft blanket underneath him because I figured his hip was bothering him."

By seven-thirty in the morning, he was crying again. Janet picked him up and he was limp. His cry was weak now, and he seemed unable to hold his head up. "I fed him a little cereal, and he took a whole bottle of formula and fell back to sleep. I thought it was strange because he usually was awake at this time in the morning. But I put it down to the shot and didn't worry."

About eight-thirty, Janet was drinking coffee, and she heard Richie give out a tremendous explosion of gas into his diapers. "I knew he was having diarrhea, but I wondered why he didn't wake up because he hated to have anything in his diapers. I woke him up and changed him. His diapers were full of light brownish diarrhea with a lot of mucus. He fell asleep again for about two hours and woke up crying. When I picked him up, he was completely soaked through two receiving blankets. I have never seen a baby soaked like that. The odor was musty and pungent, a smell I will never forget."

Janet gave Richie a bath to wash him off. "He was limp and he just stared at me with dark eyes as if he was mad at me. I noticed his little hands were ice-cold from the wrists down. It was winter, and I thought his hands were cold from the bath I was giving him or maybe I had the heat turned too low."

Janet got Richie dressed and put socks on his hands to keep them warm. She gave him eight ounces of warm water, which he drank more slowly than usual. In the afternoon, Janet changed three more diapers, all of them containing yellow diarrhea. In each diaper, however, the amount of diarrhea was less. Richie's leg still seemed to hurt him, and his fingers twitched a little while he slept.

"I did not call the doctor," Janet explained, "because Richie had the exact same symptoms as Ryan earlier had had with his shots—strange crying alternating with unusual amounts of sleeping, diarrhea, and a red, swollen leg. The only difference was that Richie slept more and did not have a fever, and I was thankful for that because I know a high fever can produce febrile convulsions. In fact, he was on the cool side, and I made sure I kept him dressed warmly after I noticed his hands were cold. The whole day I kept giving Richie his bottle. I just didn't realize what was happening to him."

At four o'clock that afternoon, Richie vomited a little. He had gagged on the nipple of the bottle, and so Janet spoon-fed him water to keep fluids in his body. "I tickled his lips with my finger, and he didn't smile at me like he usually did. He just kept staring at me with dark eyes like he was mad at me."

At eight o'clock that evening, Richie still did not have a fever and his hands were still cold. Janet's husband, Anthony, changed another diaper with a small amount of diarrhea in it while Janet was at the drugstore buying Pedialyte for Richie. At ten forty-five, she woke her baby up and started to give him a bottle.

"He took two sucks. His eyes were open. All of a sudden he stopped sucking. I shook his shoulder, and called his name. He didn't respond to me. I put my lips to his forehead, and he was ice cold and clammy. Then he started sighing. With each breath, he made a sighing sound."

With Richie in her arms, Janet ran and told her husband there was something wrong with their baby. Anthony held Richie while Janet called her doctor's answering service and explained to the pediatrician on call that Richie had had his first DPT shot the day before. She told him all the symptoms Richie had shown since then.

"I told him everything that had happened to Richie since he got his shot the day before," Janet said. "He didn't sound worried and agreed that it was probably a DPT reaction. While I was talking to him, Anthony came into the room and held Richie under the kitchen light, and I noticed Richie's pupils were not responding to the light. I told the doctor that, too. He told me that if I wanted to, I could take him to the hospital and have him checked over. I said yes, I would, and asked him if he was going to meet us there. He said, no, it wasn't necessary, that someone else would check Richie and call him back with the results.

"He didn't tell me to call an ambulance and rush him to the nearest hospital. He just wasn't that concerned about the symptoms I described," Janet recalled. She hung up with a feeling of foreboding that she could not shake.

Anthony and Janet decided they had better get Richie to the hospital immediately. Anthony hurriedly dressed and left to warm up the car while Janet rushed into Ryan's bedroom and woke him up. Then she ran into her bedroom and laid Richie on the bed so she could get dressed to go to the hospital. Five-year-old Ryan came into Janet's bedroom and watched his baby brother, who was lying on the bed staring at the ceiling and sighing.

"I picked Richie up, and he stopped breathing. I screamed for Anthony and breathed into Richie's mouth but there was no response. I ran down to the dining room and started to perform CPR [cardiopulmonary resuscitation] on him while Anthony called the ambulance. I kept doing CPR, and all of a sudden vomit started to fly out of his mouth. I turned him over and clapped him on the back to clear his breathing passages. Then I continued the CPR. The ambulance came, and the paramedics continued the CPR. I knew my baby was gone. I kept screaming he was dead. When he had stopped breathing in my arms, all of a sudden, the whole day came together like one big nightmare. He had been dying all day, and I didn't even know it."

Richie had died thirty-three hours after he received his first DPT shot. When the emergency-room doctor pronounced Richie dead, Janet told the nurses to call her pediatrician.

"The first thing I said to him was, 'Why didn't you tell me that the vaccine could do this to my baby?' And he said, 'Oh, the vaccine couldn't have done this to your baby.' And I said, 'Don't tell me that. My son Ryan had the same reactions. He had diarrhea and. . . .' He cut me off. 'The vaccine doesn't cause diarrhea,' he said. I asked him, 'If the DPT shot doesn't cause diarrhea, then why did both of my sons react with diarrhea within a day of their DPT shots?'"

Weeks after Richie had died, one of Janet's friends said to her, "Janet, if the baby had awakened that morning and he hadn't had a DPT shot the day before and he had exhibited all the symptoms he had on the day he died, would you have called the doctor?"

"I thought to myself, my God, of course I would have called the doctor in a minute if Richie had not had the DPT shot the day before and I had not assumed he was having a normal reaction to the shot. We have been told that these reactions to vaccines are normal. We are so conditioned to that idea and to the idea that our doctor's word is to be trusted without question that we don't think for ourselves. I am a nurse. I watched my son die that day, and I didn't even know what was happening until it was all over."

❋ ❋ ❋ ❋ ❋

She is model-thin, a pretty twenty-seven year old with wide-set blue-green eyes and brown hair that would fall to her waist if she didn't tie it back. There is a toughness and cheerful resilience about her if you don't look too deep. When you do, you perceive the fresh pain that lies just beneath the surface of her self-confidence.

"Richie's death was my greatest fear come true. His death took everything from me. It stripped my insides. If you have ever thought of what it would be like to lose a child, it is worse than you could ever imagine," Janet says steadily.

It has been six months since her son died and the thoughts and feelings tumble out of her, one on top of another. "If this had not happened to my baby, I would still be part of the uninformed public. I would still be taking my doctor's word as the word of God, like most mothers do."

Her story of the events following Richie's death is, in a sense, as alarming as the story of the death itself. It raises as many questions about routine autopsy procedures and findings as it does about doctors' basic understanding of the pertussis vaccine.

After Richie's death, Janet and Anthony were first told that the autopsy report would take six to eight weeks to complete. After eight weeks, Janet and Anthony started calling the coroner's office to find out where the report was.

"After the fourteenth week, I was told it could take six months to a year to get an autopsy report because of the paperwork involved. In all this time, nobody bothered to ask me exactly what happened to my son during the thirty-three hours before he died. So I called the coroner and asked him if he wanted to know the facts before he determined the cause of death. He said to me, 'Talking about babies dying over the phone really makes me squeamish,' and I asked him, 'How do you think it makes me feel?' "

When the autopsy report finally appeared, it was surprisingly brief. The final diagnosis was hyperplasia (enlargement) of the thymus gland, the gland that helps regulate the immune response in the body. Also noted were congestion and edema in the lungs and brain. Janet and Anthony then set up a meeting with the coroner to discuss the autopsy report.

When they entered the coroner's office, a nurse handed Janet an article entitled "The Pathologist and the Sudden Infant Death Syndrome (SIDS)" and told her to read it. Janet refused. Then the coroner started reading out loud to her from the article. She interrupted him. " 'My son did not die a SIDS death,' I told him. Then I said, 'Now I am going to tell you what happened in the thirty-three hours following Richie's first DPT shot.' I told him, and he listened. He then wrote down on the death certificate, 'death due to irreversible shock.' When I asked him what caused the shock, he said the best he could do was to write down that the shock was due to a 'possible' DPT reaction."

Janet asked the coroner why he could not state point-blank that Richie's death was due to a DPT shot reaction, when it was obvious. She produced the *Physician's Desk Reference* (PDR) and read him the portion pertaining to pertussis vaccine reactions. The PDR was one of the many medical references and scientific articles Janet had read since Richie's death.

"He said he couldn't write down on the death certificate that Richie had died from a DPT reaction because 'the state's standing on immunizations would be in an uproar.' Besides, he said, it would be unscientific because the autopsy report was not specific enough about the cause of death. At that point, we discussed the specific, scientific definition of SIDS. Finally, he admitted that my son had died from 'irreversible shock' due to a 'probable reaction to DPT.'"

The coroner gave Janet and Anthony a note exempting any future children they might have from receiving the pertussis vaccine. Three weeks later he gave them a signed "query of death" stating the official cause of death, which was that Richie died from "irreversible shock" due to a "probable reaction to DPT." About two and a half months later, they discovered that Richie's official death certificate had not yet been filed by the coroner at the town clerk's office.

"We kept waiting for the state to send us an official death certificate and when we didn't get one, we called the town clerk's office and discovered that the official cause of death had never been filed by the coroner with the registrar. After we gave the registrar the signed 'query of death' given to us by the coroner more than two months before, listing the cause of Richie's death, we received an official death certificate the next day."

Janet recently spoke with her county health commissioner and asked if the county was aware of the coroner's report and the official cause of Richie's death. "The commissioner told me that she was not aware of the official cause of death, although she had heard that my son died soon after a DPT shot. She admitted that there is no follow-up on reports of adverse vaccine reactions or deaths immediately following immunization by state or county health officials," Janet said.

"You see, at the time of Richie's death, my husband and I were very concerned that Richie might have reacted to a bad lot of DPT vaccine. We wanted the vaccine preserved for analysis to find out if there was something wrong with it, but to our knowledge nothing was done. We were concerned that other children might receive the same vaccine, and we felt it should be investigated."

The commissioner also told Janet that it costs the state and private pediatricians a great deal of money to spend office time to educate parents about adverse reactions to vaccines. "She told me that it costs the state health clinics fifty-five dollars per child to explain to the mothers about reactions and have them sign the consent forms that are required by law in public health clinics. But it costs a private pediatrician only twenty-five dollars to give the same vaccine to a child because private doctors are not federally required to inform parents about reactions and have them sign a consent form. She said, 'Doctors are not paid to educate parents. They are paid to give vaccinations. Besides, most parents do not want to know about adverse reactions because it puts the responsibility in their laps and they don't want to have to deal with it.' "

Janet was in a state of shock for weeks after Richie's death. She could not drive a car or make the simplest decision without help. Anxiety attacks made it difficult for her to leave the house. A person who had always prided herself on her strength and steadfastness, she was completely lost for the first time in her life.

Five-year-old Ryan was also in a state of shock. He had seen his baby brother die in his mother's arms and had experienced the anguish and terror which that night had brought to his family. In the days following Richie's death, Ryan started exploding with hysterical fits; he refused to eat unless Janet first tested his food for "poison."

"Ryan did not understand why the baby died. Everything I had taught him over the years—like not putting anything in your mouth except food—became blown out of proportion. If he touched a plant leaf, he would scream that he was going to die. He thought everything was going to kill him, and he would make me eat a bit of his food first—even ice cream—before he would eat it."

In the middle of making funeral arrangements for Richie, Janet stopped and took Ryan aside. She held him close and talked softly to him.

" 'Ryan,' I said, 'we are a special family now. We have a baby angel to watch over us. Richie is a baby angel now and he has magic. His magic will make us love each other more.' Ryan became calmer, but he still wanted to know why Richie died. So I told him, 'When babies are born, they get shots to make them strong. The shots didn't work for Richie. They didn't make him strong.' And he seemed to understand."

One morning later that winter, Ryan and Janet were looking out the window at the falling snow. Janet remembers it was a bright day and sunlight was hitting the snow just right. "It looked as if the sky was raining little diamonds that were fluttering down all around, covering the trees and grass with sparkles. Ryan said, 'Mommy, what is it?' We used to call that angel dust when I was a child, so I said, 'That is angel dust.' He looked at me with big eyes and said, 'Mommy, is Richie doing that?' I thought, well, what's the harm and said, 'Yes, Richie is doing that for you.' Well, he ran around the house so excited for about two hours. When it stopped, he said, 'Mommy, I think Richie got tired of throwing it down.'"

They laughed together. It was then that Janet knew Ryan had finally accepted Richie's death. "Ryan knows the shot didn't work for Richie, but he doesn't know the DPT shot killed him. Someday he will know. I am keeping all the records for him so he will know why his brother died."

As much as Janet and Anthony mourn the loss of their baby, Janet has come to believe that it is better that Richie died rather than survive with severe brain damage.

"If I could have struck a bargain with God, I would have given my life for my son's life. I would have gladly given my life for his, but only if God would have given my son back in the condition he was before he got his DPT shot. If God had said to me, 'I will take your life and give back your son but he will be severely brain damaged,' I would have said, 'No.' Because at least I know Richie is in heaven and has eternal peace and happiness. I would not want him to be down here suffering with half a brain. I don't know how the parents of the children who are so terribly brain damaged from this vaccine bear it. It must be a living death to see your child suffer every day."

Even though she gives silent thanks that Richie did not live to suffer, Janet admits she will never be whole again. That realization has made her determined to speak out about Richie's death so that other parents will become better informed about the pertussis vaccine.

"A part of me died with Richie. I can't bring him back. I can only continue with my life. These doctors and officials in the government, who keep talking about the benefits and risks of this vaccine, better take fair warning. My baby may be just another statistic to them, but he was my child and there is nothing more powerful than a mother's fight for her child. There is no war stronger than a mother's fight for her child. I will fight no matter what I have to do and no matter how long it takes to keep this from happening to other babies. I will not let the cause of my baby's death be forgotten."

Janet looks away. Her voice is angry, but her eyes are wet with tears. Carefully, almost lovingly, she takes Richie's autopsy report out of an envelope.

"This is all I have left of him," she says. "This report and the pictures we took the day he was christened."

She reads the autopsy report, as if reading it one more time will lead her from that dark land where a mother grieves for the child she will never hold again.

3

The History of Whooping Cough and the Pertussis Vaccine

> Cured yesterday of my disease,
> I died last night of my physician.
> *Matthew Prior*

Early Pertussis: Death and Bad Remedies

For centuries, parents struggled to nurse their children through the ravages of pertussis, or whooping cough as it is called in America. Just how long the disease has plagued humanity is unknown, but the first recognized description appears to have been made by the French physician Guillaume Baillou during a pertussis epidemic in Paris in 1578.

"The lung is so irritated that, in its attempts by every effort to cast forth the cause of the trouble, it can neither admit breath nor easily give it forth again. The sick person seems to swell up and, as if about to strangle, holds his breath clinging in the midst of his jaws—for they are free from the annoyance of coughing sometimes for the space of four or five hours, then the paroxysm of coughing returns. . . . it was resistant to every medicine. The cough was very fatiguing, upset the stomach and caused vomiting; or it shattered the veins of the brain, causing blood to spurt forth in hemorrhages. These stopped for several days, but in July and August, they returned, more violent than ever and attacked children primarily."

14

A seventeenth-century British physician, Thomas Sydenham, coined the name "pertussis" for the disease from the Latin words meaning "severe cough." Describing the disease, he wrote: "The patient expectorates but little but is taken with a long-continued act of coughing which rises higher and higher both in the straining and the hooping noise until at length the child grows black, sometimes bleeds at the nose, and foams at the mouth through the violence thereof."

Paris and Rome had ferocious pertussis epidemics as early as 1695. In Scandinavia, there was a fifteen-year epidemic in the mid-eighteenth century which took 3,000 lives every year and almost twice that number in 1755. In Glasgow, Scotland, whooping cough was the cause of nearly 12 percent of all deaths that occurred in 1809. In England, between 1858 and 1865, more than 120,000 died. In Prussia, approximately 85,000 died in the five years from 1875 to 1880.

Whooping cough was so common in all the European countries for centuries that every European language created its own folk name for the disease. In England it was called the "chincough" or "kinkough," stemming from the Dutch word *kinchin* (meaning to pant or gasp) or the Dutch word *kindt* (meaning child).

It is easy to understand why the folk names for the disease were derived from words associated with children. Whooping cough has always claimed most of its victims from among the youngest and most vulnerable portion of the population: babies and small children. In past centuries, it was particularly virulent in such places as crowded hospitals and orphanages where an infectious disease could quickly be transmitted. An American physician described a typical case in a three-and-a-half-year-old boy in the year 1872:

"Upon entering the room, I found him in a severe convulsion, and the mother about to place him in a warm bath, which was immediately done. The respiration was rapid and painfully oppressed. Mucous rales distinct over lower lobes, and in fact over the greater part of both lungs there was dullness on percussion; no respiratory murmur discoverable; pulse rapid and weak; extremities cold. Convulsions returning, he was again placed in the warm bath, when the muscles relaxed, the eyes closed, the head fell back, and respiration was entirely suspended; could feel no pulsation of either the radial or temporal arteries, but the heart beat feebly. I thought grim death was claiming a victim from that household when the child gently gasped."

The severe coughing, frequently accompanied by vomiting, could go on for weeks or months and often prevented children from eating so that they became emaciated and died. Others developed high fevers and convulsions and, if they survived, were left with permanent brain damage.

Whooping cough also attacked adults. Benjamin Waterhouse, the famous Boston physician who performed the first smallpox vaccination in the United States on his own four children in 1800, himself came down with whooping cough fifteen years later when in his sixties. He left an account for future generations of Americans who, as he wrote, "are not sufficiently apprised of the violence, and of the fatality, of this terrible distemper.

"The patient appears to gasp, and strain, and hiccup, and strangle rather than cough. In this painful action, the veins of the face as well as the eyes, appear swelled; the countenance becomes very dark; the eyes are turned upwards, and there seems danger of a fatal strangulation. Sometimes the sufferer appears as if gasping for life, without being able to make the least noise. Adults will fall down instantly as if apoplectic. It seems as if the epiglottis was shut down firmly by a spasm without the sufferer having the power, at once, of opening it. There have been instances where the power has been so totally overcome that a fatal strangulation has been the consequence."

Pertussis appears to have reached a peak incidence of mortality (death) and morbidity (illness) in the nineteenth century among families huddled in tenements in the crowded cities of both the Old and the New Worlds, where backyard privies, unclean water from public wells, and inadequate nutrition were commonplace. Every winter took its toll of sickness and death, with the following account from Zanesville, Ohio, in 1877 probably being typical:

"Six weeks or two months ago fully one half the children in the public schools were coughing away, many with unmistakable whoop . . . Several times I have noticed children stop on the sidewalk, go to the curb, have a spasmodic cough, throw up a mouthful of mucus, and then pass on. . . . Some very young children show, speedily, pneumonia or cerebral complications, or both, ending in death. But in the bulk of cases they pull through to recovery."

Those who did not die of the disease itself would often die of secondary complications. Abraham Jacobi, a mid-nineteenth-century physician, wrote, "The deaths from pertussis proper are inconsiderable when compared with the mortality of its complications." Even as late as 1916, Sir William Osler, the renowned Canadian physician, remarked, "If we include its complications, whooping cough is a very fatal affection, ranking one of the first among the acute infections as a cause of death in children under five years of age."

Pneumonia, bronchitis, and otitis media (severe middle-ear infection) were not unusual secondary complications of pertussis. Blindness, in particular, was not uncommon following a bout with the disease. It is unclear whether this was caused by some direct effect on the nervous system of the eyes or by the bursting of blood vessels in the eyes from the pressure of the cough on the circulation. A Maine physician wrote in 1811: "I saw one case in which the tunica conjunctiva of both eyes was totally suffused with blood, so that not a trace of the beautiful pearly whiteness of the healthy eye was to be discerned."

Physicians did not know how to treat or manage the disease. The common methods used by most doctors prior to the twentieth century must have only increased the death rate. Bleeding was a widely practiced therapy for whooping cough in the seventeenth century, and Thomas Sydenham has described the treatment given in that period: "The child is to be blooded and afterwards purged, upon which by degrees the cough will go off without any more ado, save that it may be necessary to let it use the open country air."

In 1793, a New Jersey doctor showed that there had been little change in a hundred years. He said bleeding was necessary but "great caution is requisite in bleeding, and particularly children, who experience mostly its bad effects."

Cathartics, causing diarrhea, were made from mercury and often administered to whooping cough victims. Vegetable emetics, causing vomiting, were also given because they were thought to "interrupt the return of the spasmodic cough. . . . they promote the expectoration of mucus." Other doctors prescribed castor oil, musk, opium, and quinine "in such quantities as the patient can conveniently bear."

When confronted with these "cures" prescribed by doctors, patients often sought alternatives. British and American folk medicine reveal a dazzling array of folk remedies for pertussis. For instance, a child with whooping cough would often be taken to the highest hill in the neighborhood for a change of air. Even in recent decades, children have been taken up in airplanes for the same purpose.

Various strong smells were thought to help cure whooping cough, such as fumes from natural gas, boiling tar, boiling vinegar, or smoke from the hooves of horses being shod. Children were sometimes placed in the midst of a flock of smelly sheep or even held upside-down through the seat of a privy.

Mice have always been thought to possess curative powers, whether roasted, baked, boiled, stewed, or burnt to ashes. In one district in England, whooping cough victims ate three mice in the morning on an empty stomach for three days in a row. In Ireland, powdered mice were drunk in milk or ale.

Other animals were also used in attempts to cure whooping cough. Soup made from an owl was sipped in Yorkshire. Kentucky folklore mentions tea made from white ants. It was believed the disease could be passed on to a pet dog by putting a hair from the patient's head between two slices of bread and giving it to the dog to eat. Sometimes a small fish was tied to the child's chest and allowed to flap itself to death. A variation of this remedy was to insert the head of a live fish in the child's mouth and then throw the fish back into the river.

Many plants were used as medicines to help cure pertussis. In Kentucky and elsewhere, a child with whooping cough was passed nine times through a bramble bush. More often, the bramble bush was made into medicine. The most common folk medicine, which the early American colonists learned from the Indians, was made from the leaves or bark of a chestnut tree boiled in water or wine. Indians and settlers also made teas from Angelica root, Indian turnip, wild thyme, red and white clover blossoms, sumac berries, black cherry stems, and sunflower seeds.

The Decline of Pertussis

Even though doctors were unable to prevent or cure whooping cough, morbidity and mortality from the disease in Western Europe and the United States steadily declined from the mid-nineteenth to the mid-twentieth century. Although many Americans still have vivid memories of the pertussis epidemics of the 1920s and 1930s, statistics show that deaths from pertussis had dropped from 210 per million in the 1870s to 21 per million in 1940, despite the fact that few Americans had received the pertussis vaccine developed several years earlier.

Other European countries had the same experience. In England, one child out of 1,000 under the age of fifteen died of whooping cough in the late nineteenth century. By 1940, this death rate had declined by 90 percent.

In Sweden, 800 children died of pertussis each year between 1911 and 1915; there were 10 deaths from 1951 to 1955 and no deaths in 19,000 cases between 1977 and 1979. In Hamburg, the mortality from pertussis was 986 out of 7,716 cases between 1901 and 1905; in the years 1951–1955, there were only 33 deaths out of 11,123 cases.

This dramatic decline in the death rate before a pertussis vaccine was used on a mass basis either in the United States or Europe is not really surprising, since the same decline in mortality was occurring with other infectious diseases such as scarlet fever, measles, influenza, tuberculosis, and typhoid. All were formerly prevalent and lethal, and all declined as causes of death during the same period.

One reason for the decline in the mortality rate of these formerly deadly diseases may have been that the populations of Europe and the United States acquired a certain degree of natural resistance to them after so many generations of exposure. Certainly, the level of exposure within any population was great. For example, in the 1920s and 1930s, whooping cough was so common in America that by the age of ten, 73 percent of all children had a clinical history of the disease.

Another reason for the decline in the death rate from pertussis and other infectious childhood diseases prior to widespread use of vaccine was the vast improvement in living standards in both Western Europe and the United States. Better sanitation, nutrition, housing, and health care resulted in a better general state of health among the infant population. In addition, the introduction of antibiotics during World War II had a dramatic effect on the control of pneumonia—often a virulent secondary complication of whooping cough. With the successful use of antibiotics to control secondary infections such as pneumonia and bronchitis, babies had a much better chance of surviving whooping cough and other serious childhood diseases.

A. H. Griffith, of The Wellcome Research Laboratories in England, commented in 1982 that mortality from whooping cough dropped ten years before the vaccination program was introduced in England "with the advent of antibiotics for treatment of complications and new treatments evolved for maintaining fluid balance in the very young, which constitute the main majority of fatal cases of whooping cough."

In one respect, the decline in pertussis morbidity and mortality differs from that of other childhood diseases. While the incidence and death rate of such childhood diseases as scarlet fever dropped simultaneously in fairly equal proportions, the deaths from whooping cough declined much more rapidly than the incidence of the disease.

Between the early 1920s and the mid-1950s, pertussis deaths in the United States declined from 70 per million to 7 per million. But at the same time the number of cases only declined from 1,300 per million to 250 per million. Whooping cough in developed countries obviously remained infectious although much less deadly.

The Mysterious Pertussis Bacterium

Part of the reason pertussis has been such a difficult disease to treat and control is because it has remained a mystery to scientists, who have not been able to define the nature of the complex bacterial organism responsible for the disease.

In 1906, the French bacteriologists Jules Bordet (who discovered the Bordetella pertussis and in whose honor it is named) and Octave Gengou reported that they had isolated the toxic bacterium responsible for whooping cough. But three quarters of a century after their discovery, scientists admit they are still confused about the bacterium that causes the disease. "Unfortunately, we do not know the toxic component responsible for central nervous system injury in pertussis disease," John Robbins, M.D., of the Food and Drug Administration (FDA) stated in 1978. "The pathogenesis of the disease is not even completely understood at this time," said Harry Meyer, M.D., also of the FDA, in 1982.

What is known today is that each pertussis bacterium is made up of hundreds or even thousands of tiny bits of protein, called antigens. The very largest can be seen under a microscope, but most are invisible. Although some scientists believe they have identified certain antigens responsible for causing neurological damage as well for stimulating immunity, much about the B. pertussis remains a mystery (see Chapter 19).

Vincent A. Fulginiti, M.D., wrote in 1980, "We do not know why children recover from pertussis nor which antigens evoke which immunologic responses related to protection. Although much is known of the antigenic composition of B. pertussis, and some information is available on specific antibody responses, no conclusive and noncontroversial link between immunity and protection has been made."

The Progression of Pertussis

B. pertussis is a fragile microbe that cannot survive outside the human body for more than a few minutes. The disease is spread by coughed or sneezed droplets of sputum or mucus containing the bacterium which enter the nasal or respiratory tract of another person. There the bacteria attach themselves by an unknown mechanism. Some researchers say that FHA, a protein component of the pertussis bacterium, is responsible for this attachment.

The microbe causes a local infection in the respiratory tract, which produces such symptoms as a runny nose and a short, dry cough, which may last for several weeks. This is called the catarrhal phase of the disease. Scientists suspect that two toxins produced by the microbe (tracheal cytotoxin or TCT and dermonecrotic toxin or DNT) are responsible for the local infection.

The next stage is the movement of the effects of the disease from the local site to the entire body. At this point, the disease enters the "paroxysmal" stage. Even though the pertussis microbe is only found at the site of the local infection, some scientists think the microbe liberates a highly toxic component (referred to as pertussigen, pertussis toxin, lymphocytosis-promoting factor [LPF], islet-activating protein [IAP] and by other names) that attacks different systems in the body and produces the more severe symptoms such as the characteristic "whoop" coughing, vomiting, high fever, and sometimes convulsions.

A mother may often not immediately recognize that her child has come down with whooping cough, because in its classic form it starts with a few ordinary symptoms that can be confused with the common cold. The child may be tired and stop eating very well, run a low-grade fever, and have a small, dry cough for about two weeks. Only when the cold symptoms disappear does the paroxysmal cough begin.

Fulginiti has described this stage of the disease (1982): "Children with this illness cough unmercifully, choking in the process and gasping for air. They often vomit and become acutely undernourished and dehydrated. They may destroy parts of their lungs and brains from hemorrhage, lack of oxygen, or both."

The characteristic whoop is caused when the child, after coughing "as if through a one-way valve" and entirely out of breath, finally succeeds in taking in some air through his partially constricted throat. The paroxysm may be followed by vomiting or nosebleed or a hemorrhage into the eyes.

This classic picture is found in children between the ages of two and six. Tiny infants, who are the most vulnerable, typically do not exhibit the whoop and may simply choke and be unable to breathe. In adults, the whoop is usually much milder and often not present at all. Adults who get whooping cough may be diagnosed as having bronchitis, influenza, or merely a bad cold.

The convalescent stage of the disease, with its sporadic coughing, may last for weeks or months. It can be complicated by secondary bacterial infections, such as pneumonia, which were major causes of death in the past when antibiotics were nonexistent and supportive medical care was less sophisticated.

The most dreaded complications are neurological, including convulsions, paralysis, coma, blindness, deafness, seizure and movement disorders, and mental retardation. Some of these may result from oxygen deprivation (anoxia) during the coughing spells. Like the characteristic whoop itself, however, they undoubtedly represent the direct effect of the B. pertussis bacterium's destructive action in the body, whether via the various toxins released by the bacteria or via a direct effect on the nervous system.

At a 1982 FDA Symposium, a Japanese scientist pointed out that the toxic substances produced by B. pertussis may be responsible for the neurological complications of whooping cough as well for those of the vaccine which contains B. pertussis: "Reactions such as fever and neurologic involvement [from the vaccine] are reminiscent of symptoms associated with infection [natural whooping cough] and suggest the possibility of common mechanisms for these physiologic conditions. Bordetella pertussis may produce a toxic substance which elicits the adverse reactions in disease and, similarly, these same toxic substances may be present to a limited extent in current whole cell vaccine and result in comparable effects."

How Vaccines Work

All vaccines work on the principle of protection by artificially stimulating the immune system to produce antibodies—small molecules of protein that attack the invading organism—to overcome a disease in the same way the natural disease stimulates immunity. In the case of the pertussis vaccine, this is achieved by injecting the child with controlled quantities of whole-killed pertussis bacteria. The theory is that periodic injections of small amounts of bacteria will compel the child's immune system to produce the antibodies conferring immunity.

But bitter experience has shown that the vaccine created to protect a child sometimes injures or even kills. As mentioned previously, medical science is still trying to define precisely which antigens in the pertussis bacterium produce immunity and which cause brain damage, or whether the same antigen does both. When Fulginiti testified before Congress in 1982, he stated: "The same chemical principles in the bacterium that produce the immune response in the host also have toxic properties, and it has been very, very difficult to separate these two elements and insure that the child is going to be protected and yet have no side effects. . . . We simply have had difficulty separating those two effects of the bacterium."

This theoretical problem has dogged pertussis vaccine research from the beginning. So scientists have gone ahead and used the whole cell with all of its components. This is why the pertussis vaccine used in the United States and nearly all other countries is known as the whole-cell vaccine. This is also why it is referred to as a "crude" vaccine.

Perhaps this is why D. L. Miller, M.D., was prompted to state in 1982: "Judged by strict scientific standards, much of the existing evidence on the dangers of the disease, the effectiveness of the vaccine, and the risks of immunization remains unsatisfactory."

The Whole-Cell Vaccine

The first whooping cough vaccine was created in 1912 by Jules Bordet and Octave Gengou, who wanted to use it in Tunisia to prevent the disease from spreading among the children of that country. They grew the pertussis bacteria in large pots, killed them with heat, preserved the mixture with formaldehyde, and injected it into children.

Bordet and Gengou took the bad with the good, the impurities with the protective antigens, because no one knew how to separate them. And this still remains true. The crude vaccine created more than seventy years ago is quite similar, in principle, to the pertussis vaccine injected every day into hundreds of thousands of children throughout the world.

In Tunisia, London, and Paris in the early twentieth century, the fact that the newly brewed vaccine was crude and impure was the last thing on anyone's mind. Whooping cough was killing infants and children by the hundreds and the first priority was to protect them. Furthermore, the early part of the twentieth century was a time of explosive interest in the development of vaccines.

In London, Almroth Wright developed a typhoid vaccine which probably saved millions of lives during World War I, while Pasteur's rabies vaccine and the diphtheria and tetanus vaccines of Emil von Behring were already a part of history. Work pressed on with pertussis vaccine as doctors tried to find a way to eliminate all infectious diseases from the earth.

In 1925, the Danish researcher Thorvald Madsen tried out a modified pertussis vaccine during a whooping cough epidemic in the Faroe Islands. He made it from the bacilli first isolated by Bordet and Gengou. He vaccinated babies and, while it did not prevent whooping cough, it appeared to make the disease milder and reduce the number of deaths.

Madsen's work stimulated other researchers to develop their own pertussis vaccines. During the 1920s, a number of them appeared on the market in Europe and the United States. The situation became so confused that in 1931 the American Medical Association (AMA) removed pertussis vaccine from its list of approved drugs.

This crisis, however, brought forward a woman who was to revolutionize research on this vaccine and make it a viable option for mass immunization. Pearl Kendrick completed her graduate work at Johns Hopkins Medical School in the spring of 1932 and went home to Grand Rapids, Michigan, to begin a lifetime of work on the pertussis vaccine. Her associate, Grace Eldering, has described their efforts:

"The early 1930s were years of the Great Depression, and we learned about the disease and the Depression at the same time. Many of the families we visited were very poor, and their living conditions pitiful. Our watchword became: 'round to the back and up the stairs.' We listened to sad stories told by desperate fathers who could find no work.

We collected specimens, by the light of kerosene lamps, from whooping, vomiting, strangling children. We saw what the disease could do. In the laboratory, we isolated the pertussis bacillus, not from every patient but from most of them in the early stages of the disease. Our findings were reported to the attending physician and to the health officer. The cultures were saved and studied in every possible way. We soon had little doubt about the cause of whooping cough."

Initially, Kendrick and Eldering gathered samples of the bacilli by holding the child's mouth open with a spatula, causing a paroxysm of coughing, and recovering sputum from the child's mouth with a cotton swab. In the late 1930s, two Danish physicians thought of having the child cough directly onto a culture plate containing a mixture of boiled potatoes and sheep's blood. It had been found experimentally that the fastidious pertussis bacterium required this kind of medium for proper growth. In the laboratory these cultures were cultured in the same medium of potatoes and blood, washed off, and then "killed" with a mixture of salt water and Merthiolate.

In the 1930s and early 1940s, scientists and physicians were feverishly trying to define the best way to prepare the vaccine, the best age for giving the first shot, how many shots were needed to protect a child, and whether or not the pertussis vaccine should be combined with others such as diphtheria and tetanus.

One of the changes made in Bordet and Gengou's original vaccine was to add an "adjuvant." These are materials, usually metal salts, which for reasons still not understood heighten the capacity of vaccine to produce antibodies. In 1943, Kendrick reported that alum had this adjuvant effect; the pertussis vaccine was more protective, and fewer pertussis bacteria had to be included. After her report, alum or alum-based substances were added to the vaccine.

Kendrick was also instrumental in having pertussis combined with the diphtheria and tetanus vaccines already in use in the 1940s. In 1942, she said, "With the multiplicity of accepted immunization procedures for children it is logical that appropriate combinations of antigens for active immunization be studied in order to reduce the number of required injections, thereby lessening discomfort for the child and family and simplifying administrative procedures."

So for the sake of "simplifying" the lives of children, their parents, and busy doctors, Kendrick urged that the pertussis vaccine be combined with the diphtheria vaccine. This logic became even more compelling when it was found that the pertussis component boosted the efficacy of the diphtheria component when the two were combined: the pertussis vaccine itself acted as an adjuvant. Shortly afterwards, tetanus was added to these other two vaccines for the same reasons. This triple combination created the DPT shot as we know it today.

When the Salk polio vaccine came on the market, pharmaceutical manufacturer Parke-Davis decided to make things even easier for children, parents, and physicians by combining the killed polio vaccine with the DPT shot. This created a new combination of four vaccines, called Quadrigen, which was licensed by the National Institutes of Health (NIH) in the spring of 1959. But the vaccine experts had evidently combined one too many vaccines because Quadrigen was found to be highly reactive. It was eventually withdrawn from the market in 1968, and several lawsuits were brought against Parke-Davis by parents of children who had been damaged by the four-in-one shot (see Chapter 16).

Problems with Production and Testing

Today the whole-cell vaccine is made in essentially the same way as in the time of Bordet and Gengou, although each manufacturer prepares it differently, and the exact formula is considered a trade secret. The pertussis bacteria are usually grown on a casein hydrolysate medium with yeast dialyzate supplemented with agar and charcoal and preserved with a mercury derivate. Other possible ingredients are hydrochloric acid, the adjuvant (usually an aluminum compound), sodium hydroxide, and salt.

In the past, human blood was often added. Today this is prohibited by federal regulations, but manufacturers are still permitted to add blood from "lower animals other than the horse."

The mixture is prepared in vats and washed, and the bacteria are then "toxoided," or killed with heat and formaldehyde. The vaccine is stored for a while at near-freezing temperatures by the manufacturer. It is combined with the diphtheria and tetanus components, poured into vials, and shipped to regional distribution centers. Then it is shipped to wholesalers before being transported to pharmacies, private physicians, and public health clinics. Finally it is injected into babies.

The whole-cell pertussis vaccine is the crudest vaccine in current use. It is also the most difficult to produce.

In 1978, Charlotte Parker of the Department of Microbiology at the University of Texas in Austin paid poetic tribute to this peculiarity of the pertussis microbe: "Bordetella pertussis is a fascinating organism to study. A certain amount of empiricism, as opposed to logic, is required for success with pertussis. Diagnostic cultures are difficult and sometimes unreliable. Different lots of vaccine, made in the same way, from the same strains, sometimes show different properties. Experimental work is not always reproducible from one laboratory to another, but this is common in biological research. The diagnostic culture problems and the unexpected variability in vaccines and in pertussis strains themselves are not easy to explain."

Charles Manclark, a pertussis vaccine expert in the FDA, stated at the 1982 FDA Symposium on New Pertussis Vaccines: "The manufacturers will tell you that they will have a vaccine produced one time that meets all the criteria for Phase I organisms, and one time it will be a good vaccine, and the next time it will not be a good vaccine." Philip Brunell, a leading American pediatrician, added, "The only time you know what the potency is is when you have finished making the vaccine."

"Serotype variation," the ability of the B. pertussis to mutate unexpectedly and change its character, adds another level of complexity. In addition, the quality of the vaccine is affected by the medium in which it is grown. John Cameron, of the University of Quebec, stated at the 1978 FDA-sponsored International Symposium on Pertussis: "A point not generally appreciated is the difference in performance, even with carefully selected strains, when they are grown on or in different media. . . . This, in effect, is another way of admitting how little we understand the metabolism of B. pertussis in spite of being able to grow it on a chemically defined medium."

A Matter of Safety and Efficacy

The pertussis microorganism is one of the most complex, unstable, and generally tricky bacteria known. It is also extremely poisonous and has a broad range of effects on the human body. In the words of Dr. Margaret Pittman (1965), who was the United States government's leading pertussis vaccine specialist for many years until her retirement in 1971, "Bordetella pertussis is unique among infectious bacteria in its marked ability to modify biological responses. Hence, there has been special concern that pertussis vaccine be as free as possible from reactive factors and yet provide adequate protection against whooping cough."

Scientists do not use direct chemical analysis to demonstrate that the pertussis vaccine is potent and nontoxic. Instead they have developed indirect tests, conducted on mice. If the vaccine can stimulate immunity in mice, it is considered to be equally effective in humans. If mice do not lose weight after the vaccine has been injected into their abdominal cavities, the toxicity level is thought to be safe for children.

Today, the FDA is responsible for testing pertussis vaccine for safety and efficacy before it is released for administration to the public. But the vaccine's notoriously unstable and difficult character often causes vaccine lots to fail FDA tests. The FDA's pertussis vaccine specialist, Charles Manclark, commented in 1976: "Pertussis vaccine is one of the more troublesome products to produce and assay. As an example of this, pertussis vaccine has one of the highest failure rates of all products submitted to the Bureau of Biologics for testing and release. Approximately 15–20 percent of all lots which pass the manufacturer's test fail to pass the Bureau's tests."

The Lab Test for Vaccine Potency

Very early in the development of the pertussis vaccine, scientists decided to test its potency (ability to cause immunity) by injecting it into mice and then exposing them to B. pertussis infection. If they became sick, the vaccine was considered to be ineffective or subpotent. Grace Eldering commented on these early experiments: "The exasperating thing was that some protection was demonstrated by nearly all methods, but the results were not reproducible with any precision, and definite end points could not be arrived at."

The need for a standard potency test became a high priority after Randolph K. Byers and Frederick C. Moll of the Harvard Medical School published an article in 1948 describing children who had become brain damaged after receiving pertussis vaccine. Their findings shocked the medical world and provided the first clear substantiation that the vaccine caused serious neurological complications in children. Doctors and scientists hurried to develop definitive laboratory tests to measure the potency and toxicity of the vaccine.

Two years earlier, in 1946, Kendrick and Pittman had hit upon the idea of "challenging" or exposing vaccinated mice to whooping cough by injecting the challenge dose of B. pertussis bacteria directly into their brains. Until then, many different ways of exposing vaccinated mice to the pertussis bacterium had been tried, including putting them into an aerosol chamber. With the new Kendrick and Pittman technique, the mice were first immunized with the experimental vaccine whose potency was in question; then, two and a half weeks later, a "challenge dose" of pertussis bacteria was injected into their brains. The vaccine's ability to protect against whooping cough (potency or efficacy) was judged by how many mice survived and how many died from the challenge dose of pertussis bacteria.

The Division of Biologics Standards (DBS) of the Public Health Service (PHS) established a national potency test in 1949, after working with vaccine manufacturers for four years. It was modified in 1953 to establish maximum and minimum potency limits, the same year that a standard pertussis vaccine was established as a yardstick against which every lot of vaccine was to be measured. Today a single potency test lasts four weeks and requires five samples of the vaccine on 350 to 400 mice.

A major weakness of this potency test is that its meaning can only be determined by comparing the results in mice with the results of a clinical trial in humans. Other inadequacies of this test led Frank T. Perkins of the World Health Organization (WHO) to state in 1978: "We subject all pertussis vaccines to the mouse protection test without knowing what antigen is involved in this somewhat complex active challenge test. The test, although having served us well for the last twenty years, may eventually be shown to be inappropriate when the active principle in immunity has been identified."

The Lab Test for Safety

The manufactured vaccine is also subjected to the toxicity test developed and refined by Pittman and others at the DBS between 1954 and 1965. It is supposed to measure the vaccine's safety, meaning how likely it is to cause severe reactions in children. This involves injecting the vaccine into the abdominal cavities of young mice to see if they continue to gain weight over a period of time. If the mice continue to gain a specific amount of weight, vaccine manufacturers and the FDA consider the vaccine safe for release to be administered to the public.

This test has also been plagued with problems. When Pittman was trying to refine it in the 1950s, some mice were seen to gain weight satisfactorily no matter what kind of vaccine was used. Mouse weight gain was also affected by the presence and types of adjuvants in the vaccine, the temperature and size of the mouse cages, the amount of light to which the mice were exposed and even the strain of mice utilized. But the most troublesome aspect of the toxicity test was that some children had and still have serious and even fatal reactions from vaccines that have successfully passed this test.

The potency and toxicity tests developed nearly four decades ago by Kendrick and Pittman were designed to eliminate the kinds of neurological reactions Byers and Moll had described in the 1948 article that stunned the medical world. During a 1968 trial involving a lawsuit against Parke-Davis by a parent whose child had been brain damaged by the 4-in-1 vaccine Quadrigen, the company's director of microbiological research testified:

"It was our opinion and I think most people agreed (see for example the reports of Dr. Pittman and others at the National Institutes of Health [NIH] and at the Centers for Disease Control [CDC] branch of the Public Health Service) that under the new regulations the encephalopathic type of reaction was no longer a problem. Factors contributing to this improvement were: (1) the decreased amount of pertussis in the formula which was made possible by the use of the phosphate adjuvants (2) the new maximum as well as minimum potency standards (3) the toxicity of the pertussis component was reduced by extra heating and controlled by the toxicity test. These precautions which are part of the standards for all pertussis [vaccine] made in this country had eliminated the encephalopathic type of reaction."

But despite the fact that all pertussis vaccine made in the United States has been subjected to these various laboratory tests, neurological reactions have continued to occur. John Cameron said in 1978, "What are we attempting to control when we do a mouse toxicity test? Clearly we are trying to decide whether or not a particular lot of vaccine is suitable for release. On the other hand, presumably every lot of vaccine released in the last 5–10 years has been safe by this standard, yet reactions are still observed in infants."

The sad fact is that after more than forty years of subjecting the pertussis vaccine to the mouse "toxicity test" children are still dying and becoming brain damaged after the vaccine has passed this test. The fact that FDA tests for toxicity are not reliable indicators of toxicity is discussed further in Chapter 16.

At What Age Should We Vaccinate?

One of the important issues being debated during the frenzied period of vaccine development in the 1920s and 1930s was the earliest age at which children should be given the pertussis vaccine. Newborns and young children were always the first to die from whooping cough, but some doctors were beginning to suspect that the vaccine did not "take" in the first months of life. Louis Sauer, M.D., of Evanston, Illinois, who developed his own pertussis vaccine and was an outspoken supporter of mass vaccination, reported in 1941 that only 27 percent of a group of eighty-nine babies developed protective antibodies when vaccinated at three months of age or less.

Sauer urged that pertussis vaccination begin no earlier than the age of seven months, observing that "most of these infants did not yet possess the power to develop adequate immunity when they were injected so early in life." He also commented that "some could not be injected during the first several months because they were 'feeding problems,' especially those born prematurely." This was a prophetic remark which has come back to haunt the medical establishment today in its effort to define children who are at high risk of reacting to the pertussis vaccine (see Chapters 7 and 13).

Sauer's view was opposed by others who felt that even partial protection of newborns against the ravages of whooping cough was better than none. Wallace Sako, M.D., of New Orleans, was one of those who disagreed with Sauer. In 1945, after conducting a trial on 4,000 infants two to twelve weeks of age and finding that three quarters of them developed antibodies to pertussis, he urged doctors to vaccinate early.

Jean V. Cooke, M.D., of the Department of Pediatrics, Washington University of St. Louis, observed in 1948 that babies produce excellent antibodies to diphtheria and tetanus toxoids and so "there appears no reason that antibodies to pertussis antigen cannot be as readily formed as those to tetanus antigen, and the justification for early pertussis immunization is strengthened."

Eventually doctors opted for vaccinating babies with DPT vaccine in the first few months of life largely because the polio vaccine was being given at this early age. They solved the problem of poor antibody response in newborns by simply giving the babies more shots.

This line of thinking was the origin of the "booster shot," first suggested in 1938, which became customary in the 1940s. Booster shots evened out any difference in antibody response between children vaccinated as newborns and those vaccinated much later. Today most American children have received five DPT shots by the time they are six years old.

The question of antibody response may not have played as important a role in deciding when children should be vaccinated as the convenience of the pediatrician who was giving the shots. A 1962 study using Parke-Davis's Quadrigen vaccine, funded by Parke-Davis and conducted in a Detroit hospital for indigent families, determined that "pertussis antibody response, as measured by agglutinin titers, was as good in the 3-month-old as in the 6-month-old infants. The response in the 2-month-old infants was relatively poor at the postprimary stage but was equivalent to that of the older infants at the post-booster interval."

The authors of this study concluded: "There are several reasons why the clinician is desirous of starting immunizations as early in life as possible. Pertussis may pose a serious threat to infants under three months of age. . . . There is also a greater likelihood of completing the recommended series of injections if immunizations can be started early in infancy and coordinated with other reasons for the baby's being brought to the physician's office or clinic. For most practitioners, the age of four to six weeks would be a convenient time to start the series of immunizations against diphtheria, tetanus, pertussis and poliomyelitis. At this age the baby is starting his series of health supervision visits, and the mother is due for her traditional postpartum examination at about this time." In the 1950s, the American Academy of Pediatrics was urging that the series of DPT shots be started at between one and two months of age.

No one called attention to the possibility that moving up the vaccination to the first weeks after birth might increase the risk of neurological reactions or sudden death. George Dick, M.D., wrote in 1967, "It has long been known that increasing the number of B. pertussis per dose of vaccine increases the frequency of reactions. It would be surprising if decreasing the size of the infants receiving a particular vaccine did not also increase the reactions."

Dick's observations suggest what appears to be a violation of a standard axiom in medicine: the lower the weight of the individual, the smaller the dose of a drug to be given. Doctors would not think of injecting a baby with the same number of units of penicillin as an adult. Yet a two-month-old baby weighing nine pounds gets the same amount of vaccine as a fifty-pound child entering kindergarten.

Dick further pointed out that "Before whooping cough vaccine was employed routinely in Britain, the Medical Research Council carried out a series of trials including a study of reactions in babies, of whom 80 percent were 14 months of age or over. It seems to have been concluded by many people that the results of these trials were definitive and were applicable to babies of all ages, for all time, with all vaccines. How did it come about that it was assumed that babies of only a few months of age would react in the same way as babies twice their weight? Why was immunization with pertussis-containing vaccines recommended in babies of a few months of age with no adequate toxicity tests having been done?"

Dick's comments reveal a very curious fact in the history of how American children routinely came to be given their first DPT shot at two months of age. The United States never conducted its own clinical trials to prove that the pertussis vaccine was safe and effective. Instead, it relied (and still relies) on data collected by Britain in clinical trials conducted in the 1950s for proof of safety in newborns. But, as Dick points out, these clinical trials were not performed on two-month-old infants. The majority of the children in the trials were more than fourteen months old!

Between 1946 and 1957, the Medical Research Council in England sponsored several large-scale fields trials of the pertussis vaccine designed to measure its ability to prevent whooping cough. The vaccine was tested on about 50,000 children between six and eighteen months of age, with the great majority of them fourteen months of age or older.

Although eight infants had convulsions within seventy-two hours of the shot, and thirty-four more had convulsions within twenty-eight days of the shot, these trials were considered a success and the vaccine was soon being administered to most children in England. Though the trials were designed to demonstrate efficacy (the ability to prevent whooping cough), not safety, the United States health authorities used them as evidence that the vaccine was safe to give to babies as young as six weeks of age.

To this day, the British Department of Health and Social Security regulations state that when vaccinating with DPT "a better general immunological response can be expected if the first dose is delayed to six months of age." A second dose is recommended six to eight weeks later and a third dose four to six months after that.

In contrast to the British recommendations, today the United States Public Health Service and the American Academy of Pediatrics recommend that a child receive the first DPT shot at two months of age, with subsequent shots given at four months, six months, eighteen months, and between the ages of four and six years.

4

Profile: Screams in the Night

> I have walked and prayed for this young
>   child an hour
> And heard the sea-wind scream upon
>   the tower,
> And under the arches of the bridge, and scream
> In the elms above flooded stream;
> Imagining in excited reverie
> That the future years had come,
> Dancing to a frenzied drum,
> Out of the murderous innocence of the sea.
>   *William Butler Yeats*

Ellen remembers the day fourteen years ago when she tucked her three-and-a-half-month-old daughter into her bassinet and drove her to the pediatrician. Sherry was a sweet, cheerful baby with bright eyes and an alertness reminiscent of her four-year-old sister when she had been a baby.

"Just that morning I had written notes in Sherry's baby book," recalled Ellen. "I described how she would raise her head up in her crib and hold her head unsupported while I carried her. I remember she was fascinated with her hands because I would catch her inspecting them with such curiosity. Whenever I was in the room, she would try to follow me around with her eyes. But, most of all, I was proud of her imitation of simple syllables such as 'ah' and 'oo,' which was something she had begun doing at two-and-a-half months of age."

That day the pediatrician gave Sherry her first shot: a DPT vaccination to protect her against diphtheria, pertussis, and tetanus. Ellen remembers Sherry cried briefly after being stuck with the needle but soon calmed down.

"When I got home, I gave her a bottle, and she took it with her usual eagerness. She never had been a picky eater. After burping her, I put her in her playpen to take a nap and she seemed to doze off. About thirty minutes later, she woke up crying uncontrollably."

For the next three hours, Ellen alternately walked and rocked her baby, trying to persuade her to stop screaming. Then she noticed that Sherry felt exceptionally warm. "I called my pediatrician. He told me that a fever and crying were normal reactions to a DPT shot and to give her a baby aspirin. So I did," said Ellen.

But Sherry did not respond to the baby aspirin. At two in the morning, she had been crying for about thirteen hours, and her fever was more than 105 degrees.

"It sounded as if she was in unbearable pain, as if her body was literally exploding inside," said Ellen, "and all I could do was to continue sponging her with cold water to try and bring down the fever. It was a terrible, helpless feeling to know I could not take her pain away."

Early the next morning, Ellen called her pediatrician again. "He told me to keep giving her the baby aspirin and sponging her. What I could not believe was that she had still not stopped crying. Her screaming was causing my neighbors to come out of their houses to see what was the matter. I just kept walking back and forth in my living room holding her in my arms and praying her agony would stop."

Sherry continued shrieking all through the second day and into the second night after the DPT shot. "I was beside myself because I was so tired and worried. I hadn't slept for more than a few hours the past two nights. I even felt guilty sleeping for those few hours because it meant I had to leave Sherry screaming in her room."

By the third morning after the shot, Sherry was still screaming and running a temperature near 105 degrees. Her face was contorted and flushed.

"Aspirin and sponge baths did not seem to touch the fever. I couldn't believe this was a 'normal' reaction to the DPT shot, no matter what my pediatrician kept telling me. I was embarrassed to call him again, but I did. And he said the same thing all over again—that she would soon stop crying and the fever would come down and I should stop worrying."

Ellen remembers that she did not think she could bear another night of Sherry's screaming. "I felt like my heart was breaking because I could not help her." Her baby continued screaming throughout that day, and then "mercifully, sometime late that night, she fell into a deep sleep." It had been almost seventy-two hours since Sherry had received her DPT shot.

"When Sherry woke up the next morning, she appeared to be okay but tired," said Ellen.

Ellen went over Sherry's reaction with her pediatrician when she took Sherry to him two months later, but he did not express concern. He gave Sherry her second DPT shot, and she suffered another high fever and bout of high-pitched screaming, only this time it was for a shorter period of time. It was soon after Sherry's second DPT shot that Ellen began to realize that her once-alert baby no longer responded to her voice or followed her around the room with her eyes the way she had when she was three-and-a-half months old.

"After her second shot, I noticed that Sherry could no longer raise her head or turn it from side to side. I had to support her head when I carried her. And her eyes started to cross. She could not imitate the sounds of simple syllables or play with her hands. Basically she was just uninterested in life. She wouldn't eat, and I had to take her off the bottle because she would gag when the nipple was placed in her mouth. And when she would cry, often she would throw her head back and her voice would rise several octaves into that high-pitched shriek that reminded me of those days and nights of hell following her DPT shots."

Ellen's pediatrician put Sherry into the hospital to have a specialist examine her throat to try to determine the cause for her high-pitched screaming. After the specialist said he could find no cause for Sherry's unusual cry, her pediatrician kept reassuring Ellen that, despite Sherry's lack of physical and mental development, there was no reason to be alarmed.

"When Sherry was eleven months old and still could not sit or hold a rattle, I took her to another pediatrician. He readmitted Sherry to the hospital for extensive tests. The tests showed she was mentally retarded but did not reveal a genetic or any other reason for her retardation. But the pediatrician chose not to tell me that the tests showed she was retarded. He kept the results from me. Instead he told me not to worry about her and to give her more time to develop," said Ellen.

When Sherry was eighteen months old, Ellen had her evaluated at a national clinical diagnostic center. It was there that, for the first time, a doctor finally admitted to Ellen that Sherry was mentally retarded.

Three months later, Sherry was tested at a nationally known rehabilitation institute. "Each time I took her to a new doctor, I mentioned her violent reaction to her DPT shots, but the doctors never commented. In fact, they often looked at me like I was crazy to even bring it up. Eventually, I just stopped talking about the shots because no one was interested," Ellen said.

After a complete evaluation, the doctors told Ellen that her daughter was severely mentally and physically handicapped. "They told me that Sherry falls into the one-percent category of individuals with no known cause for their mental retardation. They advised me to 'take her home and love her.' "

Sherry reached for her first object and put it into her mouth when she was two-and-a-half years old, a normal skill for a seven month old. She took her first step when she was seven. She was toilet-trained at age nine. Today, at fourteen, she has a vocabulary of about thirty-five words and walks with difficulty. She lives at home with her mother, who is divorced and works full time as an accountant. Sherry's eighteen-year-old sister is in college.

Sherry is enrolled in a special class for severely and profoundly handicapped children in a public school. At age twenty-one she will no longer be eligible for public schooling. At that point, Ellen will either have to find approximately twenty-five thousand dollars per year to place her in a residential home or she will have to quit her job, sell her house, and stay home with Sherry until their money runs out. Ellen maintains she will never place Sherry in a state institution for the mentally retarded. Now forty-one, Ellen will be responsible for her severely mentally retarded daughter for the rest of her life.

✿ ✿ ✿ ✿ ✿

A vibrant, quick-spoken woman, Ellen flashes one of her frequent smiles as she speaks with pride of her teenage daughter's most recent accomplishments.

"The other day, Sherry knocked over a wastebasket, and instead of just leaving the trash lying there on the floor, she went into the broom closet, got a broom and dustpan, and cleaned it up. It was hard for her and took a long time, but she didn't give up. Now the best part is that, after she was finished, she put the broom and dustpan back into the closet! I couldn't believe it! When I told her doctor about it, he agreed it was very significant for Sherry to have developed the capacity to comprehend that certain objects belong in certain places."

Ellen lights another cigarette and finishes what must be her eighth cup of coffee for the day and then goes on enthusiastically. "A few months ago, Sherry tried to get herself a drink of water for the first time. I turned the water on and she picked up her cup and put it under the faucet to fill it. I was so excited because it meant she understood that the water coming out of the faucet could provide her with a drink of water."

Sherry, who at fourteen is already as tall as Ellen, walks into the kitchen taking small, awkward steps. She has a strong, wiry body, and her long, thin arms and legs move stiffly as she inches her way over to her mother.

"Sherry is here!" she booms in a husky slurred voice, twisting her brown hair in her fingers. "Sherry is here!" she repeats cheerfully.

"Your hair looks very nice, Sherry," Ellen says with an approving nod.

Sherry beams at the compliment she wanted to hear. She is holding a toy mirror in her hand. "Sherry," she confirms, pointing into the mirror.

"Yes," agrees Ellen. "That is Sherry and she is very pretty."

Sherry grins and slowly shuffles out of the kitchen. Soon there are sounds of toy pots and pans banging together in the next room, punctuated by Sherry's guttural expressions of delight.

Ellen smiles again. "I have always tried to teach her to like herself, and she has responded by developing an outgoing personality. It tickles me to see her begin to be concerned about things like wanting people to notice her hair. And lately, she is asserting herself more. She is definitely developing a mind of her own. Even though it presents control problems, I just love it when she refuses to eat a certain food or refuses to let me help her because she wants to do it herself. Her struggle for independence means she is continuing to grow mentally and emotionally."

Sherry comes back into the kitchen and grabs her mother's arm, impulsively shouting, "Mommy! Mommy!"

"No, Sherry," Ellen says firmly as she tries to release Sherry's firm grip on her forearm. She taps her daughter's clutching fingers. "No, Sherry, not so hard. Let go."

Obediently, Sherry lets go, shakes her head, and repeats, "No, Sherry." Then she grins. After a hug from her mother, she wanders back into the next room and continues playing with her toys like any contented three year old.

"She doesn't know her own strength right now," Ellen explains. "It has only become a problem in the past year since she has grown so fast. But she is learning to be more gentle."

Ellen puffs nervously on another cigarette. She speaks with the gutsy determination of a survivor, a characteristic that unites many of the mothers of vaccine-damaged children. Still there is pain and a hint of anger in her eyes and surrounding the edges of her voice. She is a survivor who knows exactly where she has been and how far she has to go.

"It wasn't until a few months ago that any pediatric neurologist would admit that Sherry's retardation was due to the pertussis vaccine in the DPT shots. Up until then, no doctor would listen or even discuss the possibility with me. They can be so damn patronizing. You know, pat the little mother on the head and tell her to calm down. But I could never forget about Sherry's reaction to her DPT shots, no matter how many doctors said there was no connection between them and her retardation. And when I saw the television documentary 'DPT: Vaccine Roulette' I sat down and cried. It was then I knew I had been right all along.

"For a long time I was very angry with the doctors who tried to make me think nothing was wrong with her, when it was obvious to me that she had stopped developing mentally and physically at about five-and-a-half months of age. I remember asked one of them why he had withheld the truth from me. He said, 'You and your husband made such a beautiful couple. How do you tell parents their child has cancer?' My reply to him was, 'My child didn't have cancer and she wasn't going to die. She's retarded, but she's alive.' Why can't doctors honestly share information with parents? If scientists and doctors have known for thirty-five years that the pertussis vaccine in the DPT shots can cause brain damage, why didn't the doctors at the national medical centers where Sherry was tested listen to me when I told them about Sherry's severe reaction to her DPT shots? More importantly, why was Sherry given a second DPT shot after her first one produced such a violent reaction?"

Ellen goes on to point out one of the most disheartening aspects of her struggle to learn the truth about her daughter's retardation and to cope with the long-term implications.

"From my experience, most pediatricians divide mothers of damaged children into two categories: those mothers who blindly accept a pediatrician's every word and can be easily reassured or controlled; and those mothers who question a diagnosis, ask for more information, and cannot be easily controlled. I was in category number two. I was not satisfied with the answers I was getting about Sherry's condition and prognosis. Therefore, very early on, I was officially labeled a 'troublemaker' and a 'hysterical mother' in Sherry's medical records. They did not like my attitude."

Ellen and her husband divorced soon after Sherry was diagnosed as mentally retarded. Ellen's main activity outside of caring for Sherry and her full-time job is lobbying hard for better social services for handicapped children and adults.

"I am not the only single working mother who is trying to raise a brain-damaged child and hold down a job at the same time. We need help, not isolation. We need day-care centers, more group homes and decent, affordable residential placement centers for those twenty-one years and older. At the age of twenty-one, the state cuts off all public education for the handicapped. Do you know how hard it is to find a babysitter for a fourteen-year-old retarded teenager? I can't imagine what I am going to do when Sherry is twenty-five or thirty-five years old."

According to Ellen, throughout the nation there are far too few placement centers offering day programs that allow handicapped adults to return home at night. "For example, in my county there is a day placement center with 130 slots and a three-year waiting list. So the majority of American communities have handicapped adults, who may have learned simple skills in public school, but end up sitting at home vegetating after the age of twenty-one. Either that or they are put into state institutions for the mentally retarded."

When you ask Ellen about the possibility of placing Sherry in a state institution in the future, Ellen's eyes narrow with defiance. "I would never put Sherry in a state institution. They are warehouses. If I had listened to some of the doctors, who told me there was no hope for Sherry to develop intellectually and emotionally beyond the infant stage, I might have put her into a state institution and today she would probably still be a fourteen-year-old infant. Instead, today she is an often delightful teenage three year old. I don't know what I will do when I get too old to handle her, say when I'm in my sixties or seventies and she is only in her thirties and forties. But she is part of me. If I could afford it, I would consider placing her in a good residential home when she is an adult, but I will never abandon her in a state institution as long as I am still alive."

The concept of a federal compensation system for vaccine-damaged children and mandatory vaccination laws are two subjects that Ellen feels strongly about. "We need to revise our state mandatory immunization laws to allow parents the right to object to a particular vaccine. And we need a compensation system that allows a parent to either go through the government for compensation or to sue negligent doctors and drug companies for the damage that has been done to a child. Last year, the AMA and drug manufacturers supported a federal compensation system that would be an 'exclusive remedy' and would prevent all lawsuits against doctors and drug companies. That is outrageous. If you combine that kind of exclusive remedy compensation system with our country's mandatory vaccination policy, you have a situation where the government, drug companies, and doctors have absolutely no incentive for producing safe vaccines or administering them properly. It makes it easy for the government to tell us we have to get our children vaccinated with every new vaccine that is developed because if they are hurt, they will pay us for it. In effect we would be financing through our taxes the killing and injuring of our own children. Do they really think that money can ever compensate Sherry for what they took from her?"

Gazing out the window into the sun shining on her garden, Ellen's voice becomes quieter and her face looks drawn. "Sometimes Sherry will glance at me, and for just a moment, I see in her eyes the girl she might have been. What is hard to take is knowing it could have been prevented. Her life did not have to be wasted."

Then, she adds evenly, "I learned a long time ago that I would destroy myself if I let anger and fear take over my life. I'm trying to channel it. I want to try to make the lives of handicapped children and their parents more bearable. I want to get information out to parents about the vaccine to lessen the chances of other kids being hurt like Sherry was hurt."

Quickly changing the subject, Ellen holds up a package of pink leotards. "See these? These are for Sherry. She has her first ballet lesson this afternoon, along with five other retarded kids. Isn't that great? She is so excited! I wish her sister were here to see this."

The telephone rings and Ellen answers it. At the sound of the phone ringing, Sherry makes a reappearance wearing her usual infectious grin. She is carrying a brand-new ballet slipper in one hand. Impishly she gets down on the floor and crawls over to her mother, grabs one of Ellen's legs, and gives it a big bear hug. Ellen doesn't know whether to laugh or get mad. She rolls her eyes good-naturedly and groans, "Sherry! What are you doing?"

Sherry just keeps grinning with a gleam in her eye, a trace of saliva trickling down the left corner of her chin. "Sherry is here," she announces happily, still clutching the shiny black ballet slipper and holding on to her mother's leg for dear life.

5

Adverse Reactions: An Afterthought?

In medicine, sins of commission are mortal,
sins of omission venial.
Theodore Tronchin

One of the strangest elements in the pertussis vaccine story is that the vaccine was introduced on a mass scale in England, the United States, and other industrialized countries of the world without a systematic effort to evaluate its side effects. Once vaccination programs were in full swing in developed countries, almost no attempt was made to adequately monitor side effects or improve the safety of the vaccine.

In the late 1940s, government health officials and physicians were aggressively promoting pertussis vaccination throughout America as the incidence of whooping cough was swiftly declining. At the same time, vaccine researchers and physicians were becoming aware that the benefits of the pertussis vaccine were not without accompanying risks.

The vaccine's ability to kill without warning was first signaled in 1933 by Thorvald Madsen in Copenhagen. He reported that two babies, who had been vaccinated immediately after birth, had died within a few minutes of the shot.

Later in the 1930s, American researchers reported that some children reacted with fevers, convulsions, and collapse. But most doctors discounted these reports, convinced that reactions were insignificant compared to the protection the vaccine gave against the dreaded whooping cough.

In 1946, Werne and Garrow described the deaths of identical twins within twenty-four hours of their second shot. In 1947, Matthew Brody, at the Brooklyn Hospital, gave detailed descriptions of two cases involving brain damage leading to death after the shot.

But the major contribution to persistent reports of pertussis vaccine reactions was the 1948 study by Randolph K. Byers and Frederick C. Moll of the Harvard Medical School. They examined fifteen children who had reacted violently within seventy-two hours of a pertussis vaccine injection. All the children were normal before the shot; none had ever had a convulsion.

One case they described was that of an eight-month-old boy, whose first pertussis shot was given at seven months. That shot was followed by irritability and drowsiness, which cleared up in about three days. Three weeks later he was given a second shot and "rapidly became irritable, restless, febrile, and held right arm stiffly. About seventy-two hours after the inoculation had two severe generalized convulsions and was admitted to another hospital." When he was seen by his family physician eight months later, "he was blind, deaf, spastic and helpless."

Byers and Moll concluded that of the fifteen children they studied, "one child had recovered completely, three had had too short a period of observation to allow for final conclusions, two pursued a long downhill course ending in death, and the remaining nine suffered from damage to their nervous system, which in most instances promised to interfere with competitive living."

Physicians generally were surprised and displeased by this article. Byers later told a television journalist that "the report wasn't received well by the medical community at the time." The reason? For the first time doctors had to face the fact that the vaccine was not without serious risk. A 1949 *British Medical Journal* article stated, "Pertussis vaccination, whatever might be thought of its immunizing capacity, had at least been considered relatively free from side effects."

John A. Toomey wrote in 1949 that the Byers and Moll study was "disturbing, since prior to it this [vaccine] had been considered innocuous." He himself sent out questionnaires to a number of pediatricians and collected data on thirty-eight cases of severe reactions to the pertussis vaccine.

Louis Sauer made an interesting observation after Toomey presented his report at a 1948 AMA meeting, pointing out that the neurological damage caused by the vaccine resembles the damage caused by whooping cough. "In isolated cases," he said, "a customary prophylactic dose of pertussis vaccine . . . seems to elicit a chain of untoward central nervous system reactions—fever, convulsions and, in some instances, irreversible pathologic changes in the brain. These cardinal findings resemble those occasionally encountered in cases of severe whooping cough."

In 1953, S. Köng compiled a list of 82 cases of pertussis vaccine damage from the world literature. By 1958, the literature contained 107 cases, of which 93 were from the United States. J. M. Berg analyzed the 107 cases and found that 41 had recovered, 31 showed signs of permanent damage, while the fate of the rest was unknown. Berg called attention to the danger of mental retardation as an effect of the vaccine and emphasized that "ANY suggestion of a neurological reaction to a pertussis inoculation should be an ABSOLUTE contraindication to further inoculation."

In spite of these warnings, American doctors continued to insist that the damage from the pertussis vaccine was minuscule compared to the hundreds of thousands of infants who were regularly being vaccinated without any serious reactions. But upon what evidence did they base this assumption?

As mentioned in Chapter 3, no large clinical trials of any kind were ever held in the United States to measure the pertussis vaccine's safety or effectiveness. The only large-scale clinical trials ever conducted were those held in Britain from 1946 to 1957, and by the time they were completed the United States was already using the vaccine on a mass basis. Again, the British trials primarily were designed to measure the vaccine's ability to protect against whooping cough, not to determine its safety. Doctors conducting the trials reported that "special notes were kept of children who developed convulsions after vaccination."

Although eight children in these British trials had their first recorded convulsion within seventy-two hours following a shot, the doctors added, "It is impossible to say whether or not the number of cases observed was greater or less than might be expected to occur by chance in this period." Thirty-four more children had their first recorded convulsion four to twenty-eight days after a pertussis vaccine injection, but the doctors again denied a possible connection saying, "There is no reason to consider their convulsions were precipitated by the vaccine."

These trials, therefore, were used by British and American physicians as evidence that the DPT shot was safe, even though the data could well have been interpreted to suggest the opposite conclusion. And they should never have been interpreted to mean that the vaccine was safe for everyone, since they excluded infants younger than six months, those with a personal or family history of convulsions, and those who had been recently ill—categories of children who have been routinely given the vaccine in America.

As George Dick stated in 1978, "It appears that any untoward effects that may have occurred with whooping cough vaccine tended to have been minimized or disregarded for fear of upsetting the use of a vaccine against a disease which, in the late 1950's, was giving rise to approximately 30,000 to 90,000 annual notifications."

By the late 1950s, pertussis vaccination programs were in full swing in all the industrialized countries of the world, with the United States leading the way. Physicians and scientists were apparently convinced that pertussis vaccination was almost risk-free and the American and British governments aggressively promoted this concept to the public.

But in 1960, the medical world took notice when Swedish vaccine researcher Justus Ström stated in the *British Medical Journal*, "In Sweden the incidence of neurological complications after pertussis does not appear to be as high as that after vaccination." Ström also pointed out that whooping cough had become a much milder disease in his country and concluded, "The increasingly mild nature of whooping cough and the very low mortality in this disease in Sweden makes it questionable whether universal vaccination against it is justified. The same question may perhaps arise in some other countries."

In 1961, J. M. H. Hopper, a senior school medical officer in northern England, found that some parents were refusing to bring their children into the local health clinic for further DPT shots. He investigated and found the reason to be occasional violent reactions to a previous shot.

Hopper wrote, "They told, on questioning, of the child becoming ill two to four hours after the injection. Advice was sought from the neighbors, and often the family doctor was called. This, they explained, was their reason for failing to keep the appointment."

He collected information on fifty-two such cases, of whom six suffered collapse; fourteen, persistent vomiting; and thirteen, persistent uncontrollable screaming. He thought the persistent screaming showed "irritation of the nervous system" and gave the following description of it:

"Within a half to four hours of the injection the child would start to scream and could continue unceasingly for up to three, or even six, hours. The child would lie on its cot, flushed and irritable, sometimes with the head moving from side to side. No amount of nursing or lifting the child would cause this screaming to abate. One screaming bout would follow close on the heels of the next. The child, finally exhausted, would then fall asleep, to reawake in some cases with further bouts of screaming."

No one paid much attention to these warnings, even though Hopper's observations were confirmed by other physicians, in private communications as well as in occasional published articles. However, in 1963 a British physician wrote that pediatricians had become concerned about the high incidence of unpleasant reactions to the DPT shot:

"Here again there are no satisfactory figures; health visitors, clinic doctors, and parents themselves have come to be philosophical about the unpleasant effects of immunization. Evidence on these problems is largely anecdotal, but one has only to talk to health visitors to realize their worries; clinic doctors often have the same feelings, and many medical officers of health are now beginning to be suspicious about pertussis reactions. I have two children with severe encephalopathy which I believe (but cannot prove) is due to the pertussis antigen. I have admitted to hospital over the past few years several infants who have collapsed and become pale, shocked, and apparently lifeless some hours after a combined injection. All field workers are familiar with the infant who starts uncontrollable screaming attacks within an hour or two of his 'triple' inoculation and may go on without a break for twenty-four hours. These facts are all well known but often undocumented. There is need for a careful new look at pertussis immunization."

In 1967, Dick also warned that such reactions were much more common than anyone realized: "A number of doctors," he wrote, "have recently informed me that the state of affairs which Dr. Hopper described, and which we found, is not exceptional. Information about these 'major' reactions to triple vaccines is largely undocumented. This is confirmed by letters which I have recently received from parents following a newspaper report on a recent publication on this subject."

In 1967, Ström wrote that his earlier article on adverse reactions had aroused "considerable attention and also criticism," but he insisted that "the convulsions, shock, and abnormal irritability observed after triple vaccination cannot always be regarded as commonplace general symptoms but rather reflect an objectively demonstrable cerebral reaction. . . . The vaccination reactions may be regarded chiefly as manifestations of a toxic effect, an individual predisposition being of some significance."

In 1970, the American Academy of Pediatrics (AAP) reacted to this accumulation of information on adverse reactions by writing in the *Red Book* (an often-used pediatric reference), "Severe central nervous system reactions have been reported, occasionally with permanent sequelae [residual damage] or death; however, the incidence of such complications following immunization is much lower than the incidence of similar serious reactions from the disease itself."

The controversy heated up, however, with a 1974 article by M. Kulenkampff, J. S. Schwartzman, and J. Wilson retrospectively analyzing thirty-six cases of neurological illness seen at the Hospital for Sick Children in London from 1961 to 1972. All of the cases were thought to be attributable to DPT inoculation. The authors reported that out of the thirty-six cases, two died, four recovered completely, one was permanently paralyzed on one side, four were mentally retarded, three were left with epilepsy, and twenty-two were retarded and also had epilepsy. Their report later became the basis for a television program which brought the news home to British parents and is thought to have contributed to the decline in pertussis vaccination coverage in England from 80 percent to 30 percent in the following four years.

In 1974, Dick estimated that in Britain there were eighty cases of severe neurological complications annually: one third of these children died, and one third were left with residual brain damage. He admitted to being "not entirely convinced that the community benefit from whooping cough vaccination outweighs the damage which it may be doing."

In 1977, Gordon T. Stewart, M.D., of the Department of Community Medicine, University of Glasgow in Scotland, published a study analyzing one hundred sixty cases of adverse reactions and neurotoxicity following DPT vaccination. He reported that in sixty-five of the children, reactions were "followed by convulsions, hyperkinesis [hyperactivity] and severe mental defect." Among the reactions he observed were persistent crying, or fits of screaming; marble pallor, rigidity, unresponsiveness, and shock; irritability and interrupted sleep for a few days or longer; refusal or vomiting of food; pareses or localized paralysis; one or more convulsions with or without fever and turning blue (also called "cyanotic fits").

Stewart added, "In some cases, probably the majority, these symptoms subside within a few days or weeks. But in other cases, including at least 65 reported to me, the following signs also appear: hyperkinesis;

infantile spasms extending into convulsions, epilepsy, or salaam fits; progressive unresponsiveness to parents; flaccid paralysis; partial or complete amentia [deterioration of the brain]." He concluded, "It seems likely that most adverse reactions are unreported and that many are overlooked."

The Kulenkampff, Schwartzman, and Wilson article and the publicity following its publication led to the formation of the Association of Parents of Vaccine Damaged Children, which pressured the British government to study adverse reactions to the pertussis vaccine. The government responded by conducting the National Childhood Encephalopathy Study (NCES), which tested the connection between the vaccinations and neurological disease. (The NCES study is discussed in Chapter 20.)

In 1981, D. L. Miller, M.D., and others published an analysis of the first one thousand cases of neurological illness reported to the health officials conducting the NCES. Thirty-five of these cases had received pertussis vaccine within seven days of becoming ill. The reactions reported included prolonged convulsions (thirty minutes or more), encephalitis, encephalopathy, infantile spasms, and Reye's syndrome. Residual damage included minor and major delays in motor, speech, social, and global development; hemiplegia; blindness; and death. The authors concluded: "A significant association was shown between serious neurological illness and pertussis vaccine. . . ."

In 1979, the United States Food and Drug Administration funded a study representing the first large-scale attempt of the United States government to evaluate reactions to the DPT shot. The study, conducted at the University of California in Los Angeles, was coauthored by Cody, Baraff, Cherry, Marcy, and FDA pertussis vaccine researcher Charles Manclark, Ph.D., and published in *Pediatrics* in 1981.

After monitoring more than 16,000 DPT and DT (diphtheria-tetanus) vaccinations, the study found that the incidence of reactions from the DPT shot was much higher than after the DT shot, indicating that the P or pertussis component was the one causing reactions. It also found that the incidence of all DPT reactions—shock, convulsions, high-pitched screaming, fever, vomiting, drowsiness, fretfulness, persistent crying, and local reactions—was much higher than had ever been suspected or reported in the scientific literature. The UCLA-FDA study is discussed in more detail in Chapters 14 and 20.

But despite this study and more than forty years of warnings about the reactivity of the pertussis vaccine, physicians responsible for setting vaccine standards and policy in the Public Health Service (PHS), American Academy of Pediatrics (AAP), and American Medical Association (AMA) continued to promote the vaccine to American parents with confidence and with little emphasis on the risks associated with it. With little emphasis on risks, little attention was paid to identifying high-risk children or carefully observing contraindications.

The DPT shot had become a routine medical procedure in America and, instead of being informed about vaccine reactions, parents were legally required to have their children vaccinated in order to enroll them in school. When a child reacted violently to a DPT shot, parents were rarely told it was the pertussis vaccine that caused their child to die or become brain damaged. Not until reporter Lea Thompson at WRC-TV in Washington, D.C., broke the story in April 1982 with "DPT: Vaccine Roulette" were American parents made aware that their children could be permanently injured by the pertussis vaccine. It had been thirty-four years since Byers and Moll had informed the American medical establishment of that fact.

Adverse Reactions: What Are They?

Over the past half century, many millions of children have been vaccinated with pertussis vaccine. The majority do not react in any noticeable way or may simply run a low fever and experience pinkness and tenderness around the site of the injection. For these children, there does not appear to be any long-term damage. A small minority react violently and are more likely to be left with illness and handicaps that are almost totally disabling, such as mental retardation, seizure disorders, or paralysis.

There is another group of children, who react with varying degrees of severity, but whose growth and mental development may be affected in more subtle ways. These children may be plagued with chronic infections, behavior problems, or delayed development. Some of these conditions may not be readily apparent and will only show up when the child attends school and is found to be "hyperactive" or "learning disabled."

On the 1982 television broadcast "DPT: Vaccine Roulette," the microbiologist Bobby Young said, "If the child is not frankly rendered a vegetable . . . how many infants that are receiving this are in some way damaged by the vaccine and how can you prove that they haven't been, or that they have been? All of them are vaccinated."

Young was criticized by physicians in positions of leadership in the American medical establishment and the FDA for making that statement. Upon hearing his words, however, Daniel Levitt, M.D., Ph.D., an immunologist with the Guthrie Research Institute in Sayre, Pennsylvania, stated, "That is probably the most truthful statement that has been made in this whole situation. We really don't know what the effects are except in a very limited way. Is that frightening? Probably, because we are dealing with infants. Is it uncommon? I would say, no. It is common for most vaccines and drugs that we use. We really don't know with absolute certainty what many of their effects are upon the system."

Disturbing questions beg to be answered. Has the apparently normal child been affected by a vaccine which admittedly has a disastrous impact on a small group who are highly sensitive to it? Has the toxic neurological effect of the pertussis vaccine left its stamp on the mental and physical makeup of two whole generations in the modern world? If so, Stewart may well have been right in stating, "the number of well children who have suffered mental or physical disturbance as a result of vaccination may have to be counted not in hundreds, as in the United Kingdom, or in thousands, as in the rest of the Western world, but in hundreds of thousands all over the world. This is a heavy price to pay for marginal and temporary protection against a disease that seldom nowadays threatens the life or health of well children."

A pertussis vaccine reaction can occur in several stages. First, there is an acute or immediate reaction after the injection. This first reaction may be self-contained and followed by complete recovery. But an acute reaction may also lead to long-term chronic physical, mental, emotional, or neurological disturbances which remain with the child in some form for the remainder of his life.

Skin Reactions

The most common reaction is local: pain, redness, soreness, or swelling around the area of the injection. The 1984 information insert placed in packages of DPT vaccine manufactured by Wyeth Laboratories, Inc., stated, "local reactions, manifested by erythema [redness] and induration [hardness] with or without tenderness, are common. . . . A nodule may be palpable at the injection site for a few weeks. Abscess formation at the site of the injection has been reported."

The UCLA-FDA study reported that 37 percent of the DPT shots produced local redness, 40 percent produced local swelling, and 50 percent produced local pain. A 1979 survey of four pediatric practices in Colorado revealed that 72 percent of the children had local reactions, which included redness, swelling, and tenderness after a DPT shot.

Most local reactions only involve a temporary pinkness and tenderness around the injection site and cause no further problems. Some case reports have suggested, however, that a pronounced local reaction may be cause for caution when considering future DPT shots. British health officials consider a severe local reaction to be a contraindication to further injections of pertussis vaccine. All severe local reactions should be reported to the doctor who administered the shot, and he should not dismiss the reaction lightly.

One mother reported that the site of injection on her infant daughter's leg "swelled up like a giant hive. It swelled up to about one sixteenth of an inch in height and was as big as the palm of my hand. On a three-month-old baby that takes up a lot of space." This local reaction was associated with a neurological reaction that left her daughter brain damaged after her first DPT shot.

Several mothers have reported that a large, hard, red, swollen lump at the site of the injection after a shot may signal more severe reactions following future shots. A mother reported that her son "reacted to the first and second shots with a big, red, hot, swollen lump at the site of the injection that took two or three days to go away. His fever was never higher than 100 degrees, but that lump on his leg was disturbing." Within a week after his second and third shots, he suffered seizures that are now uncontrollable.

Another mother noticed that, within twenty-four hours, her son "had a knot about the size of a walnut or golf ball—it was red, hot, hard, and really large—come up on his leg. It was there for about two months." Again, this severe local reaction combined with a neurological reaction to leave the child with uncontrollable seizures and severe brain damage.

A mother on the West Coast had good reason to be disturbed about her son's severe local reaction to his second DPT shot. She said, "He had a little fever and was cranky, like he was after his first shot. But he also had a very large lump on his leg about the size of a baseball. I could put my whole palm over it. It was red and purple and hot. It took weeks to go away."

Her son appeared to recover completely, but her doctor did not consider this local reaction to be serious, and gave him a third DPT shot. In the days following this shot, he became unresponsive to stimulus and then began to have convulsions. Today he has constant seizures and is severely brain damaged.

A mother in the Midwest reported that after her son's second DPT shot, "Alan ran a fever and was irritable, and his leg got a big purple lump on it where the shot went in. It was about the size of a marble and came up within hours of the shot and was hot and sore for about two or three days."

The purple lump stayed on her son's leg for one year but did not seem to bother him. The pediatrician was convinced it would eventually dissolve. Exactly one year later, on the anniversary of the second DPT shot, Alan's temperature soared to 105 degrees and he began vomiting in the middle of the night. Then he turned blue and stopped breathing. Fortunately, his parents were with him at the time, and his father revived him with CPR (cardiopulmonary resuscitation). He was rushed to a hospital.

The skin around the purple lump on Alan's leg had begun to peel several days before his collapse. One week later, he had a fever of 104 degrees and was hospitalized again.

"The next day, Alan woke up and his leg where the lump had been had burst open and was all pussy with a lot of drainage. He went home the following day, and has not had any problems since then but he still has a purple scar where the lump was," said his mother. The pediatrician in this case was prudent enough to give Alan a DT (diphtheria-tetanus) shot from then on and may well have prevented far more serious complications.

Skin rashes have also been reported following the DPT shot. Byers and Moll described rashes in their case histories in 1948, and Ström observed rashes similar to measles, as well as edema (swelling) of the face, hands, and feet in 1967. Hennessen and Quast in 1979 found that 11 percent of a group of one hundred thirty-six children reacted to a DPT shot with urticaria (hives) and other kinds of skin reactions. One mother described the reaction of her daughter, who broke out in hives within a week of her DPT shot:

"Within a matter of hours of her first shot, she started screaming. She is number four for me, and you expect a child to be irritable after a vaccination and run a little fever. But her screaming was something else and it continued for a few days. Then she broke out into a rash. I thought maybe it was a heat rash because she did have a fever of about 103 degrees. But my doctor said it was definitely a reaction to the DPT shot and said that she should never have another one."

Fever

The next most common reaction to the DPT shot is a fever. The 1984 Wyeth Laboratories product insert stated that "mild-to-moderate temperature elevations, accompanied by malaise occurring within several hours of administration and persisting for one to two days, occur frequently" after the DPT shot. Lederle Laboratories and Connaught Laboratories also state that a temperature of over 103 F. is a contraindication to further pertussis vaccine.

The Colorado study reported that more than 50 percent of the children investigated in that survey had fevers of at least 100 F., while 4 percent had fevers higher than 102 F. The UCLA-FDA study reported that 46 percent of DPT shots produced temperatures of more than 100 F., while 6 percent produced fevers higher than 102 F.

Fever is the body's natural response to invasion by a foreign substance, whether it be live bacteria or a vaccine containing "killed" bacteria. In both cases, the body's immune system is challenged to produce antibodies to fight the invading substance.

A high fever can cause febrile (fever) convulsions in infants and because the pertussis vaccine is known to produce fevers, some of the convulsions following DPT shots may be simple febrile convulsions that do not result in brain damage or continuing seizure disorders. A nasty characteristic of some convulsions following DPT shots, however, is that they may trigger permanent seizure disorders.

A grandmother remembers how her daughter reacted to her third DPT shot in 1954. "Within nine hours of her shot, her temperature had risen to 106 degrees. She began screaming a terrible scream and then would become rigid and bend her head back. Her skin was very white and then she just lay there with her eyes wide open and unconscious all night long." Her daughter was left with petit mal seizures that weren't officially diagnosed until she was ten. Now thirty years old, she is on medication to control these seizures.

Within ten hours of his first DPT shot, a mother reported that her son "had a red and swollen leg and was crying a strange cry. His temperature was 105 degrees. I called the doctor and he told me to give him Tylenol and put him in a tepid bath. As I was putting him in the bath, his eyes rolled back in his head and he quivered all over." From that moment on, her son continued to have seizures and high-pitched screaming. Today, he is hyperactive and physically and mentally handicapped.

A boy in North Carolina, who is now three years old, ran fevers of 103 and 104 degrees after his first three shots. Within four hours of his fourth shot, he had swelling at the site of the injection, uncontrollable screaming, and a 105-degree fever. He continued to run a 103-degree fever for the next few days, and after it subsided, he was left with a peculiar and abrupt behavior change.

His mother said, "Overnight, he was turned from a brave and happy child into a trembling, fearful child who screamed in terror at the sight of balloons or at the thought of leaving the house. He wouldn't even enter a room if someone was chewing gum. He wouldn't leave the doorstep when we went out. He would just stand there and scream and shake until we picked him up. He became timid and nervous and we couldn't figure out what had happened."

Vomiting and Diarrhea

Vomiting and diarrhea are systemic reactions which can be mild or quite severe. Persistent diarrhea or vomiting can result in dehydration or shock. In 1984, Sato and his colleagues stated that pertussis vaccines "are known for their side-effects, which include . . . systemic reactions such as fever, vomiting, and diarrhea." Ström mentioned gastrointestinal symptoms in his 1967 study of DPT reactions. The UCLA-FDA investigators also found diarrhea and vomiting reactions. In the published report of the study, vomiting was mentioned but diarrhea was not.

Within a half day of her second shot, a baby girl in Michigan went into a seizure that lasted for hours. Her mother said, "Up until that

DPT shot at five months, she was such a healthy baby. After that she had diarrhea for about two or three weeks. It was a funny yellow color and smelled very bad."

Within an hour of her first shot, a two-month-old baby began high-pitched screaming that was followed by excessive sleepiness. Her mother reported that, within twenty-four hours, she "became very ill with diarrhea and vomiting. She had rarely vomited before, but now she began projectile vomiting. And her diarrhea had a really strange odor to it. We couldn't keep her in clean clothes. The diarrhea got all over everything. It lasted for six weeks after her shot."

Some babies who have died within days of receiving a DPT shot have had diarrhea within hours of the injection. The mother of Douglas, a two-month-old boy who died a day and a half after his first DPT shot, said, "I changed his pants and he moaned when I picked him up. I noticed he didn't have a normal bowel movement. It was just clumps of mucus and the stain around the diaper was a yellowish color. It looked like curds and smelled terrible. I will never forget that smell. I knew something was wrong." The events leading to Douglas's death are described later in this chapter.

The mother of a boy who reacted to his fourth DPT shot with a high fever and high-pitched screaming said, "Within two or three days of the shot he had a bad case of diarrhea. It was a green color and we finally had to take him to a gastrointestinal specialist. The diarrhea was kind of curdish in consistency and sometimes it would change colors but mostly it was green. This lasted for at least four months." The boy is now three years old, but his mother reports, "He still has a tendency to have diarrhea on and off even today."

After a three-month-old girl was given her first DPT shot, her mother reported that "Once at home, she started having terrible gas. About every couple of minutes, she would have violent, explosive gas. I have never heard a human sound like that. Maybe a 300-pound pig in a barn-yard, but never a human."

Although vomiting and diarrhea by themselves are not currently listed as contraindications to further pertussis vaccination, they should be considered systemic reactions and mothers should report them to the pediatrician. They may be accompanied by neurological signs, such as high-pitched screaming or excessive sleepiness. Justus Ström has found that children who have gastrointestinal reactions after one DPT shot are likely to suffer the same reaction after subsequent shots because "repeated injections produced the same effect."

Cough, Runny Nose, and Ear Infections

In 1945, pertussis vaccine researcher Wallace Sako wrote, "Following inoculation an occasional infant developed a paroxysmal pertussis-like cough which disappeared in a short time." This reaction was still being observed a quarter of a century later.

A mother recalled what happened to her two-month-old son in 1979: "Within twenty-four hours he started coughing really hard, like he had whooping cough. I thought maybe the shot had given him whooping cough. He would cough thirty minutes at a time. It sounded very croupy and hard and he would throw up. We had to put him in a sitting position to sleep to make sure he didn't choke."

A mother will often describe how her very healthy child became chronically ill following a DPT shot. Frequently the child will suffer an acute reaction such as a high fever, persistent crying, or a hard swollen lump at the injection site followed by a constant runny nose, bronchial congestion, and ear infections—all of which are resistant to antibiotics, antihistamines, and other medications. The mother cannot understand why her previously healthy child is suddenly "never well." The child may be sick for months with the mother taking him from doctor to doctor in search of a cure. Although never sick enough to be put in a hospital, the child never recovers his previous good health and continues to be plagued with constant "colds," ear infections, or the onset of allergies.

One mother recalled that, after his first DPT shot, her son "got an ear infection and it stayed from then on. We finally had tubes put in his ears. He also got a lot of upper respiratory infections, croup, coughing, and congestion."

A mother in Nevada took her two-month-old daughter to a hospital where she was given "a routine checkup. She was pronounced healthy and they gave her the shot. Within forty-eight hours, she was diagnosed as having a severe double ear infection. She also passed out and had severe diarrhea and projectile vomiting. The Chief of Pediatrics told us that we had a very sick child and that she probably had an allergic reaction to her DPT shot. Her diarrhea went on for weeks."

A mother in Chicago described her son's battle with constant infections after he reacted with convulsions within twenty-four hours of his second DPT shot. "After the second shot, he could not get rid of his ear infections. He had dozens of ear infections. And he had a lot of upper respiratory infections like pneumonia and then viral meningitis at eighteen months old."

Another mother, whose four-month-old daughter, Sharon, had a convulsion within twenty-four hours of her second DPT shot, watched her once-healthy baby develop a continual pattern of ear and lung infections. "She had been such a healthy baby, but from then on, she would run fevers, have ear infections and bronchial asthma problems. Finally, the doctors insisted we test her for allergies because she had so many lung infections." Now three years old, she is still on asthma medication and has pneumonia several times a year. Sharon's case is described in more detail later in this chapter.

Sean had a good appetite and a healthy constitution, even though he tended to spit up his milk and seemed to be plagued with colic the first few months of his life. In 1978, he reacted to his third DPT shot at the age of seven months with a large, hot, hard, red lump at the site of the injection which took several weeks to disappear. When his mother called the doctor about this, the nurse said, "We just found out it was a bad lot of DPT vaccine but it isn't causing any serious problems. The lump will go away soon."

His mother delayed the fourth DPT shot until Sean was required to get it in order to enter a "Mothers Day Out" program in a local church. At two and a half, Sean was a bright, happy, and exceptionally healthy little boy. He could recognize and name the upper and lower case letters of the alphabet. He could count and identify numbers up to 15. He had memorized a deck of cards and would intently play a "naming" game with them for a solid forty-five minutes at a time. One doctor suggested he might be "gifted" intellectually. Unlike so many children, his mother was amazed that he had never had a cold, cough, or ear infection in his life.

A month before his fourth shot, Sean was vacationing with his family at the beach. He suddenly spiked a fever of 103 degrees one evening and complained of a sore throat. The next morning he had diarrhea and vomiting. He had never been so ill. A doctor prescribed antibiotics and he appeared to recover within a week.

On the day of his fourth DPT shot, Sean's mother mentioned to the nurse that he had just recovered three weeks earlier from an infection that included diarrhea and vomiting. The nurse did not express concern and gave him the shot.

Later that afternoon, Sean was sitting in a chair. He stared momentarily at his mother and then, without a word, shut his eyes and fell into a deep sleep. She carried him to his bed, and he slept through dinner. When he awoke, he had violent diarrhea; it was dark green, almost black in color.

In the following weeks, Sean was transformed from a healthy, happy, and intellectually advanced child to one who was sick with constant diarrhea, ear infections, runny nose, and upper chest congestion. He lost his appetite and stopped growing. His weight dropped dangerously low. He no longer wanted to look at the alphabet, numbers, or cards. He couldn't sit still for more than a few minutes at a time. He became hypersensitive and cried easily without warning. His mother thought the abrupt personality and behavior change was due to his "never being well anymore." Doctors prescribed antibiotics and antihistamines, but nothing helped.

For eight months, Sean's health slowly deteriorated. His nose ran with clear drainage and he coughed day and night. His ears were always hurting, and the doctors kept diagnosing "recurring ear infections." Finally, his diarrhea turned yellow with a consistency that looked like attic foam insulation. He was placed on a diet of white rice, chicken breast meat, and diluted cranberry juice for a week. Still the diarrhea did not stop, and he became weaker and weaker.

Sean was admitted to a large children's hospital for testing. The pediatrician thought he might have cystic fibrosis or celiac disease. He was given X-rays, and blood and urine tests to screen for many diseases, including allergies. All tests came back negative.

Slowly the diarrhea stopped. When Sean was almost six years old, he still was having sinus drainage and coughing twelve months of the year, with increased symptoms during the spring and fall allergy seasons. He was underweight, had a very poor appetite, was susceptible to infections and prone to diarrhea. In kindergarten, the letters in the alphabet often confused him. His teacher, who works with neurologists at a children's hospital diagnosing and treating learning-disabled children, determined he was dyslexic with a visual perception problem, auditory processing deficit, fine motor delay, and an attention span deficit.

High-pitched Screaming and Persistent Crying

Two of the most frequent and most ignored serious reactions to the pertussis vaccine over the past thirty years are the ones described as "high-pitched screaming" and "persistent crying." The first is a thin, eerie, wailing sound quite different from the child's normal cry and very much resembles the so-called *cri encephalique* (encephalitic scream) found in some cases of encephalitis. It can go on for hours or days. The second describes a condition in which the child cries relatively normally but inconsolably, also for hours or days at a time.

Doctors have routinely told mothers to expect that their baby will be fussy or irritable for several days after the DPT shot. When anxious mothers have called their pediatricians or health clinics to report that their baby has been crying uncontrollably after a shot, doctors have often been quick to reassure them that crying is a "normal" reaction to a DPT shot.

The experience of a mother in Montana is a perfect example of how doctors often confuse unusual forms of crying with normal crying. "Three to four hours after the second DPT shot, Mark's leg turned bright red from his knee to his hip, and he started screaming this high, piercing cry. Nothing we did could get him to stop. It would go on for a good thirty minutes or more, and then he would just kind of pass out. After he would wake up again, he would start screaming. All night long he would scream. And his cry was different, not like he was hungry. It was like there was something severely wrong. If you tried to feed him, he just pushed it away. He didn't want to be rocked or held. And while he cried, he would arch his back, especially when we held him," said his mother.

When this worried mother called her child's pediatrician, his reaction was typical. "He said, 'Don't worry. Just give him Tylenol and he'll be fine.' So I didn't call him back again, because I thought, well, this is the way it is supposed to be."

Although Mark continued to scream shrilly two or three times a night for the next three months, the doctor still was unconcerned. "Whenever I called the doctor, he told me Mark might be having 'night terror' like some other babies. But, in addition to screaming, Mark stopped eating and wouldn't play or do anything. By the time I took him to the doctor when he was seven months old, he only weighed fourteen pounds and was anemic."

Even though the doctor was shocked at how underweight and weak Mark appeared, he still wanted to give him the third DPT shot. "I wouldn't let him give it to him," said his mother. "Prior to the second shot, the only problem Mark had ever had was colic until he was about a month old. I was breastfeeding him and had to stop drinking cow's milk and orange juice, which stopped the colic. Up until that second DPT shot, Mark was a perfect height and weight and had never screamed that strange cry that he had within three hours of that shot. It seemed very clear to me that the shot caused his health to deteriorate."

Today, almost two years old, Mark only weighs twenty pounds, but he appears to be developing normally mentally. He still occasionally wakes up at night with high-pitched screaming and is still on soybean formula for his milk allergy. The pediatrician was finally convinced that Mark should not have more pertussis vaccine, but only after his own son reacted to a DPT shot with high-pitched screaming. Mark had no reaction whatsoever to the DT shot he was given at eighteen months of age.

"My pediatrician believes me now," his mother said, "because his own son reacted to a DPT shot. Up until then, he kept telling me he had never seen a DPT shot reaction. I am just so thankful I didn't let him give Mark more pertussis vaccine. The only way I knew about the reactions was because I had seen a television show on it once. If I hadn't known, my son could be brain-damaged today."

As already mentioned, many authorities consider high-pitched scream-ing to be neurological in origin. Vincent Fulginiti wrote in 1982: "Many infants cry and fret after pertussis vaccination; a few adopt a pattern of consistent crying for periods of an hour or longer; the crying is often of unusual pitch and intensity and the baby is inconsolable. This syn-drome of screaming is believed to be encephalopathic in origin. . . . Chil-dren who experience such episodes are to be considered as having CNS [central nervous system] complications and further pertussis vaccine should not be administered."

The 1984 product information insert of Wyeth Laboratories agreed, describing the reaction as "screaming episodes characterized by a pro-longed period of peculiar crying during which the infant cannot be comforted" and listing it as a contraindication. Today both remaining pertussis vaccine manufacturers consider it an absolute contraindica-tion to further pertussis vaccine, as do the Advisory Committee on

Immunization Practices (ACIP) Recommendations of the Public Health Service.

However, the American Academy of Pediatrics' 1982 *Red Book* stated that infants who have excessive screaming (persistent crying or screaming for three or more hours) are not absolutely contraindicated from receiving more pertussis vaccine but only "probably" should not receive additional doses.

One mother described her son's high-pitched screaming after a DPT shot. "It was a blood-curdling scream like someone was stabbing him, and he never, never cried like that. Then he became unresponsive. His arms dropped to his side, and he became flaccid. About an hour later, the same thing happened again. His arms dropped to his side, he let out this terrible scream and became flaccid."

"What brought us into her room was her scream," said another mother of her daughter's vaccine reaction. "It sounded like something was attacking her. But we couldn't rouse her from the scream. It was like she was fighting it."

Another mother described her two-month-old son's screaming reaction after his first DPT shot. She said, "We live about thirteen miles from our doctor and I didn't even get five miles away from his office when my son began screaming like he was hurting very badly. About five hours later, he started to have a convulsion in the lower half of his body. And his fever went up to over 104 degrees."

Another little girl's mother said, "Within fifteen hours of her first DPT shot, she started screaming like she was in terrible pain. I went to my mother's house with her because it scared me so bad. Nothing we did would stop her screaming. She acted like she was falling . . . like she thought she was falling and screaming as she fell. She screamed like this off and on for two weeks during the day and night. Sometimes she would turn dark blue to black, and then she would start that screaming like someone was going to drop her."

The pediatrician ignored the reaction and gave the child two more DPT shots, which were followed by convulsions. Now two years old, she is on medication to control a seizure disorder.

Babies, of course, cannot explain why they are screaming. Mothers and fathers who listen in frustration and anxiety while their babies shriek into the night can only guess how they are feeling. But one mother, whose son, Brian, reacted to his fifth DPT shot, knows it was because he had a blinding headache.

Brian ran a fever, cried, and had swelling at the site of the injection after his first four DPT shots. He had been a colicky baby who was severely allergic to milk, orange juice, pollens, and several different drugs. He was prone to ear infections during the first five years of his life. When he was five years old, he was given his fifth DPT shot in order to attend school. He and his mother did not even get home before he started screaming hysterically.

"Because my son was five when he reacted, he was able to verbalize what he was feeling. He could just as easily have reacted when he was two or four months old and would have been unable to tell me how he was feeling. I didn't even get him home from the doctor's office before he started writhing on the floor of the car, screaming that he had a headache. By the time we got home, his fever had reached 104 degrees. He vomited, ran around the house, and hid in corners as if he was frightened to death."

Brian's mother telephoned the doctor on weekend call for her pediatrician. He examined Brian and, finding nothing wrong, sent him home. That night, Brian continued to run a high fever, scream, and hallucinate. He was finally admitted to the hospital.

"They did all the tests, including a spinal tap, and could find nothing wrong with him. That is when the resident doctor told us Brian must have taken LSD. I couldn't believe it. Because the nurses at the hospital thought Brian was hallucinating from LSD, they wrote down everything he said. You can imagine the hostility we experienced from the hospital personnel because they thought we had given our son LSD."

Brian's pediatrician was notified. "Our pediatrician stopped by the hospital the next morning and told us he had spent all night researching his medical books and came to the conclusion my son was reacting to the pertussis vaccine. Neither he nor the doctor on call had any idea that Brian could be reacting to the shot before he researched the vaccine that night."

Brian's mother believes her son should have been watched carefully by the doctor after the shot because of his history of severe allergies. "I am a nurse, and in the hospital we are taught not to give a drug unless we know each and every possible side reaction so we can be prepared. They say that with any patient who has a history of allergies, you should keep them there twenty to thirty minutes for observation. But with these vaccines, they give the child a routine exam, stick in the needle, and send you home. I had been in to that doctor almost every week with my son because of his severe allergies. He should never have been given that shot and sent right home."

After his reaction, Brian was left with a "tremor of intensity" in his hands and feet as well as learning disabilities and a tendency to hallucinate whenever he runs a fever.

The nightmarish experience of screaming in pain and hallucinating may leave a mark on a child's emotional development and cause unusual fear and nervousness for some time after the shot. A mother in Kentucky observed what happened to her eighteen-month-old daughter, who reacted to her fourth shot.

"In the next few days, she started crying a lot and her crying started to get peculiar. We called them 'crying spells' when she would arch her back and scream. It was a different kind of cry than she had done before and she began acting very afraid. She would be playing and all of a sudden stop and run over to me to be held. When we took her to the neurologist for testing because we were concerned about her strange behavior, the neurologist said that our daughter was experiencing a feeling of doom that older children had been able to describe. She said they don't know what they are afraid of, but it is a great feeling of anxiety and doom."

Some children may have episodes of high-pitched screaming for weeks or months afterwards. This was the case with Belinda, who began high-pitched and inconsolable screaming within seven hours of her first shot. "It was a pain cry," said her mother, "and she kept it up for a couple of hours. She had the very same reaction after her second and third DPT shots."

But after her third DPT shot, Belinda's sleep pattern changed, and she would alternate brief periods of sleep with long bouts of screaming. "I started going crazy," said her mother. "At night, she would only sleep for an hour at a time and during the day she would sleep for two or three hours at a time. And in between she would scream that horrible scream. She kept this up until she had her first seizure about three months later."

Belinda was put on anticonvulsant medication. Now three years old, she still has seizures about every six weeks. She will still go into fits of screaming in what her mother calls "uncontrollable temper tantrums."

Collapse or Shock-like Episodes

The terms "collapse" or "shock" or "hypotonic hyporesponsive episode" are used to define a reaction that was described in vivid detail by Dick in a 1967 British study of DPT vaccine reactions. He wrote:

"About three hours after inoculation, the baby suddenly becomes marble white, cold and collapsed and remains like this for about 15 to 30 minutes; after recovery, it often remains pale and listless for a few hours. Some mothers have said that their babies became unconscious at the onset of the collapse, others thought their baby was dead. When babies developing this syndrome were followed up a year later, they seemed healthy and appeared to have passed the usual milestones normally. It is, however, difficult to exclude the possibility of permanent damage. On observing these reactions, parents quite naturally urgently summoned a doctor, but by the time he arrived the baby had usually recovered from the severe episode and some mothers were quite unable to convince their physician that anything really serious had happened."

Charlotte A. Hannik, M.D., a pertussis vaccine researcher from the Netherlands, mentioned the collapse/shock reaction in 1969: "When describing the appearance, all mothers used expressions like 'white as a sheet' or 'ashen'; moreover, all mothers admitted, more or less frankly, to have been in fear for their child's life."

According to E. A. Mortimer, M.D., of Case Western Reserve University School of Medicine, the collapse/shock syndrome following DPT vaccination is "poorly understood in terms of pathogenesis and clinical significance." But, nevertheless, it is considered to be a severe reaction, and further pertussis vaccine should not be given, according to the commercial manufacturers of DPT vaccine, the AAP, and the ACIP Recommendations of the Public Health Service. It is extremely important that parents be aware of the physical symptoms which signal a collapse reaction and immediately report them to their pediatrician.

Within twenty-four hours of each of her three DPT shots, a baby in Mississippi collapsed. Her mother described her reaction: "She would turn blue and you couldn't even tell she was breathing. We would shake her and she would start breathing again."

Some babies who die shortly after a DPT shot have had collapse reactions before their death. Within seconds of receiving his second DPT shot, five-month-old Kevin collapsed. Because he reacted within seconds, this might more appropriately be termed "anaphylactic shock."

His father recalls what happened: "Instantly, after the nurse gave him that shot he turned blue and stopped breathing. She immediately got hold of the doctor and got him breathing again. We waited maybe thirty minutes there in his office, and then he told my wife, 'Well, Kevin just wants to act up. Some kids react a little more than others and he will probably be very fretful tonight.' And he sent us home."

Kevin never fully recovered and died after three days and nights of high-pitched screaming alternating with episodes of collapse. His death is described later in this chapter.

Within one week after each of her three DPT shots, Sandra was found in a state of collapse. Her mother described what she saw after the first shot: "I went in and she was not breathing. She was white and around her mouth she was very blue. The back of her head was drawn back. I screamed and her Daddy ran in and picked her up and breathed in her mouth. He said he could feel something give as he breathed in her mouth. She started breathing again, and even as young as she was, she seemed to be dazed and not know where she was. She seemed totally exhausted. She went to sleep and slept for four hours."

After her fourth shot, an eighteen-month-old girl collapsed. Her mother said, "The day after her shot, her leg got really stiff, and she couldn't walk on it. She couldn't move her leg. I took her back to the doctor because I thought she was crippled. The next night, she woke up screaming. It was a terrible, fearful kind of scream. My husband picked her up, and she got very silent and turned white with a purple-blue tinge around her mouth and went completely limp. We thought she was in the throes of sudden infant death syndrome."

The UCLA-FDA study concluded that 1 in 1,750 DPT vaccinations results in an episode of collapse. But, as Dick theorized in 1967, "It is possible that it is more frequent than generally believed, for it could well pass unobserved even by the mother."

Excessive Sleepiness

Although the drug manufacturers, the AAP, and the PHS seem unable to agree on the definition or significance of excessive sleepiness (somnolence) after a DPT shot, this reaction has been described in the scientific literature for decades. In 1949, Globus and Kohn told of one baby who suffered brain damage following a pertussis vaccination:

A six-month-old boy given his second DPT shot "shortly thereafter became alternately irritable and drowsy; for the first time since birth he slept through the entire night. There was no rise in temperature. An abrupt change in the child's behavior was noted by his mother. Before the second injection, he had played and reacted normally, but afterward he no longer played, would not reach out for objects, became indifferent to his environment, and slept for long intervals during the day. On the tenth day after the second injection he was seized by repeated convulsions. . . ."

Connaught Laboratories and Lederle Laboratories list somnolence (excessive sleepiness) as a contraindication to further pertussis vaccine in their DPT product inserts. But the 1981 guidelines published by the ACIP do not mention excessive sleepiness, although they do list "severe alterations of consciousness" as a contraindication. The AAP's current 1982 *Red Book* says only that infants who experience excessive somnolence "probably" should not receive more pertussis vaccine.

Children displaying this reaction usually lapse into a deep, stuporous sleep from which they cannot be awakened no matter how hard their parents may try. One mother described her daughter's excessive sleepiness after her first shot: "Within one hour of the shot, Linda went to sleep for twenty-four hours and I couldn't wake her at all. Just before she went to sleep, she acted very strangely and had a strange shrill cry that I had never heard. Then she passed out. She would not wake when her diaper was changed or when you flicked her feet or tried to feed her. We took her to a military hospital at the end of twenty-four hours, but she had started to come out of it by then. The doctors told us we were overanxious parents and to take our well child home. They were very indifferent."

Because the hospital doctors did not perceive it as an adverse reaction to the pertussis vaccine, Linda received four more DPT shots. She continued to lapse into periods of unconsciousness until she was three years old, but not one military doctor gave a reason for her "spells," and she was never put on medication. Although she was hyperactive, she did not lose consciousness again after the age of three. When Linda received her fifth DPT shot, which was required for her to enter kindergarten, her mother began to suspect the shot may have been responsible for her daughter's strange condition as a toddler.

"Immediately after she got her fifth shot, Linda became a totally different child for about twenty-four hours. Although she was usually hyperactive to the point of being out of control, she became extremely passive. We took her to an amusement park, where ordinarily she would be hard to handle. But that day she just stared and acted like she was in a daze, like she was sleepwalking."

Allergy testing revealed that Linda, now eleven, is allergic to many different pollens as well as milk. Her mother does not have enzymes to digest milk and cannot drink it. Hyperactivity, an emotional disorder, and an attention-span deficit are all continuing to cause problems for the child.

"There are days when we can't send her to school because she has such an explosive makeup. She is emotional dynamite. We have been through hell. Linda was so hyperactive as a little girl that she was always full of bruises and cuts because she would run aimlessly and crash into things. By the time she was three years old, I was a physical and emotional wreck trying to cope."

Seizure Disorders: Convulsions, Epilepsy, and Infantile Spasms

Perhaps the most frequently reported serious reaction to the pertussis vaccine in the scientific literature is the convulsive seizure. The UCLA-FDA study found that 1 in 1,750 DPT shots resulted in a child suffering a convulsion within forty-eight hours. Many parents do not know how to recognize a convulsion, and unfortunately, apparently many doctors do not either. Convulsions can range from rapid blinking of the eyes, twitching of the fingers, or staring episodes to violent jerking of the entire body. Simply defined by *Webster's New Third International Dictionary* (1976), a convulsion is a "spasmodic contraction of the muscles."

One mother described a type of seizure that her daughter had following a DPT shot. "She would stare straight ahead with her eyes dilated and her mouth frozen open. Her lips were blue and her body was stiff. The right side of her body would tremble and sometimes she would make sucking sounds while she was having the seizure."

If a child reacts with a convulsion to a DPT shot, the pertussis vaccine is absolutely contraindicated in the future. As of 1984 the American commercial vaccine manufacturers, the AAP, and the PHS all agreed on that recommendation. In the past 45 years, however, these vaccine policymakers have never determined how soon a convulsion must occur after a DPT shot in order for it to be labeled a "pertussis vaccine reaction."

Therefore, grassroots physicians have been left to make that determination themselves. Having been taught that vaccine reactions are extremely rare, many refuse to believe a DPT shot can cause a convulsion unless it occurs within minutes or hours of the inoculation. When a seizure occurs in conjunction with a fever shortly after a DPT shot, many doctors dismiss it as a harmless febrile convulsion brought on by the pertussis vaccine's ability to produce a fever. Still others are unaware that a DPT shot can cause a convulsion at all.

This widespread confusion and ignorance, combined with America's past tragic policy of not considering a history of convulsions to be an absolute contraindication to the vaccine, may have resulted in countless numbers of convulsive children becoming brain damaged from repeated injections of pertussis vaccine. There is no way of knowing how many children and adults are suffering from medication-resistant seizure disorders, epilepsy, mental retardation, learning disabilities, and other neurological abnormalities because health officials responsible for setting vaccine policy have not been clear on this issue.

In 1983, when the AAP and Dissatisfied Parents Together jointly developed the National Childhood Vaccine Injury Compensation Act, the AAP agreed that convulsions occurring within seven days of a DPT shot could be considered related to the shot. However, there are cases in the scientific literature linking convulsions occurring up to two weeks after the DPT shot to the pertussis vaccine.

Post-pertussis vaccine convulsions can occur with or without a fever. Those occurring in conjunction with a fever, known as febrile convulsions, are common in infancy and tend to run in families. As mentioned earlier, because the pertussis vaccine can cause a fever, some of the convulsions occurring after the DPT shot may be simple febrile convulsions which are self-contained and do not result in permanent damage. Occasionally, however, febrile convulsions may lead to a seizure disorder. Perhaps the most disturbing fact about post-pertussis vaccine convulsions, however, is that they are often not associated with a high fever but are "afebrile," and can also lead to long-term seizure disorders which are difficult or impossible to control with medication. Uncontrollable seizures are associated with various degrees of brain damage.

In October 1982, Jerome V. Murphy, M.D., a pediatric neurologist and clinical professor at the Medical College of Wisconsin, presented a study at a Child Neurology Society meeting in Salt Lake City on recurrent seizures with onset within twenty-four hours of a DPT vaccination. He concluded that "seizure disorders with an onset immediately after DPT immunization are generally tonic-clonic, resistant to routine anticonvulsant therapy, and have poor intellectual prognosis." Murphy's conclusions are consistent with many cases appearing in the pertussis vaccine literature during the past thirty-five years as well as with current reports by parents of vaccine-damaged children.

As mentioned earlier, Byers and Moll in 1948 found that "recurrent convulsions, either grand mal, petit mal, or localized in type, continued over variable lengths of time in thirteen children." A quarter of a century after Byers and Moll notified physicians about medication-resistant seizures following the pertussis vaccine, Kulenkampff and her coworkers repeated that warning with case history examples in their 1974 study.

But many doctors still fail to make the causal connection between convulsions, by whatever name they are called, and the DPT shot. Some are simply ignorant because they have not read the scientific literature and have not been taught about vaccine reactions in medical school. Others may know and deliberately conceal or obscure the connection because they fear lawsuits. Whatever the reason, the result is the same. Parents are not told that it was the DPT shot that caused the convulsion and are left to wander from doctor to doctor seeking the "cause" of their child's uncontrollable seizures and retardation. Often their children are given more pertussis vaccine, making the seizures worse.

Some children will exhibit neurological signs, such as excessive sleepiness or high-pitched screaming, after an earlier DPT shot before they finally react with major convulsions following a subsequent shot. Such is the story of Sharon. If her doctors had recognized the significance of Sharon's first neurological symptoms and had only administered DT from then on, she might have been spared a lifetime of uncontrollable seizures.

Sharon began screaming shrilly, staring, and holding her body rigid within seven hours after the first DPT shot. Then she fell into a deep sleep which lasted sixteen hours. When she awoke, she appeared to be perfectly normal. Her mother reported her reaction to the pediatrician, yet he proceeded to give Sharon another DPT shot, even though it was only a half dose.

"They gave her a one-half strength DPT shot because the clinic didn't carry DT at the time. I have since found out that one-half strength doesn't make any difference in the reaction. I've learned a lot since then," her mother said.

Within twelve hours of the second shot, Sharon let out a shrill scream and went into a tonic-clonic convulsion lasting four and a half hours; she had to be rushed to two different hospitals before doctors were able to stop it. Immediately after this, she developed diarrhea, otitis media, a runny nose, bronchial infections, and asthma, in addition to an allergy to all milk products.

Despite anticonvulsant medication, Sharon continued to have up to twelve three-minute seizures every day. They would increase in frequency during the pollen season or if she drank milk. She did not have another major convulsion, however, until the doctors tested her for allergies and she went into an hour-long tonic-clonic seizure.

"We've mentioned the DPT shot as the cause of her seizures quite often and the doctors just clench their jaws. We've only had two young residents at this teaching hospital who have been interested in her case. They are behind us in our efforts to have the doctors check out the DPT shot connection, but nobody will really listen to us. Most of the doctors keep telling us 'She must have an underlying seizure disorder.' I can't believe that because she didn't even have a sniffle up until her second shot. The only health problems we have in our family are severe food allergies on my husband's side. However, it is interesting that the doctors have agreed that our son will only be getting DT from now on."

Today, Sharon is three years old and continues to have seizures as well as asthma and bouts of pneumonia. She is developmentally delayed.

Because most physicians refuse to consider the possibility that convulsions occurring days or weeks after a DPT shot are connected to the shot or could be made worse by further injections of the vaccine, many children are repeatedly revaccinated. Again and again parents report that their children were given more pertussis vaccine despite previous seizures, and it was the readministration of the vaccine which did the most harm. Rick is a good example of what can happen when doctors do not consider a history of convulsions to be important.

Rick was a beautiful, normal baby until his second DPT shot at six months. His only health problem was an allergy to milk which caused him to spit up and have diarrhea from birth. After trying many different formulas, he was put on whole milk at the age of six months. Two weeks after his second shot, he began screaming uncontrollably and running a high fever. Soon after he went into a thirty-minute grand mal convulsion. The doctors diagnosed a "touch of pneumonia" in his lower lobes.

Rick was given the third DPT shot barely two weeks after being discharged from the hospital, even though he had suffered another small seizure after he went home. Within twenty-four hours of his third shot, he had a much more severe grand mal convulsion. From that moment on, Rick developed a pattern of up to fifty convulsions a day until he was five years old, even though he was taking more than two thousand milligrams of anticonvulsant medication every twenty-four hours. Now eight years old, he has "cerebral palsy," a behavioral disorder, and is mentally retarded.

"A neurologist has told me that Rick's cerebral palsy is a result of the severity of his uncontrollable seizures. He used to have petit mal seizures so bad that he couldn't walk across the room without falling and had to wear a helmet to protect his head. He's had spinal taps, blood work, CAT scans, and they all come back negative," his mother said.

Some babies, like Marie, immediately react with high-pitched screaming or extreme sleepiness and appear to recover within twenty-four hours. But then, within a matter of days or a few weeks, they will be found in a state of collapse or in the throes of a convulsion. To make matters worse, mothers find that doctors will not take them seriously when they try to explain what happened to their baby. Marie's mother could not even get her pediatrician to believe that there was something very wrong with Marie after her second DPT shot. He preferred to think she was "choking on her milk."

Marie had no reaction to the first DPT shot, but within six hours of her second one, she started high-pitched screaming. "I had never heard her cry like that," said her mother, "and I felt so bad for her that I began crying myself. She sounded like she was in bad pain." She screamed for five hours, but appeared to be fine the next morning.

Seven days later, Marie's mother found her baby in the crib apparently lifeless: "She was totally still and silent, not breathing or moving. I thought she was dead. I quickly picked her up and she responded. Even so, I felt something was wrong."

Three weeks later, Marie's mother watched her daughter open her eyes and mouth and give a brief shout shortly after she had fallen asleep for the night. "Looking back on it now, I realize she had a very mild seizure. But, at the time, I didn't know what seizures were. When I called my doctor, he told me to use a humidifier because it was the time of year for respiratory infections."

Marie continued to have "spells" just after falling asleep and her mother continued to call the pediatrician and tell him about them. "He kept telling me she was just choking or regurgitating milk. He said she would grow out of it." At her six-month checkup, Marie was given the third DPT shot.

"Within thirty minutes of the shot, while we were on our way home, Marie had a bad seizure where her eyes were twitching and her chin was shaking. For the next five days she had constant seizures. We took her back to my pediatrician, and he said I was really overreacting and Marie would grow out of it."

Finally Marie's parents took her to a hospital where doctors admitted Marie was having seizures but maintained that no cause could be found for them. At the hospital, Marie's mother met another mother whose child was in the neurology ward. "She told me that after her baby got her first DPT shot, her eyes started twitching. The doctors were doing all sorts of tests on the baby and couldn't find any reason for the twitching. The mother kept telling me, 'Nobody will believe me. Nobody will listen to me. My baby's eyes started to twitch right after her DPT shot, but they won't believe there is a connection.'"

Infantile Spasms

Seizure disorders can be caused by many factors, including head injuries, birth trauma, certain infectious diseases, and vaccinations. Many are of unknown origin. Over the years they have been given various names and classifications such as cerebral palsy, convulsions, epilepsy, and grand mal and petit mal disorders. The different names obscure the fact that all types of seizures are manifestations of a central nervous system disturbance. Nearly every form of seizure has been associated with the pertussis vaccine at one time or another, and all have been the subject of debate over whether or not they are actually caused by this vaccine. But no category of seizures believed to be caused by the pertussis vaccine has been more controversial than infantile spasms with hypsarrhythmia.

In 1946, Douglas Buchanan, M.D., a professor of neurology at the University of Chicago School of Medicine, called attention to a neurological disorder which he believed was often being misdiagnosed. He wrote, "a type of major convulsion in young infants which is frequently not recognized as such is one in which there is a sudden forward dropping of the head with adduction and flexion of the arms. These attacks are extremely brief and tend to occur in bursts. They are really *lightning major convulsions*. They are most common in children less than two years old. They are notoriously difficult completely to control and are most often found in association with severe degrees of cerebral agenesis and mental retardation."

Buchanan did not suggest their cause but said, "Obviously there must be some other chain of events which periodically and irregularly run in specific sequences and which terminate in a seizure. The nature of this chain remains a mystery." This particular type of convulsion would later be described as infantile spasms, although it was first named West's Syndrome in honor of the British physician W. J. West, who mentioned it in 1841 after observing the condition in his own son. Until Buchanan wrote about it in the mid-1940s, it had been a very rarely reported condition.

A striking aspect of the syndrome was that it nearly always occurred in the first year of life and in infants who had previously appeared in perfect health. Today, infantile spasms are also sometimes called "jackknife seizures" or "salaam convulsions," because the child often looks as if he were "bowing" as he violently bends at the waist and throws his head to his knees or brings his knees up to his chest.

Dr. Buchanan was from Chicago. Since 1933, a municipal whooping cough vaccination clinic had been operated in Evanston, a northern suburb. Chicago was also the home of Dr. Louis Sauer, a pioneer in the research and development of one of the first pertussis vaccines used in America. By 1944, nearly every infant born in Evanston was being vaccinated with pertussis vaccine, and two years later, Sauer reported that whooping cough in that area had been virtually eradicated. Thus, Buchanan was observing infantile spasms in Chicago at a time when neighboring Evanston had one of the most comprehensive pertussis vaccination efforts in America.

The next description of infantile spasms appeared in 1951 in Buenos Aires, Argentina, where mass pertussis vaccination had been instituted a few years earlier. Vazquez and Turner reported on ten cases of a new epileptic syndrome, which they called "generalized bending" (*flexión generalizada*), and which occurred in infants less than a year old. The convulsions consisted of a sudden flexion of the head and limbs, with or without shouts or cries. They lasted only a short while, occurred many times each day, and could not be controlled by medication. In most instances, they also produced a highly unusual electroencephalogram (EEG).

The abnormality of the EEG was given the name "hypsarrhythmia" in 1952 by Frederic and Erna Gibbs of the University of Illinois College of Medicine in Chicago. The word means "exceedingly disorderly" and was used to describe the lack of a regular EEG pattern in infants with a history of infantile spasms. Instead of the rhythmically repetitive and organized pattern that characterizes normal epilepsy, the EEG accompanying infantile spasms often consists of random, high-voltage slow waves and spikes spreading to all cortical areas and varying from moment to moment in both duration and location.

While infantile spasms could be present without hypsarrhythmia and vice versa, the two usually came together. The Gibbses noted that when hypsarrhythmia was present, the seizures were characterized by "sudden jerking of the head, rolling up of the eyes, upward flinging of the arms, or quivering of the entire body." The prognosis was usually severe mental deterioration. The Gibbses suggested that the cause might be "bacterial or virus disease in the mother during gestation."

During the next decade, more reports appeared defining this new syndrome and stressing the puzzling fact that it occurred in infants who had previously appeared completely healthy. R. S. Illingworth, M.D., in England wrote in 1955, "From experience at the Children's Hospital, Sheffield, I believe that there is a clear-cut group of cases in which a child develops normally up to a certain age, and then practically simultaneously develops fits and mental deterioration. I have not found a reference in the literature to this type of case. . . . The absence of an abnormal birth history, and the fact that all the babies were full term, is striking."

It took several years for scientists to realize that this increasingly frequent neurological condition, which usually struck healthy infants when they were about six months old, might have something to do with a new procedure administered at about the same age—namely, the pertussis vaccination. Evidently, it was not an obvious or easy correlation to make.

Up until 1950, infantile spasms were extremely unusual. All of the medical literature between 1841 and 1948 contained only 62 cases. Between 1950 and 1963, 1,453 cases were reported. By 1964, more than 3,000 cases were known to medical science. In France, Gastaut and Grimaud attempted to obtain more concrete estimates of the frequency of infantile spasms in 1963 and found that, in one center, half of the children diagnosed as "epileptic," who were younger than three years, had infantile spasms.

The first researchers to actually point a finger at the DPT shot were Henry Baird and Leatrice Borofsky of Philadelphia. In 1957, they wrote: "The observation that a number of patients with infantile myoclonic seizures had histories suggesting normal development prior to the time of their immunization with diphtheria, pertussis and tetanus antigens prompted a review of our experience with this type of convulsive disorder."

They examined a sample of eighty children with hypsarrhythmia and reported that "pertussis immunization should be considered as an etiological possibility." A description of their findings was published in the 1957–58 *Yearbook of Pediatrics*. By 1958, however, the medical profession was committed to the campaign to get every child inoculated with pertussis vaccine, and there was no systematic follow-through on Baird and Borofsky's findings.

This was surprising because in 1955 Niels L. Low, also of the University of Illinois School of Medicine, had shown that the EEG of infants was sometimes altered by the DPT shot. He concluded that "mild, but possibly significant, cerebral reactions occur in addition to the reported very severe neurological changes."

During the next decade, several articles appeared in the British and Scandinavian press on the relationship between the DPT shot and infantile spasms. In 1964, Jeavons and Bower analyzed 112 cases of infantile spasms and concluded: "Enough has been said to suggest strongly that in certain of our patients the syndrome resulted from an allergic encephalitis due to triple immunization [that is, the DPT shot]."

Kringelbach and Senstius described three cases in 1966. The following year, Ström reported on 167 cases of severe reactions to the DPT shot in Sweden. Two of the children developed hypsarrythmia within three days of vaccination, and two more developed hypsarrhythmia within a week after the shot.

In 1969, Melchior described twenty-two children in whom there was a close temporal connection between various vaccinations, especially pertussis, and infantile spasms. In 1971, he observed, "all agents giving a cerebral reaction might be suspected as etiology thus including immunization," but concluded that the only connection between the two events was temporal.

Other physicians played down the relationship between infantile spasms and the DPT shot. In 1972, Gomez and Klass mentioned encephalopathy due to "pertussis immunization" as one of sixteen "disorders" associated with infantile spasms and hypsarrhythmia and concluded: "At present the etiology can be established as presumptively determined for only about half of the patients with this clinical-electrographic syndrome of infantile spasms and hypsarrhythmia."

A major work on myoclonic seizures by Maurice Charlton in 1975, which devoted a chapter to infantile spasms, stated: "The most important question here is the relationship of infantile spasms to inoculation with pertussis vaccine." But having come in like a lion, the author went out like a lamb, concluding, "It is difficult to produce acceptable evidence of a serious risk [of infantile spasms] from whooping cough immunization, sufficient to advise against the use of the newer vaccine adsorbed on aluminum hydroxide." He then darkly theorized that "unsuspected inborn errors of metabolism and storage disease of insidious development" may be the cause of infantile spasms.

In 1979, Gordon T. Stewart found that among the pertussis vaccine-damaged children he studied, "In 25% of cases, the pattern of convulsions corresponded closely to clinical descriptions of West's syndrome or infantile myoclonic seizures in which, according to Jeavons and Bower (1964), about 17% of cases are strongly associated with injections of DPT."

And by 1979 many American researchers were acknowledging that infantile spasms and hypsarrhythmia were indeed connected to the pertussis vaccine. The authors of the UCLA-FDA study, which explored the rate of reactions between DPT and DT shots occurring within forty-eight hours after vaccination, said, "No infant developed infantile spasms. This may be in part due to the brevity of follow-up in this investigation. In an attempt by Melchior to relate infantile spasms to pertussis immunization, a period of two weeks was discussed."

Also in 1979, Jeffrey P. Koplan at the CDC and others published a benefit-risk analysis of the pertussis vaccine which noted: "The rate of severe reactions is one in 34,000 vaccinees; they consist of repeated convulsions, hypsarrhythmia or serious meningitis. . . ." In 1980, the British Committee on Safety of Medicines reported that an examination of data on pertussis vaccine-damaged children suggested that infantile spasms were one of the possible consequences, together with chronic epilepsy and acute encephalopathy. And the AMA Drug Evaluations of that same year mentions "infantile massive spasm" and hypsarrhythmia as possible central nervous system (CNS) reactions to the DPT vaccine.

But in 1983, Bellman, Ross, and Miller published a study of 269 cases of infantile spasms reported to the National Childhood Encephalopathy Study (NCES) which returned to the position that infantile spasms are unrelated to the DPT shot. Although they found "some clustering of cases immunized with either diphtheria-tetanus-pertussis or diphtheria-tetanus vaccines in the 7 days before onset," they concluded that the vaccines "do not cause infantile spasms but may trigger their onset in those children in whom the disorder is destined to develop."

After more than thirty-five years of reports in the scientific literature linking certain cases of infantile spasms to the DPT shot, physicians who recommend vaccine policy for America are still officially disputing a connection between infantile spasms and the pertussis vaccine. When members of Dissatisfied Parents Together were discussing the formulation of a compensation bill for vaccine-damaged children with members of the AAP Red Book Committee, the AAP steadfastly refused to explicitly recognize that the pertussis vaccine could cause infantile spasms and/or hypsarrhythmia. Citing the Bellman, Ross, and Miller study, among others, as proof that the vaccine does not cause infantile spasms, they declined to add infantile spasms to the list of conditions compensable under the bill.

One needn't ask parents of some vaccine-damaged children whether or not there is an association between the DPT shot and infantile spasms. A mother in Massachusetts, whose son reacted to his third DPT shot with infantile spasms, knows there is an association. She said, "Within 48 hours of his third shot, Patrick began staring, dropping his head to his chest, and falling asleep without warning. He also would just lay in his crib and sleep with his eyes open, which he had never done before. He kept this up for about two weeks before he had his first salaam seizure. When he had it, he would start to stare and all of a sudden he would violently jerk his whole upper body forward. A neurologist who saw him do it said he had atypical salaam seizures because he didn't fling his arms out or make a grunting noise while he did it."

Patrick was put on the powerful steroid ACTH for three weeks to try to stop the seizures, and during this period he became bloated and accumulated rolls of fat around his neck. He also developed diarrhea, thrush, and ear infections, but the ACTH did stop his infantile spasms.

"We were lucky that Patrick did not have the classic infantile spasms with hypsarrhythmia. We understand that combination is devastating and results in profound brain damage. Patrick never had an EEG reading show hypsarrhythmia. He still drops his head to his chest occasionally but the neurologist has assured me it doesn't mean anything."

Patrick's mother did not notice that her son had any reaction to his first or second DPT shots. "He was a big healthy baby up until he was six months old. I have three other boys, and I know what healthy is. I have always thought there was a connection with the shot, but my pediatrician tried to put me off. The neurologist told me it was probably due to the shot and that Patrick should not have the pertussis vaccine again. They are going to have to monitor his growth and development very carefully."

Another child was not so lucky. Laura was born a month early and weighed only four pounds, two ounces. Because of her low birth weight and prematurity, she did not get her first DPT shot until she was three months old. Her mother does not recall that Laura had a noticeable reaction to this shot. But after the second shot, which Laura's pediatrician gave just one month after the first, she did have a reaction.

"Even though I started giving Laura Tylenol immediately after her second shot, she ran a fever for twenty-four hours and it peaked at 103 degrees," said Laura's mother. "She also screamed on and off for twenty-four hours. And it was a high shrill cry like I hadn't heard before. After that shot, whenever she cried it was high and shrill."

Laura appeared to recover from her reaction, and by her third DPT shot four weeks later, she could hold her head up and roll over. But three hours after this shot she began the first of many infantile spasms.

"She got the shot at about eleven-thirty in the morning, and by two o'clock Laura started these strange movements where her hands would go straight up in the air, her feet would go straight out, she would clench her fists and hold her breath for two or three seconds, and then she would cry that shrill cry. About ten seconds later, she would hold her breath again and start all over. She could do twenty-five of these in a row."

Laura's mother called the doctor, and took Laura in to see him two days in succession. "The doctor listened to what I described and said she might have a stomach ailment. He took her off all formula and put her on Pedialyte. Finally, six days after her shot, I took her to him again, and we sat in his office for three hours waiting for her to do it so I could show him. She didn't have one so he sent us to the hospital for an EEG, and she had one while they were taking the EEG. The reading showed a very bad hypsarrhythmia, and they diagnosed infantile spasms."

Laura's doctor denied that the infantile spasms were due to the shot. "He told me that Laura would have gotten infantile spasms anyway, and that if they hadn't been triggered by the DPT shot, they would have been triggered by something else. My husband and I believed him."

ACTH therapy stopped Laura's infantile spasms, but she continued to have a mild hypsarrhythmia, and, despite anticonvulsant medication, had several seizures when twelve months old. When thirteen months old, she was at a six-month level in gross motor skills and an eight-month level in intellectual ability.

"She has very low muscle tone," said her mother. "She can't stand. She can't get up on her knees so she pulls herself around with her arms. She doesn't babble as most babies do, and we suspect she may have learning disabilities. She still cries shrilly a lot. But we continue to be encouraged that she will continue developing and won't have more seizures."

Laura's mother would like to know the batch and lot number of the DPT vaccine given to her daughter, especially after learning that another child in her pediatrician's office developed infantile spasms following a DPT shot during the same month Laura reacted. "As far as I know, Laura's reaction was not reported to anyone. When I called up recently to find out the manufacturer, batch, and lot number of the vaccine, all they could tell me was the manufacturer's name. They don't write down the batch or lot number."

She wishes her doctor had told her about reactions. "If I had known that high-pitched crying was an important reaction, Laura would not have gotten more pertussis vaccine. If I had known to look for seizure activity, Laura wouldn't have had to suffer six days of infantile spasms before she was admitted to the hospital and put on medication to stop them. Parents and doctors have to be better informed about vaccine reactions."

Loss of Muscle Control

Loss of muscle control, which manifests itself in such disorders as hemiparesis (slight paralysis on one side of the body), hemiplegia (paralysis of one side of the body), paraplegia (paralysis of the lower part of the body including the legs), quadriplegia (paralysis of all four limbs), or simply poor coordination, has been reported in the scientific literature to be a side effect of the pertussis vaccine.

In 1954 Miller and Stanton described the case of a baby girl who reacted to her third shot: "Seven days after her third injection of a combined diphtheria-pertussis vaccine, this previously healthy baby developed a severe attack of screaming, followed by drowsiness. During the subsequent two days the child remained alternately drowsy and restless, though she was able to take her food. At the end of this period the parents noticed that she was not moving her right arm and leg. Examination revealed a right hemiplegia involving face, arm, and leg . . . Two years later right hemiparesis persists. There is difficulty in using the right hand, but the child can walk. General development and intelligence appear to be unimpaired."

In 1970, Hannik discussed the case of a child who was found "in his cot with a left hemiplegia the fourth morning after vaccination. Two years later a slight paresis of the left leg is still present and the left leg is shorter than the right one."

In 1977, Stewart published a study evaluating 160 cases of adverse reactions occurring after a DPT shot and included "pareses or localised paralysis" and "flaccid paralysis" among the reactions he studied. In 1978, A. H. Griffith wrote about a child who "became lethargic and had convulsion on fourth day; admitted to hospital on fifth day with total left hemiplegia and partial paralysis of the right; became quadriplegic for six weeks; residual moderate left hemiplegia and mental retardation."

In 1983, Cindy was given her first DPT shot at the age of six months. Her mother, an occupational therapist, had delayed the shot because Cindy had been five weeks premature, and she had been concerned about the side effects of the pertussis vaccine. In her job, she has worked with brain-damaged children, most of whom have reacted to smallpox vaccinations. In addition, her first daughter had reacted to the DPT shot with a two-day fever that climbed to almost 105 degrees.

"I kept putting the shot off," Cindy's mother said. "But finally, at six months, my doctor told me that Cindy was more at risk of getting whooping cough than of having a reaction. He convinced me that her prematurity and her sister's severe reaction were not significant enough factors to warrant not giving the shot. The doctor cited statistics about whooping cough and how the disease could cause irreparable damage. In the end, I just gave in."

Cindy ran a fever of 102 degrees that night. It wasn't until the next morning that it became evident to her mother that Cindy was not able to sit up or roll over as she had before. "Her arms were bent and held against her body. She clenched her fists and could not lift her arms up to reach. The muscles in her legs were tight and it was difficult to spread them apart to change her diapers."

Cindy's mother called her pediatrician immediately. "I described Cindy's condition and told him of my fears of central nervous system damage. He kept telling me not to worry. That was hardly possible since Cindy wasn't doing any of the things she had done before the shot. He said, 'I'm sure it will go away in a week or so.' But I made him see her immediately, even though he didn't want to see her. I wanted it documented on her medical records."

Because Cindy's mother is a trained occupational therapist, she was able to immediately begin therapy with her daughter for several hours a day. Now one year old, Cindy is starting to walk, and does not appear to be mentally impaired.

"When your child is damaged from a shot you let the doctor give to her, you feel so much guilt. You go over and over in your mind asking yourself, why did I let him do it? Thank God she didn't have a seizure because then the damage could have been even worse. Her muscle tone improved a little at a time during the therapy. Her motor coordination, although not where it was before the shot, was much improved. The one thing I am worried about is the possibility of future learning disabilities."

Cindy's pediatrician has agreed not to give either Cindy or her sister more pertussis vaccine. Their mother is still afraid of the possibility that they could get whooping cough.

"I live with the fear that they might get whooping cough. It's scary. But until they come up with a purer vaccine, I will have to live with these fears. Doctors should start weighing the risks of giving a dangerous vaccine to children who appear to be at risk, such as preemies, kids with central nervous system damage, and children whose siblings have had severe reactions."

Heather weighed less than ten pounds when she got her first DPT shot at two months of age. She had been five weeks premature, and her mother had had gestational diabetes during the pregnancy. "The second day after her shot she ran a low-grade fever and started projectile vomiting," said her mother. "She also screamed a scream I had never heard before—it was shattering. She screamed for two days and nights. She was finally hospitalized and they said she had an ear infection. At that point we noticed that her left foot was arched, curved. The doctor said, 'Oh, she's going to be a ballerina.' "

Heather received her second DPT shot at four months of age. Again, within forty-eight hours, she was running a fever, had projectile vomiting, and high-pitched screaming. The hospital diagnosed another ear infection. Her left foot was still curved inward.

"I kept bringing up the left foot arching and my doctor said again, 'I told you she is probably going to be a ballerina.' It was after the second shot that we noticed she wasn't using her left hand anymore. She was still using her left hand after the first shot but after the second one, she quit using it. When I told my doctor this before her third shot and mentioned the foot again, he was not concerned."

When it came time for Heather's third DPT shot, her mother objected. "I told the doctor, 'Look, this child is not tolerating these shots well.' So he gave her a one-half dose. Again, she had a temperature but only slight vomiting this time."

At nine months of age, Heather's mother again pointed out to her pediatrician that Heather was not using her left hand. "They did a CAT scan and told us that a small portion of Heather's right brain had never formed properly. But when she was a year old, she fell off her chair one day and was limp but mentally alert. They did another CAT scan and this time said that her brain was completely formed but she had a lesion. They said she had had an insult to the brain—like a stroke—at some point."

Heather has a left hemiparesis. Her mother said, "She is three years old and appears to be mentally and intellectually gifted. But she looks like a stroke victim. The left side of her body is curled and crippled."

Inflammation of the Brain

Inflammation and swelling of different parts of the brain after a DPT shot are variously referred to as meningitis, encephalitis, encephalomyelitis, and bulging fontanelle. Some children do not withstand a bout with meningitis or encephalomyelitis and die.

In 1978, Griffith studied severe reactions occurring after fifteen million doses of pertussis vaccine were administered to children in England. He stated that one child "was admitted to the hospital with pyrexia, signs and symptoms of meningeal irritation; transferred after three days with provisional diagnosis of encephalomyelitis but died thirty days after vaccination; necropsy showed no specific changes; recorded cause of death: encephalopathy due to injection of triple vaccine."

In 1979, California physicians Jack Jacob and Frank Manning wrote in the *American Journal of the Diseases of Children* about the case of a child who experienced a "bulging fontanelle associated with increased intracranial pressure as measured by lumbar puncture" within twenty-four hours of a DPT shot. This seven-month-old girl (the daughter of a pediatrican) began running a fever after her third DPT shot, and nine hours later her parents noticed the soft spot on her head was bulging and pulsating. She became very irritable and also had redness and swelling at the site of the injection.

She was admitted to the hospital, and all tests came back negative, but the bulging did not stop until about forty hours after the shot. The doctors concluded, "The clinical symptomology in this patient, consisting of fever and irritability, are symptoms frequently associated with DPT immunization. The bulging fontanelle was accidentally noted by the child's parents who recognized its importance. It is, therefore, conceivable that this complication may be missed unless specifically looked for."

Children who suffer brain inflammation may recover completely or only sustain a minor permanent injury. Steve was one of the lucky ones. Within twenty-four hours of his second DPT shot, Steve started running a fever. Two days later, he was in the hospital with spinal meningitis. His mother said, "The morning we put him into the hospital, I found him in his crib laying there with his eyes wide open. He started dry heaving and then he had a terrible cry. I have never heard anything like it. It was about three octaves higher than it normally was and there were no tears, just a constant scream between breaths. And his neck was real stiff. In the hospital, his fever went up to 105 degrees."

Although the doctors diagnosed spinal meningitis, his mother suspected the DPT shot may have been connected with Steve's condition. "My doctor told me the shot couldn't possibly be related to the meningitis. But I told him, 'You gave him a clean bill of health the day of the shot. He was perfectly fine. How could he suddenly be in the hospital with spinal meningitis three days later if it didn't have something to do with the shot?' "

Steve was given a third DPT shot, even though his mother was worried about what might happen. "The doctor told me there was nothing to worry about. So, at six months, right on schedule, they gave him his third shot. And within twenty-four hours, it started. He ran a 104-degree temperature and vomited for three days. I thought we were going through meningitis all over again."

At two years of age, Steve appears to be developing normally. The only residual damage he sustained was a slight loss of hearing in the right ear. After he reacted to the MMR (measles, mumps, rubella) shot with a two-day 104-degree fever and aching joints, his father said, "That's it. No more shots. I'd rather he take his chances with the diseases. There must be something in his system that just can't tolerate what is in the shots."

Six-month-old Jake was hospitalized with meningitis within a week after his third DPT shot. "Before we took him to the hospital, he began sleeping a lot and running a 104-degree fever. At the hospital, they first thought it was an ear infection and then they said they thought it might be meningitis. The doctors wouldn't admit that it might be due to his DPT shot, but the nurses told me that a lot of times a child will get a DPT shot and a week later come down with meningitis."

Jake recovered with no permanent damage but another little boy was not so lucky. Richard reacted to the second DPT shot at the age of five months with a large, red, hot lump at the site of the injection, which stayed for three to four weeks. One month later, he got another DPT shot. His mother told the doctor at the public health clinic about the lump.

"She told me that she would bury the shot deeper, that maybe the other doctor had hit a muscle. When we got home, Richard just lay in his crib moaning and kicking one leg. For the next few days, he lay in his crib with his eyes open. Before the shot, he had been trying to pull himself up, so when he just lay in his bed totally out of it, it was a radical behavior change."

Eight days after the shot, Richard had his first focal seizure: he dropped his head to his chest. As days went by, these "head nods" became more frequent. He was admitted to a hospital nearly two weeks after the third DPT shot with a temporary diagnosis of "allergic encephalitis."

A lawyer specializing in defending vaccine-damaged children commented on Richard's story: "As is the case with many pertussis vaccine-injured children, none of the treating physicians would commit themselves to a final etiological diagnosis. It is strange that parents of pertussis vaccine-damaged children often can only get an etiological diagnosis by hiring an attorney and seeing one of the few recognized experts in the U.S. on post-pertussis vaccine encephalopathy."

Today, Richard is eleven years old and has been evaluated at a two-year-old level. He cannot talk. At various times in his life he has had to wear a helmet to protect his head from injury during seizures. His mother must watch him constantly and take care of all his personal needs.

"He is a very loving, gentle boy. If he were violent, as some of these children can be, I think my heart would be broken more than it has been. About three years ago, my husband and I began to realize that he was going to need care for the rest of his life, and that we were not always going to be alive to provide it. That is when we decided to see a lawyer. I know we might lose our case and not have money to provide for him after we die. When I die and leave him to the world, nobody will take care of him or love him like we have. The state will have the power to put him into a state institution and drug him or put him in restraints and tie him to a chair. He has lived with love all his life. It is a terrible thought to know it would be kinder if he could go with me."

Blood Disorders: Thrombocytopenia and Hemolytic Anemia

Whooping cough is characterized by an apparent increase in the number of lymphocytes (a type of white cell) in the blood. Researchers have suggested that this is due to the lymphocytosis-promoting factor (LPF) mentioned in Chapter 3—which is a synonym for "pertussis toxin" and is also found in the pertussis vaccine. Two blood disorders that have been associated with the pertussis vaccine are thrombocytopenia and hemolytic anemia.

"Thrombocytopenia" means a reduced number of platelets circulating in the blood. This sometimes causes "purpura," blotchy red patches on the child's body caused by the thinned blood seeping into the tissues beneath the skin. The 1984 product inserts of Wyeth, Connaught, and Lederle Laboratories all listed thrombocytopenia as a contraindication to further pertussis vaccine.

Hemolytic anemia is characterized by premature death of the red blood cells and inability of the bone marrow to produce more blood cells quickly enough to replace those that have died. *Dorland's Medical Dictionary* states, "it may be hereditary or acquired, as that resulting from infection or chemotherapy or occurring as part of the autoimmune process." The 1984 DPT product insert of Connaught Laboratories listed the development of hemolytic anemia after a DPT shot as a contraindication to further pertussis vaccine, citing a 1978 Scandinavian study linking the vaccine to this dangerous blood disorder.

During discussions between the American Academy of Pediatrics (AAP) and Dissatisfied Parents Together in 1983, while the two groups were developing the National Childhood Vaccine-Injury Compensation Act, the AAP would not agree that hemolytic anemia could be a reaction to the pertussis vaccine. And in April 1984, the Advisory Committee on Immunization Practices (ACIP) announced that "although hemolytic anemia and thrombocytopenic purpura have previously been considered contraindications by the ACIP, the evidence of a causal link between these conditions and pertussis vaccination is not sufficient to retain them as contraindications."

A Connecticut family has no trouble believing in a connection between the vaccine and hemolytic anemia. Six days after his fourth DPT shot, Paul became very irritable. Then he stopped eating. In the next seven days his symptoms became increasingly alarming. He developed a high fever and started vomiting. His skin turned yellow; his lips were colorless. He began sleeping for long periods during the day.

Fourteen days after the shot, he was so weak that he would fall to the ground and remain unconscious for twenty minutes at a time. His parents took him to their pediatrician. His father said, "The doctor thought it might be leukemia or cancer, so we rushed him to a hospital. We went through six days of hell there. They were taking blood samples from my little two-and-a-half-year-old son every fifteen minutes. Paul was shell-shocked and terrified. My wife was a wreck and I was a wreck. The doctors told us they had never seen a child with a hemoglobin of three and a hematocrit of ten survive before. His blood was literally as thin as water. They told us he would probably die. But, after three blood transfusions, somehow Paul pulled through. I think the fact that he was such a strong, healthy kid made the difference."

The doctors diagnosed hemolytic anemia and told Paul's parents they must not be feeding him properly. A nutritionist was assigned to teach Paul's mother how to improve his "iron-poor blood" by preparing meals that were high in protein. The hospital prescribed some vitamins and sent Paul home.

He returned to his usual state of good health until the fifth DPT shot. Six days after this shot, Paul became irritable. Then he stopped eating and started running a fever, vomiting, sleeping for long periods of time, and losing consciousness. Exactly fourteen days after the shot, he was back in the hospital with hemolytic anemia.

"He was near death again," said his father. "But this time his hemoglobin was only down to four or five. It could have been because he was a lot bigger and heavier than he was at the time of his fourth shot. This time he had to have two transfusions to pull him through. When I got home from the hospital, I went over to my neighbor's house and borrowed some medical books. That's when I discovered the connection with the pertussis vaccine and hemolytic anemia."

After he had done his research, he called the pediatrician, who told him to call the hospital. "My pediatrician wouldn't admit there was a connection with the DPT shot. Every doctor I confronted at the hospital walked away from me when I suggested it was the DPT shot that caused my son to almost die twice. I even showed them the book and page number and sentence, and they wouldn't listen to me. They told me I was nuts and walked away from me. There wasn't one comment like, 'We'll look into it,' just flat denial. I would say they are covering it up."

Paul's father would not let the matter drop. The hospital referred him to a pediatric hematologist, who took six vials of blood from the infant in order to try to find a cause for his two bouts with hemolytic anemia.

"She took six vials of blood from my son, and when I called her for the results, she would not answer my calls, my paging at the hospital, or my letters," Paul's father said. "We have never heard from her. She sent me a bill later, and I sent her a letter back telling her I would send her the money if she would contact me. I never heard from her again. Like I said, nobody would admit it was the shot. When I would mention it, the doctors would get really belligerent. I might not have a college degree, but I am not ignorant. I read. When I read those medical books, I did my own little term paper. The doctors just didn't like a layman learning their business."

Paul did not suffer any permanent damage. He is five years old and a big, healthy boy today. His father knows how fortunate they were.

"I look at Paul sleeping sometimes and think back to how we almost lost him. Thank God he is okay. Parents should be told the shot could take the child's life. At least doctors should give parents a list of symptoms of reactions so they know when to get him to the hospital before it is too late. It should be a law."

Diabetes and Hypoglycemia

The body's glucose (sugar) metabolism is regulated by insulin, a hormone which is secreted by the pancreas. Insulin helps "burn up" or store away for later use excess sugar in the blood. If too much insulin is secreted by the pancreas, the body's blood sugar level drops. This condition is known as hypoglycemia.

Another name for the LPF, or pertussis toxin, is islet-activating protein, or IAP, so called because it has been shown in laboratory animals to provoke excess production of insulin by the pancreas. Researchers have also detected increased insulin production in infants injected with the pertussis vaccine.

In 1970 Pittman stated, "The infant whose blood sugar level is influenced by food intake may be especially vulnerable to vaccine-induced hypoglycemia should a feeding be missed because of a feverish reaction following vaccination. . . . the vaccine induces hypoglycemia in mice and rabbits." Stewart observed in 1977 that "more than any other vaccine in common use, pertussis vaccine is known pharmacologically to provoke . . . hypoglycemia due to increased production of insulin."

Hannik and Cohen stated the same in 1978 and drew the conclusion: "Infants who show serious reactions following pertussis vaccination suffer from a failure to maintain glucose homeostasis." And Hennessen and Quast in West Germany found that 59 out of 149 cases of adverse

reactions to the pertussis vaccine developed symptoms corresponding
to the hypoglycemic syndrome.

An equally serious issue, about which less information has been
developed, is the relationship between the vaccine and diabetes. Diabetes has been reported to be a complication of a very serious case of
whooping cough.

Four researchers in France, West Germany, and Great Britain published an article in 1982 detailing the role the DPT vaccine played in
causing diabetes in a sixteen-month-old girl who was genetically predisposed to diabetes and who suffered from a viral infection that
attacked her pancreas. They concluded that "an insulotropic variant
virus, genetic predisposition, and perhaps some uncontrolled adjuvant
factors, e.g. steroid therapy and DPT vaccination, may have determined
insular damage and anti-islet antoimmune reactions, leading to insulin-
dependent diabetes mellitus."

Death and Sudden Infant Death Syndrome

Death was the first reaction to be associated with the pertussis vaccine.
Thorwald Madsen, the Danish vaccine pioneer, published an article
in 1933 describing the deaths of two babies a few hours after they had
been vaccinated. One had hiccups and convulsions, while the other
had nothing more visible than a bluish tint of the skin.

Following his report, other physicians added their own case histories
of infant deaths immediately following pertussis vaccination. As mentioned earlier in this chapter, Werne and Garrow in 1946 described
deaths of identical twins within twenty-four hours of their second shot.

But what about the baby who dies a few days after the DPT shot?
This raises the issue of Sudden Infant Death Syndrome (SIDS), which
is sometimes known as crib death or cot death. According to the FDA,
one in every five hundred live births in the United States today results
in a death which is labeled SIDS. That means that some seven thousand
babies, out of the three and a half million born in the United States
each year, die for unknown reasons. Premature, low-birth-weight, and
black infants appear to be at particular risk of dying from SIDS.

The incidence of SIDS increases after the first month of life, rises to
a peak at two and three months, and declines after the age of four
months. More than one researcher has been impressed with the co-

incidence between the peak incidence of SIDS and the months in which most babies receive their first DPT shots.

Vaccine manufacturers mention the connection to SIDS in their product information inserts. Wyeth Laboratories stated in their 1984 insert: "The occurrence of sudden infant death syndrome (SIDS) has been reported following administration of DTP. The significance of these reports is unclear. It should be kept in mind that the three primary immunizing doses of DTP are usually administered to infants between the age of two and six months and that approximately 85 percent of SIDS cases occur in the period 1 through 6 months of age, with the peak incidence at age 2 to 4 months."

Some of those who suspect a link between what coroners classify as SIDS and the DPT shot maintain that the vaccination is merely the last straw in a series of events which overwhelm a baby who may not be well prepared for life in the first place. E. M. Taylor and J. L. Emery wrote (1982), "In our experience, most unexpected deaths have a multifactorial aetiology, and we cannot exclude the possibility of recent immunisation being one of several contributory factors in an occasional unexpected infant death."

Many researchers believe that certain cases of SIDS are caused by the impact of additional stress on the infant's cardiovascular or respiratory system. In 1982, Daniel C. Shannon, M.D., and Dorothy H. Kelly, M.D., stated, "In general, the hypothesis is that infants who die suddenly, unexpectedly, and without having a sufficient cause detected at post-mortem examination share an abnormality in the autonomic regulation of cardiovascular or respiratory activity, or both: the abnormality can be triggered or exaggerated by a normal stimulus, such as inflammation of the respiratory tract. This is generally called the apnea hypothesis." (Apnea means a cessation of breathing.)

In this sense, some cases labeled by coroners as SIDS can resemble the "collapse" syndrome known to follow pertussis vaccination, in which the baby becomes limp and either stops breathing altogether or breathes with difficulty. In "near-SIDS" or "interrupted SIDS," parents or doctors are fortunate enough to be present when the infant stops breathing and are able to resuscitate him. Descriptions of near-SIDS have included the sudden onset of apnea and cyanosis (bluish tint of the skin) or pallor, which prompts parents to try to revive their apparently lifeless babies.

The lungs and respiration are under direct control of the nervous system, and breathing difficulties plus a bluish tint of the skin or pallor have often been reported by parents of infants who collapsed after a DPT shot. One mother, who was fortunate enough to discover her son when he had stopped breathing, said, "He reacted to his first shot at two months old. Right afterwards he had a fever and a hot red lump where he got the shot, which stayed there for weeks. Five days after the shot he went into cardiac respiratory arrest. We went in, and he was white and not breathing. We tried to revive him before the ambulance came. What it appeared to be was an interrupted SIDS."

Researchers have observed that infants prone to SIDS have difficulty breathing when they sleep. A "breathing monitor" has been developed which can be hooked up to the child; an alarm goes off if the heart rate drops below eighty beats per minute or if there is more than a ten-second lapse in breathing.

On March 19, 1979, a special meeting was called by the FDA on the Relation Between DPT Vaccines and Sudden Infant Death Syndrome. Daniel Shannon, M.D., who is director of the Pediatric Pulmonary Unit at Massachusetts General Hospital and a principal investigator of SIDS, spoke about his research:

"We do have a number of parents whose infants . . . have been doing entirely well after their initial near death spell who then go to the doctor, get a DPT and a polio and that is usually the two combined on the same day, and within twenty-four hours have either prolonged apnea with the alarm going off or the need for resuscitation, having not needed one since the first time, perhaps a month preceding. Whether we would advise the parents to not have any further immunizations or not at that point does not really matter. They will not. Until we tell them that we feel the infant is out of danger, perhaps six or seven months later, you could not get them near the pediatrician's office."

He added, "We do have this data. It is all recorded on tabular sheets and we have it on nearly 200 infants that we have evaluated this way. It is in a capacity that it can be pulled."

In 1982, when Shannon published an extensive two-part study on SIDS in the *New England Journal of Medicine*, a study which was financed in part by the Public Health Service, he did not once mention his data on the near-miss SIDS infants who had prolonged apnea after their DPT shots. When questioned about this omission, he replied in a letter, "I did not mention DPT shots in my review article on SIDS in the *New England Journal of Medicine* because there are no data collected in a scientific way that support an association (this includes Dr. Torch's report)."

William C. Torch, M.D., to whom Dr. Shannon referred in his letter, was formerly director of Child Neurology, Department of Pediatrics, at the University of Nevada School of Medicine. Torch also trained under Shannon at Massachusetts General Hospital. At the Thirty-fourth Annual Meeting of the American Academy of Neurology in 1982, Torch presented a study suggesting a link between the DPT shot and certain cases of SIDS. After observing four sudden deaths within nineteen hours of DPT vaccinations in Nevada, Torch studied the relationship between this shot and SIDS in over two hundred randomly reported SIDS cases.

In a preliminary report on the first seventy cases, Torch stated that two thirds had been vaccinated prior to death. Of these, 6.5 percent died within twelve hours of vaccination; 13 percent within twenty-four hours; 26 percent within three days; and 37, 61, and 70 percent within one, two, and three weeks, respectively. He found that SIDS frequencies peaked at age two months in the non-DPT group and had a biphasic peak occurrence at two and four months in the DPT group.

Torch added, "Cot death occurred maximally in the fall/winter season in the non-DPT group, but was nonseasonal in the DPT group. Death occurred most often in sleep in healthy, allergy-free infants following brief periods of irritability, crying, lethargy, upper respiratory tract symptoms, and sleep disturbance. Autopsy findings in both groups were typical of SIDS (e.g. petechiae of lung, pleura, pericardium, and thymus; vascular congestion; pulmonary edema; pneumonitis; and brain edema)."

But it was Torch's conclusion that infuriated neurologists and government health officials attending the meeting: "These data show that DPT vaccination may be a generally unrecognized major cause of sudden infant and early childhood death, and that the risks of immunization may outweigh its potential benefits. A need for reevaluation and possible modification of current vaccination procedures is indicated by this study."

At a press conference during the meeting, Torch was vigorously criticized for his "non-prospective" study, his use of "anecdotal data," and his conclusions. Gerald M. Fenichel, M.D., chairman of the Department of Neurology at Vanderbilt University Medical Center, wrote an editorial in a 1983 issue of the *Archives of Neurology* entitled "The Pertussis Vaccine Controversy: The Danger of Case Reports." He stated, "Public alarm, already considerable, was further increased when . . . Torch presented a paper at the annual meeting of the American Academy of Neurology in Washington, D.C., suggesting that diphtheria-pertussis-tetanus (DPT) immunization was a potential cause of sudden infant death syndrome."

In the editorial, Fenichel implied that Torch's data and conclusions should be dismissed because, "Fortunately, a prospective study on risk factors in sudden infant death syndrome had been established already by the National Institute of Child Health and Development, Bethesda, Maryland. The findings reported the following month excluded DPT as a causal factor in sudden infant death syndrome."

Yet how does one convince a young couple that the death of their first-born child was unexplained and was not related to the DPT shot he received just hours earlier? Darren began sleeping through the night at eight weeks old, but he usually cried for an hour and a half after his nine-thirty feeding until he finally fell asleep around eleven o'clock. Sometimes he would projectile vomit his formula. Darren's mother was allergic to cow's milk as a child, and his father is still allergic to milk, but Darren was never placed on soybean formula by his pediatrician.

"When I told my doctor about Darren crying for more than an hour after his nine-thirty feeding, he just said I was lucky my baby only cried an hour and a half every night because most babies cry a lot longer," said Darren's mother.

The day before nine-week-old Darren received his first DPT shot, his mother noticed he was fussier than usual. The night before he had awakened several times crying and had to be rocked to sleep, which was unusual because he generally slept for a solid ten hours once he got to sleep.

"He was unusually fussy the whole next day. Then I noticed his nose was congested and I heard him cough for the first time. I thought he was coming down with something, especially because I had a really sore throat myself," said Darren's mother.

Darren was scheduled for a checkup and his first DPT shot at six o'clock that evening, and his mother thought about canceling the appointment but she didn't. "I told my doctor Darren hadn't been himself and hadn't slept well for twenty-four hours and that I thought he was getting sick. My doctor looked in his nose and said, 'He looks fine to me.' Then the nurse gave him his DPT shot. All the doctor told me was to give him some Tempra if he got fussy."

About an hour later, Darren started crying uncontrollably. "I gave him some Tempra but he kept crying and then he started screaming really badly. We put him to bed still screaming at eleven-twenty that night. Although we were used to putting him to bed crying, we had never heard him scream like that. We didn't know what to do. We thought he was just more uncomfortable than usual because of the shot."

At seven the next morning, Darren's father went into his son's room and found him dead. "He had been dead for a while because he was blue and stiff," said his mother.

When Darren's parents arrived at the hospital with their son's body, a nurse met them and they asked her if their son's death could have been caused by the DPT shot he received twelve hours before. "She told us that the shot does not cause death and that it appeared my son had succumbed to Sudden Infant Death Syndrome.

"I called the coroner's office and talked to the doctor who performed the autopsy and asked if they could determine the time of his death because he was so discolored and stiff when we found him in the morning. We feel he must have died soon after we put him to bed that night, which would have meant it was within five or six hours after his shot. But they said it couldn't be determined."

Darren's mother doesn't understand why she wasn't questioned by anyone about her son's death. "Nobody ever asked us what happened to our son in the hours before his death. I really expected the coroner or somebody to ask me if I noticed anything unusual before he died. At least someone should have asked about whether or not he had recently been given a DPT shot. Shouldn't medical examiners care about those things if they are going to try to find the cause of death of a perfectly normal, healthy baby?"

Tami's death, like Darren's, was also diagnosed as SIDS. Tami weighed a little over ten pounds and was almost twenty-three inches long when she was born. Despite a tendency to spit up her formula, she was "healthy as an ox" according to her father.

"Tami was our second daughter, and she was a beautiful, big, healthy girl. She did spit up her milk formula both after and between feedings, and she did tend to cry herself to sleep at night. We now realize she may have had a milk allergy that was not recognized at the time. We have a history of milk allergy in my family. My brother had such a bad milk allergy that he had to be put on goat's milk until he was two years old. He also reacted to his series of DPT shots with asthma attacks. In fact, the doctors had to stop giving him DPT shots, because within twenty-four hours of a shot he would have to be taken to the hospital and receive medication to bring him out of the asthma attack."

Tami received her first shot at a public health clinic when she was almost three months old. "At the time, Tami had a runny nose," said Tami's father. "The nurse noticed her runny nose and even mentioned it to me. But Tami was given the shot anyway."

"That afternoon," said Tami's mother, "I had to run a few errands and I left Tami with a babysitter for fifteen minutes. Within three hours of her DPT shot, Tami woke up with really strange crying. The babysitter told us that Tami screamed like she was in terrible pain with a kind of shrieking sound she had never heard a baby make before—very high pitched and abnormal. Nothing would stop her crying and this went on for about five or ten minutes but eventually she calmed down."

When Tami's mother returned from running errands, she put Tami in her crib for a nap. About thirty minutes later, she went into Tami's room and found her in a state of collapse.

"Tami was very limp and heavy. I brought her out into the hall and realized she wasn't breathing. She looked pale and her eyes were closed. I ran to our neighbor's house and we immediately called the ambulance and started CPR and mouth-to-mouth resuscitation until the ambulance got there. Tami was taken to the hospital, but about ten minutes later our baby was pronounced dead."

Tami's parents were told that their baby died of Sudden Infant Death Syndrome. "The day after she died," said Tami's father, "the pediatrician told us Tami might have died from the DPT shot. We tried to get the coroner to look into it but three weeks later we were told it was not the shot, that it was just SIDS."

It wasn't until a year later that Tami's parents saw a local television program about DPT reactions and discovered that there was good reason to believe that their baby died from the effects of the pertussis vaccine. "Tami had a runny nose when she was vaccinated," said her father. "We have a history of milk allergy, asthma, convulsions, and severe reactions to DPT vaccine in our family. We now know that Tami had classic symptoms of a DPT reaction within a few hours of her shot—high-pitched screaming and collapse—and she died within four hours of her shot. If we had been informed about the pertussis vaccine before Tami received it, at least we would have understood the risk involved in giving it to our daughter."

A Georgia couple will always believe that their first son died from the aftereffects of a DPT shot. Kevin had a hernia operation at the age of two months. When he was four months old, he was admitted to a hospital for a "nervous stomach" because he had had colic since birth and could not keep his formula down. After the doctors put him on soybean formula, his colic disappeared, he stopped spitting up, and he began to thrive. Twelve days later, just before his fifth-month birthday, Kevin was given his second DPT shot.

Within seconds, Kevin's parents saw him turn blue and stop breathing. (A description of his collapse reaction was described earlier in this chapter under the heading "Collapse or Shock-like Episodes.") After the doctor had revived Kevin, they were all sent home. Once at home, he started shrieking continuously. His mother said, "Kevin would just scream and be all tight and then go limp when he couldn't scream any longer and had worn himself out. I had to hold him on a pillow because he would get so limp. While he was screaming, he would stare."

Kevin screamed for two days and nights. On the third day, the pediatrician took a chest X-ray and found that his heart had enlarged by 20 percent. Kevin's parents got in their car with their baby and drove over a hundred miles to a major medical center.

"Kevin screamed all the way in the car. When we got about forty miles from the hospital it was dark, and I told my husband 'We'd better go a little faster because he is real sick.' He felt real limp and lifeless to me. When we got to the hospital, I took him in, and I took his little sunsuit off and he just stared at me. There was no movement. He was alive but he just stared. They started to take his temperature and they were asking me a lot of questions, and then I noticed that everybody was real still in the room. I turned around and looked, and he had already turned blue."

Immediately after his collapse, Kevin was put on a respirator. Within three hours, he was dead. The autopsy report was vague, his mother said.

"After the autopsy the cardiologist said it looked like a virus had attacked his heart. They have never told us what exactly was wrong with him. On the death certificate it says 'cardiac arrest, possible myocarditis,' but the doctor said they really don't know what happened. They said his lungs were scarred from all the crying. The doctors kept telling us they were almost positive it wasn't the DPT shot whenever we would bring it up. But, you see, the minute after he got the shot he stopped breathing. Then he started screaming and was never the same again."

Kevin's parents are glad they took him to the hospital that night. "After our pediatrician X-rayed Kevin's chest and found his heart was enlarged, he told us we could take him to the medical center either that night or the next morning. We didn't want to wait. I am glad we didn't, because if we had stayed at home Kevin would have died in his bedroom."

For the next year, Kevin's mother kept hearing him screaming. "I would walk into this house, and I could hear him screaming those final nights, and I could see his little face. I would go into hysterics. He was our first child, and he was such a beautiful baby. He had been cooing and laughing and smiling a lot after we got him on soybean formula. Evidently he was allergic to milk, and he was able to digest the soybean formula better. But from the minute he got that DPT shot, he never smiled again."

The pertussis vaccine claimed the life of two-month-old Douglas after he and his twin sister received their first DPT shots. From birth, the only problem the twins had was spitting up their formula. Both had projectile vomiting of their formula after feedings, just as their older sister had when she was a baby and was put on soybean formula. But, at two months of age, both twins were still on regular milk formula despite their projectile vomitings.

Both twins were pronounced healthy by the pediatrician and given the first DPT shot. Five hours later, Douglas's mother noticed that he would not open his mouth to drink his evening bottle. When she woke him for his four A.M. feeding, he still would not open his mouth to drink.

"At nine A.M., I realized he was very pale. Then his eyes were rolling back and forth in his head. I opened his mouth for him and he guzzled the milk down so fast that I thought he would choke," his mother said.

After she changed his diapers and found a mass of strange-colored diarrhea, she rushed him to the hospital. There, doctors stuck tubes down Douglas's throat to pump out his stomach because they thought he must have swallowed something. He started gagging and went into cardiac arrest.

"They couldn't get him breathing for three minutes and when he did start breathing, he had a blue mark on his head so we knew there was already brain damage done. He went into a coma and never came out of it."

Douglas was rushed by ambulance to another hospital and had cardiac arrest several more times on the way. His right side became paralyzed. After several hours at that hospital, he was rushed by ambulance to a third hospital where he again went into cardiac arrest.

"They couldn't get needles in his arms because they said his veins had collapsed. So they had to put the needle in his head. They even tried to exchange bad fluids for good through his navel. Finally, they came in and said, 'He's not doing any breathing on his own at all.' Then he died. It had been about twenty-eight hours since he had gotten his shot."

Douglas's mother is still confused about the autopsy report: "See, my pediatrician swears Douglas did not die from the shot. They told me he died of bronchial bilateral pneumonia. One day earlier, my doctor had pronounced him totally healthy. And just before Douglas died, I remember the doctor coming in and saying to us, 'I want you to know that spinal meningitis was setting in and he wouldn't have had a chance at all if he had survived with all that was wrong with him.' But spinal meningitis is not mentioned in the autopsy."

A state official of the CDC told Douglas's mother over the telephone that her son had died from a reaction to the DPT shot. "But he told me that he would not say that to anybody else. He said, 'Between you and me, he died from a reaction to the DPT shot.' He also said that Douglas's death was only one of three in the last three years that was due to the DPT vaccine."

Douglas's parents cannot find a lawyer to take their case. "Every lawyer we have talked to has said that a judge only allows so much money on a death because there are no future expenses involved as there are in raising a brain-damaged child."

Some babies, like Andrew, do not die within twenty-four or forty-eight hours of their DPT shot but slowly deteriorate until death finally comes a week or more later. These deaths are the most difficult for doctors to recognize as related to the pertussis vaccine.

Andrew was an active, advanced baby for his age and could roll over at two and a half months. His mother says, "We feel that God gave us a very special baby because he was trying to pull himself up at two months of age. He was doing everything early."

Within an hour of his first DPT shot, Andrew was running a fever of almost 104 degrees; his leg was red and swollen, and he had started to scream. "He got the shot at one and by two o'clock, all he did was cry. He would give this piercing scream of pain. Andrew had colic from birth, but this scream was different from his colic cry. We tried giving him baths to break his fever but nothing would break it. I called the doctor two or three hours after the shot because he was having such a reaction. His leg had become so swollen that he would not use it at all. At the puncture mark it was red and swollen about the size of a fifty-cent piece. It was hard like there was a golf ball underneath it. The doctor's office told me they must have hit a muscle. They told me not to worry about his reaction until it had been twenty-four hours."

Within twenty-four hours, Andrew's fever came down but he continued to scream on and off and was unresponsive. "He had always been a very active baby before the shot, but afterward he wasn't interested in doing anything but crying. We were scheduled to go on a vacation immediately following Andy's shot. We really noticed that his temperament had changed. He just never was the same again. He cried a lot more and was listless. When we got home from our vacation, I changed his diaper and noticed blood in the bowel movement."

Andrew was admitted to the hospital for observation. His mother fed him a bottle at the hospital, and afterward, he began screaming. She hurried home to get some crib toys and clothes so she could sleep beside him at the hospital.

"Andy was screaming when I left. I was only gone an hour and forty-five minutes. When I got back at 6:45 P.M., the nurses had found him dead in his crib at 6:30 P.M. They really don't know what happened because, evidently, nobody checked on him while I was gone. Anyway, they called his death a SIDS death." It had been two weeks since Andrew received his DPT shot.

In 1983, Larry Baraff, M.D., who was a principal author of the UCLA-FDA study, published an article on SIDS deaths in Los Angeles County. He and his coauthors contacted the parents of 145 babies who were reported to have died from SIDS in Los Angeles County between

January 1979 and August 1980. Fifty-three had received a DPT immunization; out of these, six died within twenty-four hours and eleven more died within seven days of the DPT shot.

They concluded that "These SIDS deaths were significantly more than expected were there no association between DPT immunization and SIDS." They added, "If further studies substantiate our findings it seems prudent to consider rescheduling DPT immunization until after the period of highest risk of SIDS, i.e. the latter half of the first year of life."

How many deaths will it take? Vincent Fulginiti commented (in *Pediatric Infectious Disease*) on Baraff's 1983 SIDS study and said, "In the search for biological truth we must not disregard or scorn potential clues to enlightenment. . . . we do not know what causes SIDS; we do not know if DTP does. We should attempt to find out; it is not a trivial question."

But, just nine months later, Dr. Fulginiti wrote a letter to the *American Journal of Diseases of Children* about the 14 deaths of children who contracted whooping cough in Britain in 1982. He said, ". . . 14 deaths is not comforting to me, nor to those families in which they occurred." And he added that those who view the pertussis vaccine as dangerous "cannot conceivably estimate that 14 deaths would result from immunization."

6

Profile: An Unknown Future

> I will use treatment to help the sick according to my ability and judgment but never with a view to injury or wrongdoing. . . . Now if I carry out this oath, and break it not, may I gain forever reputation among all men for my life and for my art; but if I transgress it and forswear myself, may the opposite befall me.
>
> *Hippocrates, The Physician's Oath*

Soon after her third DPT shot, which she received at six months old, Alison had one ear infection after another and bouts of bronchitis that never seemed to clear up. Her pediatrician suspected a milk allergy and switched her to a soybean formula until she was fifteen months old.

Alison's mother, Katherine, cannot recall that her daughter had an acute reaction such as a fever or screaming immediately following her first three DPT shots at two, four, and sixth months of age. "All I remember is that Alison seemed to be sick a lot with ear infections and bronchial congestions after her third shot. Other than that, she was a very bright little girl and was developing just like any other child."

Alison was due for her DPT booster at eighteen months, but she came down with a cold. "Her pediatrician gave her some cough syrup," Katherine said, "and put off giving her the booster. But when I came back approximately two weeks later, he didn't examine her again. The nurse gave Alison the DPT shot, and we never saw his face."

Katherine will never forget what happened in the next twenty-six hours as she watched her daughter come close to death.

"About two or three hours after her shot, she started running a fever of 102 degrees, and it stayed there through the whole afternoon and night. The next morning I called her pediatrician and told him about her fever, and he said I shouldn't worry unless the fever goes over 102 or lasts for more than forty-eight hours. So I tried not to think anymore about it."

When Alison woke up from her morning nap at noon, she acted strangely. "She was wiggling all over. I picked her up, and her right arm started jerking and then it spread to her whole body. We live in a rural area so I had to call a helicopter ambulance. While we were waiting for the helicopter, I got a wet cloth and patted her face because I didn't know what else to do. When the helicopter arrived, she was still jerking. Her seizure must have lasted ten to fifteen minutes."

The helicopter ambulance was barely large enough to hold the pilot, the paramedic, Katherine, and Alison. "I had to get in and lay Alison on my lap. I noticed she was turning blue, but I didn't realize she had quit breathing. I could hear the paramedic talking to the pilot through his headphone. Suddenly he grabbed a bag and put it over her face and started pumping. It was then I realized she had stopped breathing. If that paramedic hadn't been there, she probably would have died. I was scared to death."

Nurses with a stretcher were waiting for the helicopter to land, and as soon as it touched down, they grabbed Alison and ran to the trauma room. "They left me outside to wander in by myself. When I saw them running with her, I started praying to God to just let her live. Before I was worried about what the seizure had done to her brain. But then I just prayed that she would live. I didn't care if she could never talk or if she was retarded. Given the two choices, I wanted her to live."

Katherine was not allowed to see her child for nearly four hours. "I just wanted to see her, to touch her but they wouldn't let me go in. The doctors kept walking in and out of the trauma room. They did request permission to do a spinal tap and that scared me. Finally, they told me they didn't know what was wrong with her or what would happen to her."

Katherine entered the room where Alison was laying on a bed. She was not prepared for what she saw. "Alison was unconscious and her little right arm and leg were all crooked up, all twisted like an old person who had had a stroke. And she was smacking her lips. I can't forget the lip smacking. I don't know why that shocked me so."

Katherine spent the night in intensive care, sitting next to her unconscious child. At midnight, miraculously, Alison woke up. "She suddenly was awake and singing 'Rock-a-bye Baby in the Treetops,' which was one of her favorite songs. I couldn't believe it. Neither could the doctors."

The following day, tests revealed that Alison had a slight touch of pneumonia in her right lung. All the other tests, including an EEG and brain scan, came back normal. "The neurologist came by and was really impressed that she was feeding herself and using her spoon. The only thing he noticed was that she staggered when she walked. He never told me why she had the seizure. My pediatrician told me her seizure was caused by the 102 fever she had been running and that the pneumonia was caused by the fever and the seizure. Neither one ever mentioned the DPT shot."

Alison was placed on the anticonvulsant Dilantin as a precaution to prevent more seizures. Although she did not have more convulsions, she dragged her right foot and would rarely use her right hand.

"If she ran and tired herself, her right side would give way. Her knee wouldn't bend and she would fall. She also began using her left hand for eating and everything else," said Katherine.

Five months after her seizure and collapse, Alison's father was killed in an automobile accident. With his death, Alison and her mother lost their right to remain on his company's group health insurance policy.

"They switched us from the group policy to an individual policy. Because Alison was on seizure medication, our insurance premiums went up to $235 per month, which is more than I pay for my mortgage. When I tried to get cheaper insurance, three insurance companies turned me down. Nobody would insure Alison because she was on anticonvulsant medication."

In April 1982, Katherine's mother saw an excerpt from "DPT: Vaccine Roulette" on the *Today* show and she told Katherine about it.

"The next time I took Alison in to the pediatrician, I asked him if the DPT shot could have had anything to do with her seizure. He looked kind of scared and then shrugged and said, 'Oh well, some people think that, but I don't think there is much to it.' But I told him I didn't want her to have any more pertussis vaccine. He said, 'That's no problem. I will just write it in her record.' He opened up her chart and there written in big, black-felt-tipped marker were the words NO PERTUSSIS. He knew I saw it and said, 'Oh, it is already down here.'

He just brushed it off as best he could." At that point, Katherine felt that Alison's pediatrician must have already suspected the pertussis vaccine had had something to do with her daughter's seizure and collapse.

Alison continued to have what her pediatrician diagnosed as bronchial infections. Finally, her chest congestion became so bad that she was unable to sleep. "Every night I would get up with her at two-thirty in the morning and rock her until daylight because she couldn't breathe. I was working all day as a teacher and trying to take care of her at night, and all the money I was making was going to health insurance and doctor bills."

Katherine left the teaching job she loved to stay at home and take care of Alison. "I love teaching and I feel better mentally when I work. But I couldn't stand the stress of going to work and leaving her, knowing she was sick, or staying at home with her and feeling guilty about missing so much work. Always, there was the threat that she might go into another seizure. I just had to quit my job to take care of her."

Katherine decided to consult another doctor, who gave Alison a chest X-ray and found that she had pneumonia and asthma. A pediatric allergist confirmed that she had asthma as well as allergies to many pollens and other airborne substances. Tests showed she was the most severely allergic to milk. She was started on weekly allergy shots and given medication to counteract her asthma attacks.

Katherine called her previous pediatrician and requested that Alison's records be sent to her new doctor. "His secretary called me and wanted to know why we were seeing another doctor. She said the doctor thought so much of us that he wanted us to come back to him. At the time I thought it was so sweet of him to be concerned about us. But he never sent Alison's records even after we asked him again to do it."

Anxious to take her daughter off Dilantin so she could obtain cheaper health insurance, Katherine consulted Alison's neurologist. This time, the EEG came back abnormal, showing seizure activity. "I told him the pediatrician had said Alison's seizure was due to her fever, and I asked him why a fever seizure would make her have an abnormal EEG. He said, 'Oh, no. What she had was more than a fever seizure. You don't get a seizure like that from a fever. She either had a reaction to her DPT shot or she had a pulmonary infection when she got the DPT shot.' It was the first time any doctor had come right out and admitted that Alison had reacted to her DPT shot."

Alison was three years old by now, and it had been almost a year and a half since the night she almost died.

* * * * *

Alison's light blonde hair is tied back in a ponytail. She is wearing blue jeans and tennis shoes. Her little legs look sturdy, but there is something slightly unsteady about her walk and her beautiful, wide-set blue eyes cannot hide the effects of the medication she must take.

At four years old, she is very verbal and is already trying to write her name. Holding the pencil in her left hand, she writes Alison perfectly, except that it is spelled backwards; every letter is turned the wrong way.

"She is very young to be writing and I know kids often turn their letters around when they start. We'll just have to wait and see if she turns out to be dyslexic or has other learning disabilities. Everybody tells me Alison is so bright, but that doesn't mean she won't be writing backwards when she is in school. I am a teacher and I have seen plenty of kids who are bright, but they can't read or write because everything in the world is backwards to them."

Katherine speaks softly and slowly with a slight Southern drawl. In a quiet voice she speaks of her determination to win financial security for her daughter's uncertain future.

"I have a lawyer. I don't like the idea of a lawsuit and I don't want to go through it. But I don't want to wait until she is eighteen and can't get a job because she has epilepsy or can't get into college because she can't read or write properly. I don't want her to look at me one day and ask me why I didn't do something, why I missed the opportunity to get financial support for her by not pursuing a court case. I want to know I did everything I could for her."

Katherine is disappointed by the attitude of doctors toward the issue of educating parents about vaccine reactions. "It is really a deception. I feel like they deceived me by making me believe there was no risk connected with the DPT vaccine. They never mentioned the slightest chance of its making Alison sick and certainly not as sick as it did make her. What really bothers me about the pediatrician who gave Alison the shot is that he never warned me not to give her more pertussis vaccine. In fact he tried to deny there was a connection. She is due for another DPT booster before she goes to kindergarten. We could have moved to Timbuctoo by then and taken her to a clinic for her DPT shot. He would have let me risk Alison's life and make her go through all that pain again just to save his own neck."

If Katherine had known that it was dangerous to give Alison a vaccination when she was sick, she would have insisted that the pediatrician give Alison an examination first. "What I regret most about what happened to Alison is that I was so ignorant. If I had been educated about the vaccine, I would have known enough to insist that the pediatrician give Alison a thorough exam prior to the shot. Since tests showed that she had pneumonia the day after her seizure, it is entirely possible that she had pneumonia the day of the shot. And it is evident now that she probably had asthma and severe allergies before that shot. My sister died with asthma. I am just really angry that I didn't know more about the vaccine."

When Katherine connected the DPT shot to her daughter's seizure in conversations with neurologists, she encountered resistance. "I took her to a pediatric neurologist, and the minute I mentioned her DPT shot he started defending the vaccine. Then he acted like he wanted to get rid of me. He reacted to everything I said with hostility and would jump on me before I could finish a statement. He didn't even examine Alison. He told me I shouldn't come back."

Katherine sadly echoes the sentiment that many parents of vaccine-damaged children hold. "I feel like I have been lied to by those I trusted. People look up to doctors and think they're godlike. At least down here in the South, doctors are powerful socially and are given a lot of respect. You think your doctor is always someone you can turn to, but I have lost that image. I see many doctors more as businessmen now, instead of people who care. Their business cames first with them, not their patients' welfare.

"As far as the mandatory vaccination policy goes, I think parents should be told how dangerous a medical procedure such as a vaccination is and then have the right to decide whether or not their child will be vaccinated with a particular vaccine. I am not against all vaccines. Alison had the MMR shot and the polio vaccine, and I will give her diphtheria and tetanus when she is due for her booster before kindergarten. I think people are intelligent enough to weigh the benefits and risks after they have been educated about the vaccine and the disease it protects against and make a choice which will benefit their child as well as everyone else. I don't like the government and doctors treating us like we are too stupid to make our own decisions."

Alison shows her mother the picture she has colored and, after getting a big hug, leaves to color another one, her paper and crayon clutched in her left hand. Katherine watches her apprehensively.

"I am afraid if she has another seizure, she won't be as lucky as she was the first time. The doctors have said she has a 90 percent chance of having another convulsion if she goes off her medication. They can't assure me that, if she goes into another seizure, she won't stop breathing again or won't be brain damaged. I don't know if the worst is over or the worst is yet to come."

7

Long-term Damage

We are accustomed to look for the gross and immediate effect and to ignore all else. Unless this appears promptly, we deny the existence of hazard. Even research men suffer from the handicap of inadequate methods of detecting the beginnings of injury. The lack of sufficiently delicate methods to detect injury before symptoms appear is one of the great unsolved problems in medicine.

Rachel Carson

L ocal and systemic reactions, such as a fever or slight redness and pain at the site of the injection, have occurred in millions of children after DPT shots, and most of them develop into normal adults. But, in an unknown number of children, the reaction passes to a stage involving more vital organs.

Severe Neurological Damage

One of the characteristics of the pertussis vaccine is its affinity for the brain and central nervous system. Pertussis bacteria have been used in a variety of research experiments to help provoke brain inflammation (encephalitis) and brain deterioration (encephalopathy) in mice. It is not surprising that the vaccine produces brain deterioration in some children.

In 1954, Miller and Stanton described several cases of severe reactions to the pertussis vaccine and commented: "One of the most serious features of these complications is the evidence of residual damage to the nervous system. Continued epileptic fits, residual hemiplegia, blindness, mental defect, behavior disorders, and reversal of sleep rhythm have been reported, and it appears that about two-thirds of the patients who recover from the acute phase are liable to such residua."

In 1960, Justus Ström described cases of pertussis vaccine damage which included progressive mental deterioration, cerebral palsy, deafness, and epilepsy. In 1979, Gordon Stewart analyzed 197 cases of children with neurological reactions to the DPT shot and concluded, "In all but a few of the cases studied here, these signs were followed in a few days or weeks by arrest or loss of mental development and by varying degrees of physical handicap ranging from spasticity to complete paralysis of all but the vital reflexes."

Today many parents of damaged children sadly confirm what Miller and Stanton and other researchers have said about the vaccine's ability to affect the brain. They have described their children's neurological reactions to this vaccine, and the mental and physical deterioration that followed, with a clarity that no doctor or scientist has equaled.

After Michelle was born, she could not keep her cow's milk formula down. Finally placed on goat's milk, she stopped spitting up. After the first DPT shot, which she received when six months old, she began running a fever. Then, within twenty-four hours, she went into a convulsion.

Her father remembers that day. "I had no idea what she was doing. I thought she was dying. She turned blue, and I tried to give her mouth-to-mouth resuscitation because I thought she was choking on something. We got her to the hospital in a matter of seconds because it was only a block away. She was in a grand mal convulsion. The doctors gave her Phenobarbital and she went to sleep. While she was sleeping, she couldn't move her left side. But when she woke up, she got up on all fours and appeared to be okay."

Michelle did not have another seizure until the second DPT shot just one month later. Again, within twenty-four hours she started a fever and went into a grand mal convulsion. Again, she was hospitalized.

"Then she started having hundreds of petit mal seizures a day," her father said. "One doctor counted her petit mal seizures for fifteen minutes and estimated she was having about 144 per hour. She has been on every combination of medication, and although her petit mals are now controlled, she still has grand mals in spite of the medication."

Unbelievably, Michelle was given a third DPT shot. She is now eighteen years old, and the quality of her life is still marred by her uncontrollable seizures.

"Her grand mal seizures have reached a point where she strains every muscle in her body, and you can hear her little joints crack because there is such a violent contraction of the muscles. Yesterday we visited friends, and they have a stone entrance to their home," said her father, "Michelle had a seizure and fell and hit her head on the stone. And today she had a seizure and fell and hit her head again. I thought she had fractured her skull she fell so hard. We usually catch her before she falls because we try not to let her get ten feet away from us."

Michelle's parents must help her take a bath and use the bathroom because she might have a convulsion at any time. "My wife bears the brunt of the responsibility. There are wet bed sheets in the morning because when she has a seizure at night, she loses control. We can't put but a half inch of water in the bathtub, and her mother has to stay with her because she could have a seizure and drown."

A pretty, dark-haired girl with big brown eyes, Michelle is about five feet tall and weighs only seventy-five pounds. She is extremely thin because eating causes her pain.

"Her anticonvulsant medication has ruined her teeth and her ability to chew food. It hurts her to chew so she takes large bites and is liable to choke when she swallows. Her teeth are not loose, but they haven't formed properly."

Michelle is visited by a teacher who is helping her learn how to read and write. She can print her first name in block letters and recognize Stop and Go signs. Her parents take her with them when they travel, if at all possible.

"We worry about what would happen to her if something happened to us," her father said. "We are afraid to fly without her. We have no plans to put her in an institution because we don't want her in a situation that would threaten her safety. She is a very loving child and we protect her. I keep asking myself, 'Why did it have to happen to Michelle?' It was so unnecessary."

Will Paula's future be like Michelle's? Paula is only three-and-a-half years old. Within ten hours of her first shot, she had a one-hour grand mal seizure. Her mother said, "They had to use Valium to bring her out of what was a status epilepticus seizure. But they gave the Valium to her so fast that it put her into respiratory arrest. That did stop the convulsion."

Paula has had fifteen status epilepticus seizures in her young life. When she was two, she had a status seizure that no amount of drugs would stop. "This time, the doctors had to deliberately put her into respiratory arrest with a large dose of Valium to bring the convulsion under control. Then they put her on a respirator."

Paula has twenty to thirty seizures a month. She is on high levels of Depakene and Tegretol. She can walk but she cannot talk. Her mother is afraid that the high levels of anticonvulsant medications are delaying her development as much as the seizures.

"She got toxic on Depakene, but they have lowered the dose now. The medication has prevented her from having status seizures, which is good because status seizures can be fatal. But as she grows older and her medication is increased, she is having more frequent regular seizures. I would like to cut down on her medication, but I am afraid of her going into a status seizure and dying."

Status epilepticus seizures can be fatal and seizures which occur after the DPT shot have been known to eventually result in a child's death. Peter's mother describes the brief life of her only child.

Peter did not react to the first two shots. But within three hours of his third DPT shot, he had a grand mal seizure. His mother rushed him to the pediatrician while he was in the middle of the convulsion.

"They gave him a shot to stop the convulsion, but it didn't work. After a second shot, it finally stopped. Peter's convulsions were resistant to the medication, and every time he had a seizure he would end up in a hospital emergency room. Sometimes he would be there for two or three hours at a time. The doctors think he suffered more brain damage because the convulsions were so long."

By the age of seven, Peter had been evaluated and treated at several major medical centers on the East Coast. Although he no longer went into three-hour seizures, he still had grand mal convulsions that were not controlled, even by a combination of four or five anticonvulsants.

"By the time he was seven, the seizures came less frequently. In fact, he was probably better than he had been in his whole life as far as the seizures were concerned. Physically, he was just fine in that he could run and shoot baskets and hit a golf ball. The major delay was in his speech. He had a good vocabulary, but he couldn't string the words together. He understood much more than he could communicate. Even though he was only about a three year old intellectually, he was interested in everything. He thought he had the world by the tail and was happy as a clam. His sweetness had such a positive impact on so many people who knew him."

But Peter's parents did not know that his condition was to trigger his premature death without warning.

"We were used to his seizures," his mother said. "He would usually fall to the floor and have them. One day, he was standing in front of me, as usual, with a smile on his face. Then he fell, and I immediately knew this seizure was different, more violent. I thought maybe he had aspirated something. We gave him mouth-to-mouth resuscitation. But his fingers were already turning blue by the time the rescue squad arrived. There is no question that his little heart was not pumping. The doctors said he might have had an aneurism in the part of the brain that controls the heart. Whatever it was, he died instantly."

Peter's mother has always believed that her son had a rare seizure disorder and that his death was an unusual consequence of the disorder. "Of course, we always felt, and it was explained to us, that his condition was connected with the DPT shot because it occurred within hours of the shot. We had a well-known neurologist at a national medical center tell us he thought Peter's condition was probably related to the shot. We understood it was an allergic reaction because whenever Peter would get a vaccine, such as polio, he would go into seizures. But we really always thought what happened to Peter was a very rare occurrence. The way he died was highly unusual. I have never heard of another case like it to this day."

Michelle, Paula, and Peter were left with medication-resistant seizures after their DPT shots, but they continued to develop, even if that development was delayed. Other children stop developing altogether and remain stuck at the age when their brains were so profoundly damaged. Debbie was one of these.

She had been developing just like any other newborn until her first DPT shot. Her mother told what happened: "Up until her first shot, she had been doing so well nursing and sleeping and cooing and smiling. Within a week of her shot, she started crying a very annoying, strange cry unlike she had done before. She had been such a contented baby before the shot. I didn't know what was wrong. Nothing would comfort her. Then she started petit mal seizures."

Debbie's parents took her to a neurologist, and although her EEG came back abnormal, no cause could be found for her seizures. She was referred to a major teaching hospital, and there a second neurologist confirmed that her condition might be related to the DPT shot.

"He told us that they were seeing children come in with seizures a week to ten days after the DPT shot. But our doctors were appalled that we had been told by a neurologist that her condition was DPT related. They absolutely denied it and insisted on giving her a second DPT shot."

Within an hour of the second shot, Debbie went into much more violent seizures. "I saw a more involved seizure, much stronger, almost immediately after the shot. Her seizures were now longer and involved her arms and legs and lots of rapid eye movement. I could see a definite worsening of her condition."

Now eight years old, Debbie still has seizures, and her development has halted at the three-month level. "She is severely retarded. She doesn't talk. She sits up fairly well. She is still in diapers, and we still have to feed her because she can't feed herself. She lives at home and goes to a school for retarded children every day. It is very hard to be strong sometimes. The hurt never goes away," her mother said.

Minimal Brain Damage, Learning Disabilities, and Hyperactivity

Today few vaccine experts will deny that pertussis vaccine can cause severe brain damage. But the connection between the DPT shot and "minimal brain dysfunction," or learning disabilities, is much more controversial.

While the number of severely brain-damaged children is a small portion of the general population, the number of learning-disabled children in America is growing at a phenomenal rate. Schools are increasingly burdened with the need to set up special education programs. The learning-disabled population in the public schools of America has risen from 830,000 in 1958 to 3,234,000 in 1980, according to the National Center for Educational Statistics, and their number is increasing even as school enrollment declines. Is it a coincidence that this dramatic rise in America's learning-disabled population occurred precisely during the three decades when the pertussis vaccine was being extended to include virtually all American children?

Vincent Fulginiti stated in testimony before a Senate subcommittee in 1982, "I know of no evidence linking learning disability as an isolated condition to DPT." Then he added, "Of course, if a child develops encephalopathy, one part of the possible residual from that might be a learning disability."

Reports in the scientific literature and by parents suggest that pertussis vaccine damage covers the spectrum from death and severe retardation to such milder forms of neurological damage as learning disabilities. Stewart has stated, "It would be out of keeping with other adverse reactions to other substances if the only cases were severe ones. More likely there are numerous cases of lesser damage and lesser disability."

The federal law used as a guide to funding special education programs in the public school system defines children with learning disabilities as "those children who have a disorder in one or more of the basic psychological processes involved in understanding or using language, spoken or written, which disorder may manifest itself in imperfect ability to listen, think, speak, read, write, spell, or do mathematical calculations."

Clements and Peters of the Department of Psychiatry, University of Arkansas for Medical Sciences, have defined "minimal brain dysfunction" as "a medical designation for certain aberrations of behavior and/ or cognitive functioning resulting from milder forms of central nervous system (CNS) dysfunction or developmental deviation." Most often a child with minimal brain dysfunction has a normal or above-average I.Q. But he seems to suffer from some impairment of the ability to transmit information from the senses to the brain, and to process this information in order to initiate speech, action, and behavior. Authorities have given various names to this impairment, such as "delayed integration" (Richard J. Schain), "defects in comprehending abstractions," or "central processing deficits" (Clements and Peters).

The origin of learning disabilities is no better understood today than it was in 1966, when the government-sponsored National Project on Minimal Brain Dysfunction in Children: Task Force I, stated, "These aberrations may arise from genetic variations, biochemical irregularities, perinatal brain insults or other illnesses or injuries sustained during the years which are critical for the development and maturation of the central nervous system, or from unknown causes. . . . During the school years, a variety of learning disabilities is the most prominent manifestation of the condition."

A noted authority on minimal brain damage, Richard J. Schain, M.D., of the University of California School of Medicine, defined the syndrome in 1977 as "acquired minimal damage of areas of the brain which is not extensive enough to result in gross neurological deficits but is sufficient to produce language, perceptual and motor disturbances."

In addition to specific learning disabilities, children may have a short attention span; inability to concentrate; poor memory; hyperactivity; clumsiness; sleep disturbances; impulsiveness and emotional lability; hearing and speech difficulties. Most children have a combination of these symptoms; and one type, known as the "mixed type," involves "moderate reading and spelling difficulties [dyslexia], a short attention span, and mild to moderate hyperactivity," according to Clements and Peters.

The concept of minimal brain damage syndrome was first brought to the attention of doctors in the 1920s, when a mini-epidemic of a disease called "von Economo's encephalitis," or "encephalitis lethargica," swept through Europe and America. Physicians found that those who recovered were often left with a marked change in their behavior, restlessness, insomnia or disturbance of sleep patterns, irritability, short attention span, and emotional disorders. Sometimes they exhibited destructive behavior or had seizures, tremors, and tics.

In 1934, Kahn and Cohen described a group of children with hyperkinetic activity, the inability to sit still, and poor attention span, which they also attributed to an encounter with encephalitis of the von Economo variety. Finally, in 1947, Gerhard Gesell, the famous child psychologist, developed the concept of "minimal cerebral injury" to explain certain behavioral disorders in preschool and elementary school children. He emphasized speech, reading, visual, and hearing difficulties, and difficulty in distinguishing between left and right.

The study of what is now called "minimal brain dysfunction" has become a growth industry. Schain states with some wonderment, "The early workers who described the brain damage syndrome consequent to epidemic encephalitis would be surprised at its present prevalence, albeit in an attenuated form."

Problems with reading are a common feature of the minimum brain damage syndrome. Parents whose children have had serious reactions to the DPT shot describe their subsequent problems with reading and writing.

Brian, whose reaction was described in Chapter 5, ran a high fever and suffered high-pitched screaming and hallucinations within an hour of his fifth DPT shot. He was left with learning disabilities and tremors that affected his writing. "He was dyslexic at six," said his mother. "He had mirror handwriting in the first grade. If you held his writing up to a mirror, it was perfect. He would make a calendar with every number backwards."

Now a teenager, Brian can read and write but has not lived up to his potential. "He has never gotten it together in school," said his mother. "He does well on tests but is a poor student. They tested him and found him to be gifted but not productive. And he has tremors in his hands and feet. He'll never be a surgeon or hold any job that requires a steady hand."

Susan had several collapse/shock episodes after her second DPT shot. She appeared to recover and did not have another one until the fourth shot at eighteen months of age.

When Susan was five, a child psychiatrist told her parents that she was exhibiting learning disabilities. "Everyone who knows her can't believe it because she seems so bright, but the psychiatrist told us that she is right-handed and right-footed but with left-eye coordination. When she writes her name, she starts on the right-hand side instead of on the left-hand side. We have to do exercises with her that first start clockwise and then counterclockwise. She is extremely sensitive, very emotional, and often fearful. She will be sweet and happy one minute and crying the next."

The learning disability known as dyslexia is associated with "disturbances in eye movements" according to Norman Geschwind, M.D., of the Harvard Medical School, or with "deficits in visual perception" according to Clements and Peters. The vaccine is also known to affect the nerves and muscles of the eyes. One of Byers and Moll's cases became blind, and Justus Ström in 1960 found that pertussis vaccine can cause paresis (slight paralysis) of the ocular muscles, conjugate deviation of the eyes, and nystagmus (involuntary jerky movements of the eyeballs).

The mother of a baby girl who had seizures after her second DPT shot and is learning disabled said, "Another thing that happened after her second shot is that her eyes started crossing. I took her to the doctor, and he said, 'Oh, that's normal with babies. Don't worry about it.' To this day, her eyes still cross sometimes."

"Her eyes stick to the left sometimes, and she has to shake her head to make them straight," said the mother of a girl who reacted at eighteen months to her fourth DPT shot.

Vision is only one of the senses that can be affected by the pertussis vaccine. Minimal brain damage is also associated with auditory processing deficit and hearing problems. Byers and Moll mention an infant who became deaf from the vaccine, and Ström also mentions a case of deafness. Hearing loss can also be caused indirectly by otitis media, or chronic inflammation of the inner ear, with continuous discharge of pus. Many parents have mentioned their babies became sick with inner ear infections shortly after a DPT shot.

Ryan was given his first DPT shot at six weeks, and within an hour was running a fever of 105 degrees. His mother remembers his violent reaction: "His leg was swollen to triple the size it was normally. We were up all night giving him tepid baths and Tylenol to try and get his fever down. He screamed helplessly off and on for three days and three nights. My doctor said he was just having a reaction, and that it was not unusual."

Within a week and a half of the shot, Ryan had developed bronchitis. His ears also became inflamed. In addition, he began spitting up his breast-milk, which he had not done since birth. He continued spitting up until he was eight months old, and he had colic until he was about two.

Two months after the first DPT shot, Ryan was given a half dose of DPT vaccine. "He had the same reaction all over again. Within an hour, his fever climbed to 105 degrees and his leg was swollen to an incredible size. Like before, the lump stayed in the leg for about two weeks. He screamed and screamed again on and off for three days and three nights."

Ryan did not get the third DPT shot, which was also a half dose, until about a year later because his mother "dreaded giving it to him. I didn't want him to have another shot, but the doctors really pressure you. I've always been very respectful of doctors and medicine. You just want to do the right thing." Again, Ryan ran a fever of 105 degrees and had a swollen leg. Soon afterward, he began waking up at night screaming in terror.

"We couldn't figure out what was wrong with him. He would scream like he was frightened to death or in terrible pain. It would last for about thirty minutes and nothing would comfort him. It was awful.

We decided it was night terror. Sometimes he would wake up every night screaming. This lasted a couple of months."

Ryan continued to have upper respiratory infections and inflamed ears. He was frequently on antibiotics. He was also not yet talking. He was given a fourth DPT shot when two and a half years old. Still, he was not talking. Again he ran a 105-degree fever and had a swollen leg. A year later, doctors put tubes into Ryan's ears and discovered that the inner ear was bulging with fluid. They also found he only had 40 percent of his hearing, which was most probably caused by the constant otitis media infections that had gone undetected since he was several months old.

Today Ryan is five years old and has difficulty talking. He has continual ear and upper respiratory infections. "He is very bright, but he has a hard time talking and putting phrases together. I suspect he has a learning disability. He definitely can't hear well, and the older he gets, the more frustrated he becomes. He is very emotional and can't handle stress well at all."

Allergy testing has revealed that Ryan is allergic to milk. He has also been diagnosed as having hypogammaglobulinemia, an immune deficiency that his mother, grandfather, and aunt also have. "I begged the doctors to test Ryan when he was a baby for the disease, but they wouldn't do it. I wish they had, and I wish I had known more about the pertussis vaccine," his mother said.

The voice and speed can also be affected by the vaccine. In 1947, Byers and Moll were the first to draw medical attention to this problem when they mentioned several children who either failed to develop the power to speak or had delayed language development after a pertussis vaccine reaction. Various speech difficulties, including stuttering, are common in the minimal brain damage syndrome.

Mark was a healthy toddler who had learned to talk by the age of sixteen months, when he received his first DPT shot. Within twenty-four hours, he stopped talking altogether. His mother described his reaction. "Right after the shot, when we got home, he got very sleepy. When he woke up, he shrieked and screamed. Then, he would stare off into space. And he wouldn't talk at all, not even babble like he had when he was a baby. He just kept screaming."

A week later, Mark started running a 107-degree fever. He still would not talk. His mother called the doctor. "He said I should give him Tylenol. But when the 107-degree fever wouldn't come down, I took him to the hospital, and they gave him ice baths and finally brought it down."

Mark continued to have high-pitched screaming during the night, and his temperature would shoot up to 107 degrees twice a month for no apparent reason. Even so, he was given the second DPT shot one month after the first one. His mother cannot remember his reaction because he had not stopped screaming or running fevers. "He was sleeping a lot during the day and he seemed uninterested in everything. He was just never the same after that first shot."

Nine months later, he was given a third DPT shot. Because, by this time, high-pitched screaming and fevers were part of his normal behavior, his mother does not know whether or not he had a reaction. He still could not talk. The doctors who had been treating him finally ordered an EEG.

"They said he had expressive aphasia and that the portion of his brain where speech is centered had been damaged by an early insult to his brain. They also said he had cerebral palsy. What really bothers me is that up until sixteen months of age, he was a perfectly healthy baby who hadn't even had a cold."

After the third DPT shot, Mark's mother found him on the couch with blue lips and fingernails. He had stopped breathing, and she revived him. She was told by the doctors that he had had a seizure. Despite this history, Mark was given his fourth and fifth DPT shots.

"I didn't want him to get his fourth and fifth DPT shots," his mother said. "But our state is really strict about all kids getting their shots before they go to school. The school officials said he absolutely couldn't get into school without both of them. They never came out and said they would force him to have the shots, but they implied it. So I gave in and he had the fourth shot at five years old and the fifth shot one month later."

His mother will always regret that she gave in to the state and agreed to let her son have more vaccine. "A few days after the fifth shot, he lost control of his bowels and urine. He had been totally toilet-trained since the age of three, but now he was urinating and having diarrhea in his pants. He was very upset. He told me he couldn't tell when he had to go to the bathroom."

In addition to speech and coordination difficulties, Mark also developed severe emotional and behavior problems. "After the fifth shot, he became very whiny and much more emotional. One minute he would be smiling and the next, angry and mean. This past year, he went to kindergarten, and one day the teacher left the room. When she got back, the room was in a shambles. My son and another boy had destroyed the room."

At six years of age, Mark still has difficulty controlling his bowels and bladder. He requires speech therapy and continues to have emotional and behavioral disturbances. "He is very frustrated and angry. He can understand what you are saying but he can't translate it into speech. It's the same with his physical movements. He knows how to tie his shoes, for example, but can't make his body do it. He has gone through such a lot and will continue to go through a lot for the rest of his life. I don't know what will happen to him, and it makes me very sad to think of what his life will be."

A mother who lives in Nebraska and has been labeled a "slow learner" all her life knows what it is like not to be able to express yourself verbally or physically. Her father has told her that she had a 104-degree fever and suffered nine to twelve grand mal convulsions for about thirty-six hours within two days of her first pertussis vaccination.

"The town doctor told my father, 'We are going to vaccinate every child in town, but we won't ever vaccinate Anne again.' I was put on Phenobarbital for a year and didn't have any more seizures until after I was married and began taking birth control pills."

Anne expresses the same frustration that is felt by many children with minimal brain damage: the feeling of being imprisoned in a broken body that will not respond.

"All my life I have been told I was 'slow,' even though I got B's and C's in high school. I can think faster than I can speak or move. My mind comprehends everything, but I can't keep up with it physically. I speak very slowly. My mother was a dance teacher, and I used to watch her and I knew every step. But I couldn't move the way I knew was right. All my life I have been frustrated. It's as if I'm imprisoned in a body that won't do what I want it to do."

The mother of a daughter who reacted to her fourth shot said, "She talks but she has a difficult time. She is in speech therapy. She understands everything you tell her. That is her problem. She is angry and frustrated when she can't communicate back to us what she wants us to know. You see, the harder she tries to do something, the more frustrated she gets and that sets her off into a tantrum."

Another mother spoke similarly about her vaccine-damaged daughter. "She is not really retarded. She is just slow. What has always bothered me is that she understands everything, but she can't get it out. You can see it in her little eyes. It's all there, but she can't get it out the way she wants to. Sometimes her little voice quivers because she tries so hard. You can see she's got it but it's trapped."

This breakdown in the ability of the brain to process and translate understanding into speech or action may be carried so far that a child is labeled autistic. Bradley had a grand mal seizure within twenty-four hours of his second DPT shot and now has five to six uncontrollable grand mal seizures each month. His mother described his disabilities.

"He can't talk. He can repeat what you say, but he can't have a conversation with you. They like to give kids a label, but it is hard to give Bradley a label. I've been told he is autistic and retarded and all sorts of things. Yet he can put a hundred-piece puzzle together and count to twenty in Spanish. He can sing commercials and songs from tapes, but he can't speak unless you tell him what to say, and then he can only repeat the words you say. He can't initiate speech."

Bradley, who is now ten years old, has been evaluated as at about a six-year-old level. "He used to make the letter R, but he can't do it anymore," his mother said. "His hand shakes a lot. Sometimes he makes a letter by accident. He doesn't do well with a change in routine. Like if he doesn't ride the school bus in the morning as he usually does and I take him somewhere else, he gets really nervous. I can put my hand on his chest and feel his heart thumping away."

Bradley's case raises the question of a possible relationship between the pertussis vaccine and autism. The phenomenon of early-infantile autism was first observed and discussed by physicians in the early 1940s, a few years after the pertussis vaccine became more widely used in the United States.

Medical science has yet to find the cause of autism, which is defined by *Dorland's Medical Dictionary* (1980) as a condition in which the individual is "dominated by subjective, self-centered trends of thought or behavior which are not subject to correction by external information" and which cause "developmental language disorders, and inability to adjust socially." In other words, the brain appears to be isolated from the senses in autistic children. The parallel to certain cases of pertussis vaccine damage is striking.

The mother of Richard, who was diagnosed as having "allergic encephalitis" after his third DPT shot and whose case was described in Chapter 5, described her son's autistic tendencies: "Although Richard is not the classic autistic child, he does exhibit certain types of autistic behavior and he does periodically attend a program for autistic children. For example, he is nonverbal and likes to play and relate to material things rather than people. He can put puzzles together but can't put his shoes on properly. He will repeatedly practice turning around on one foot for one week or he may play with a single toy, such as a top, for six months. There is a definite information processing problem there, and I am convinced there is a connection between autism and the pertussis vaccine."

Both autism and minimal brain damage, as discussed previously, suggest a breakdown in the brain's ability to receive and process information through the senses. The relationship of autism to pertussis vaccine damage deserves further investigation.

Some autistic children share another trait with the minimally brain damaged—a tendency to be hyperactive with all of the associated emotional and behavioral problems. As part of the minimal brain damage syndrome Richard Schain mentioned "distractability, hyperkinesis, lability of mood" and another described the "classical symptoms of a hyperactive, distractable, impulsive . . . child." Clements and Peters mention "lability of emotions," "impulsivity," "short attention span," and, above all, "hyperactivity."

Today, at least one American child in twenty-five can be considered "hyperactive." As J. Gordon Millichap, Professor of Neurology and Pediatrics at Northwestern University Medical School, said, there is "at least one in every classroom."

Some doctors believe that these behavioral difficulties result from the child's frustration in trying to deal with his learning disabilities. But Samuel Torrey Orton, M.D., who first discovered dyslexia in 1925, maintained that emotional disturbances can be a direct result of changes in the brain. According to Geschwind, "This observation was . . . a particularly remarkable and perceptive one, and was so revolutionary that it was almost entirely neglected, and continues to be neglected even today."

Whatever the cause of hyperactivity and other behavioral problems typical of the minimal brain damage syndrome, they are often exhibited by vaccine-damaged children. This was even noted in 1948 by Byers and Moll: "All showed defects of attention, irregularities of mental development most marked in relation to abstract behavior, and difficulty in organizing material." Miller and Stanton reported "disturbances in behavior" in their analysis of pertussis vaccine damage, and Stewart noted "hyperkinesis" in many cases of vaccine damage he investigated in 1977. Parents report their children became emotionally hypersensitive, occasionally violent, and often hyperactive after reacting to a DPT shot.

The mother of a baby boy who was given four DPT shots despite high fevers, convulsions, and collapse reactions knows what it is like to have a hyperactive child. Now twelve years old, her son is learning disabled, hyperactive, and still has grand mal convulsions despite medication. She said, "My son is in a learning-disabled class and has some mainstreaming classes. He loves to read, and the teachers have done a fantastic job with him. Still, I worry because he can have a violent nature. He is very emotional and can be very depressed, hyper, and negative when he is off his medication. He will be mean and pull the cat's tail and start fights. I had one doctor who would put him on medication during school and take him off in the summer and he would harass everyone in the family. The whole neighborhood was angry at him because he was doing abnormal things and getting into trouble."

His mother could not find a babysitter to stay with her son because he was so hyperactive. "Before his reaction, he was a happy, normal baby. Then when his seizures started, he became very restless and active and hard to keep up with. I could never get a babysitter who wanted to stay with him. He does try hard to be good, but I worry about him, about what may happen to him as he grows older with his behavior. He is like two different kids at times."

Hyperactivity and occasional violent behavior are a problem for another little boy who reacted to a DPT shot. Within one hour, George's leg became swollen and red. He began high-pitched screaming and ran a temperature of more than 105 degrees. Then he started having convulsions.

"From that day on, George would arch his back like a rainbow with only his head and the back of his heels touching the surface of the floor, and he would scream while he was doing this," said his mother. "It happened about five times a day until he was four and a half years old.

My doctor shrugged his shoulders and acted like it was nothing to worry about. The only thing I could do was put him in a corner somewhere so he couldn't hurt himself. One day he had a convulsion that lasted for five hours."

Unbelievably, George received two more DPT shots. His mother could not tell if he had a reaction "because he was having seizures and screaming so much all the time I couldn't have separated a reaction from his usual behavior. The doctor who gave him all three shots never recognized that he was having seizures. He told me I just had to live with it."

George was never put on anticonvulsant medication but spontaneously stopped having seizures when he was five. When he was six, he learned to feed himself and to hold a pencil. Now seven, he has no reflexes or sense of balance, so that when he falls, he lands flat on his face. He is highly allergic to milk, as he has been from the time he was put on cow's milk at six months old and developed croup and eczema. He is also susceptible to ear infections. But his mother is particularly disturbed by his hyperactive, sometimes violent behavior.

"It is difficult for people to accept his erratic behavior. One doctor told us that he was just hyperactive, and so we sent him to a normal preschool for two years. We know now that was the worst thing we could have done for him because the normal children told him he was a 'retard' and 'dumb' and, of course, he couldn't do the work they were doing. He can't write because the motor skills are not there. We took him to a diagnostic center and he was labeled multihandicapped and learning disabled. We have him in a school for handicapped children now, and when he started, he would bite and kick and hit the other kids. The teachers had to put him in isolation whenever he became violent. But he is doing better each day and his behavior is getting less and less violent."

Like many learning-disabled children, George is dyslexic and favors his left hand. He cannot read or write and is seeing a speech therapist because he is still unable to make certain sounds.

The mother of a little girl who reacted to the fourth shot spoke of her daughter's Dr. Jekyll/Mr. Hyde behavior: "The most difficult aspect to cope with right now is her behavioral problems. There are days that she comes out of her room and starts screaming. And we have no idea what brought it on. And it will go away as fast as it came. Then she will be as sweet and wonderful as any other little kid. But there are other times when you can't even get close to her."

Learning disabilities and aggressive behavior are characteristic of Kathy, who started fluttering her eyelids within hours of the first shot, and five days later, began rolling her eyes and having seizures. Her mother was unable to convince the doctor that there was anything wrong with Kathy.

"It took me a month to convince him she was having seizures. In the meantime, they got worse every day until she was having them for fifteen minutes at a time. After he saw one, he told me she must have been having them before the shot. I positively know she was not, because I have five children and I know what a normal child is like."

Kathy received all her DPT shots, despite the fact she was having uncontrollable seizures. "My doctor kept telling me there was no connection with the vaccine. Besides, you can't get a child into school without the shots. They absolutely refuse to take a child that hasn't had them. Since my doctor didn't believe the shot caused her seizures, there was no way," her mother explained.

Now eight years old, Kathy is in a special education class. She is dyslexic and unable to memorize. Her mother said, "her attention span is so short it is pathetic." Although her parents, sister and brothers are right-handed, Kathy is left-handed. Her behavior tends to be aggressive.

"She is a real little scrapper," said her mother. "She will pick a fight at a moment's notice. She would as soon tackle her older brother as fight someone her own size. She is an agitator. She will make trouble where there wouldn't be any if she would leave it alone."

It appears that a higher than expected proportion of minimally brain-damaged children are ambidextrous or left-handed. Sometimes a parent senses that the child is confused about which hand to use, or has "poorly defined unilateral dominance," as Schain has stated.

Dr. Jerre Levy, professor of behavioral sciences at the University of Chicago, suggests that one cause of left-handedness is stress on the brain during the prenatal period or during the birth process. Geschwind and Behan completed a study in 1982 showing that left-handed persons have a much higher incidence of dyslexia and stuttering than right-handed persons, as well as a much higher incidence of allergies.

While more research is needed, enough information has already accumulated to suggest a connection between pertussis vaccine and minimal brain dysfunction, including hyperactivity and behavioral disorders. It is difficult to understand the reluctance of medical researchers to accept this as a possible connection, since it has been known for decades that whooping cough is capable of causing changes in intellectual capacity and behavior.

In June 1942, Louis A. Lurie, M.D., and Sol Levy, M.D., reported at an AMA meeting that whooping cough, which had long been recognized as a cause of brain damage, may also, through a less dramatic but equally serious injury to the brain, cause a wide variety of behavior disturbances. They stated that there appeared to be "a definite relationship between the neurologic sequelae of the whooping cough and the behavior disorders and personality changes shown . . . in later life."

The doctors went on to describe a study they conducted on five hundred "problem children" housed in the Child Guidance Home of the Jewish Hospital in Cincinnati. Almost half had suffered from whooping cough in childhood, although this fact was not highly significant because probably at least half of *all* children in the late 1930s and early 1940s had experienced whooping cough. Lurie and Levy focused on fifty-eight children who had whooping cough before the age of two years. They found that sixteen were later delayed in walking and talking; nine suffered convulsions; one continued to have convulsions; nine had speech difficulties; fifteen had nerve deafness; and five had abnormal EEG tracings.

The doctors described these children as exhibiting "hyperactivity, extreme restlessness, destructiveness and short attention span." In summary, they said, "whooping cough occurring early in infancy may lead to development of severe behavior problems . . . [and] personality distortions."

More than one scientist has pointed out the similarity between permanent damage caused by the pertussis vaccine and that caused by whooping cough itself. Louis Sauer, in 1949, reinforced Lurie and Levy's conclusions. He stated, "In isolated cases a customary prophylactic dose of pertussis vaccine seems to elicit a chain of untoward central nervous system reactions—fever, convulsions, and in some instances, irreversible pathologic changes in the brain. These cardinal findings resemble those occasionally encountered in cases of severe whooping cough."

The reports of Lurie, Levy, and Sauer more than three decades ago are just several more pieces of evidence that the B. pertussis, whether it enters the body via the vaccine or via the disease, can cause a variety of neurological damage ranging from the profound to the more subtle forms of learning and behavior disorders.

Allergy and Hypersensitivity

As discussed in Chapter 3, another name for LPF or pertussis toxin is HSF, or "histamine sensitizing factor," meaning that it increases the body's sensitivity to the action of histamine.

Histamine causes dilation of the capillaries, constriction of the muscles in the lungs, and increased gastric secretion, all of which are elements of the allergic or hypersensitive reaction. That is why antihistamine drugs are prescribed for children or adults suffering from allergies.

A child with severe allergies has a hypersensitive immune system— one that is ready to react instantaneously to contact with any allergenic substance, whether food, drug, plant, or environmental pollutant. When one of these is introduced into a hypersensitive child's body, it stimulates a violent reaction which is aided by the presence of histamine. Any substance which increases the production of histamine, or heightens the body's sensitivity to it, will intensify an allergic reaction.

Pertussis vaccine is known to stimulate the production of IgE antibodies, which mediate the allergic response. Many physicians and scientists have noted the relationship between allergy in the child and a severe pertussis-vaccine reaction.

As early as 1947, Matthew Brody, M.D., described the gross mental deterioration of two children repeatedly inoculated with pertussis vaccine and concluded: "It would seem most likely that what is involved here is some sensitization phenomenon. Neither child had a previous history of sensitivity, although in both cases there was a family history of allergic disturbances."

In 1953, Köng stated that one contraindication to the pertussis vaccine was the existence of "allergoses of the child or family (under no circumstances should vaccine be given in the acute phase of the special allergoses!)." In 1961, Hopper found that "Infants with a family history of fits or allergic conditions are more likely to become ill after vaccination than those without such a history." He added that his study suggests "the cause of this illness following pertussis vaccination is handed down from the preceding generations, just as many other traits are."

In 1969, Dr. Charlotte Hannik found a history of allergies in twenty out of thirty-five children who reacted with persistent screaming, shock/collapse, or convulsions to the DPT-Polio vaccination.

Many parents of pertussis vaccine-damaged children have reported their child had allergies, particularly to milk, or that there was a history of severe allergies in the family. Some children, like Sharon, whose case was described in Chapter 5, develop allergies after a DPT shot.

Sharon had high-pitched screaming and excessive sleepiness after her first shot and a four-and-one-half-hour convulsion after the second one. Her mother said: "She was such a healthy baby until that shot at five months. She was on Similac from birth and did fine with no spitting-up or diarrhea. But after her shot, she had diarrhea, which was a funny yellow color and lasted for two or three weeks. We had to put her on soybean formula. She also came down with otitis media, which lasted about seven months until they put tubes in her ears. Then she began having a constant runny nose and cough. Now she has constipation, and she is virtually off all milk products. For example, she gets sick every time I feed her yogurt and either starts wheezing or goes into a seizure. We have severe allergies like hay fever and eczema coming down on my husband's side of the family, mostly to foods."

Many other children have severe allergies from birth, and their mothers or fathers are likely to have a history of allergies, too. Theresa reacted within fifteen hours of her first DPT shot with a fever, high-pitched screaming, and collapse. Within twenty-four hours of the second shot, she started screaming, collapsing, and having convulsions. Within twenty-four hours of the third shot, she again had high-pitched screaming, collapse, and increased convulsions. Her eyelids became red and swollen.

"Theresa had a milk allergy from the time she was born and has been on soybean formula since then," said her mother. "As long as I keep her on soybean, she is okay. I had a milk allergy when I was a child until I was about two years old. I can drink it now. Theresa has had hay fever since she was born. We would take her outside and her eyes would get red and watery if she was around freshly cut grass. I have always been that way. There is a lot of hay fever in my family. Theresa is also highly allergic to medications, just like I am. And she not only reacted to her DPT shots, but she also had a terrible reaction to her MMR shot. She ran a 106-degree fever for two days and had a red, bumpy rash.

Her eyes were watery and swollen and she started jerking her head much more."

Babies who have died have had symptoms of milk allergy. Douglas, whose death was described in Chapter 5, died within twenty-eight hours of a DPT shot. His twin sister, who had been vaccinated at the same time, developed a severe inner ear infection within forty-eight hours of the shot and survived.

Douglas's mother remembers that her twins would projectile vomit after drinking their formula. "I couldn't nurse the twins and they went on the bottle soon. They had trouble with throwing up. The vomit would fly out of their mouths and across the room. I have another daughter, who used to vomit like that with her milk, and the doctor put her on soy formula and that seemed to stop it. When I took Douglas and his twin sister to their blessing at the church, both of them threw up and it flew out onto the floor. My new baby, Tanya, also tends to throw up her milk across the room."

Brian, who reacted to his fifth shot with high-pitched screaming, a fever, and hallucinations (described in Chapter 5) and is now learning disabled, had a history of severe allergies from birth. He continues to be highly allergic to a variety of foods, medicines, pollens, and chemicals, and has been given allergy shots to try to help his system cope with his hypersensitivity.

"Brian is allergic to a lot of different foods and several different drugs like Tetracycline," his mother said. "He had outbreaks from orange juice, and he is allergic to milk. I breast-fed him, and he was very colicky. At four or five months, I took him off breast milk because it wasn't agreeing with him. I put him on formula. What a mistake! He would vomit it up all the time and scream with colic.

"He tolerated soybean formula a lot better. But he reacted to everything. He would get rashes all the time. If I put Clorox in the wash, he would be red wherever the clothes touched his body. Today, if he goes into the outfield when he plays baseball, he comes back with his eyes swollen shut. And he had four strep throats last year."

Brian's mother is highly allergic, too. "I have allergies. My sister has allergies, and so does my niece. I have skin allergies, and once I was hospitalized with anaphylactic shock from taking penicillin tablets. I could not see. My eyes were swollen shut. I went through allergy tests, and it showed I was allergic to milk, feathers, and a lot of other things."

Those children who have a personal or family history of allergies or develop allergies and susceptibility to a variety of infections are demonstrating fragile and hypersensitive immune systems. Whether the pertussis vaccine causes the hypersensitivity or makes an already hypersensitive immune system even more so, the outcome is the same. The child is left with a variety of medical problems or, as in the case of Douglas, robbed of life.

In 1983, Lawrence Steinman, M.D., and his colleagues at the Stanford University School of Medicine and London Hospital published a study in *Nature* suggesting that some children with allergies may be genetically predisposed to reacting to the pertussis vaccine. Steinman found that mice with a particular set of genes (occurring at the H-2 locus on the chromosome) who had been pre-sensitized to the milk protein known as BSA (bovine serum albumin found in cow's milk, most infant formulas, and also in the breast milk of mothers who drink cow's milk) died shortly after being injected with pertussis vaccine and manifested a clinical syndrome resembling post-pertussis vaccination encephalopathy. The control group of mice that did not have the genes and were not pre-sensitized to BSA did not die.

Steinman concluded that "genes acting at the level of the major histocompatibility complex may control susceptibility to B. pertussis immunization in humans. While susceptibility to many human diseases and to some allergic conditions has been linked to histocompatibility locus antigens in humans, the possibility that adverse reactions to routine immunization may be under genetic control seems novel."

While the whole story is not yet in, there is clearly a connection between allergies, especially milk allergy, and the tendency to react severely to the pertussis vaccine. It is immaterial whether the child is born with a genetic predisposition to react to the pertussis vaccine or becomes allergic as a result of vaccination. Both scenarios are possible. The point is that the vaccine interacts with the mechanisms in the body that are involved in allergy or hypersensitivity. Identifying those children at high risk of reacting to vaccine, such as those with genetic predisposition, should be a number one priority of vaccine research.

8

Profile: Hyperactive and Learning Delayed

Doubt grows with knowledge.
Goethe

When Steven was born, he was neurologically advanced. He could hold his head up, and instead of clutching his thumbs tightly in his fists as most newborns do, his thumbs were relaxed in the turned out position normally taken by much older babies. "Boy, is this one going to be crawling soon," was the comment his mother, Jo, remembers nurses in the hospital making.

Although Steven had colic and was put on soybean formula, it was not until Jo stopped mixing his formula with boiled tap water when he was five weeks old that his colic suddenly disappeared. He was a cheerful baby from then on. Jo was especially proud of how bright and alert he was and was pleased when friends would talk about his beautiful big, blue eyes.

Steven received his first DPT and oral polio shots at an Air Force Base clinic when he was two and a half months old. "The doctor told me that he would probably run a fever and be irritable but that it was nothing to worry about. They told me to give him Tylenol," Jo recalled.

Jo and her husband were not prepared for their baby's reaction. "That night he ran a 104-degree fever and just wailed. It was a different cry from the one he had when he had colic. He would arch his back and scream like an animal in terrible agony. This screaming went on four days and four nights. We walked the floor with him. We held him. We gave him Tylenol and sponged him. We called the clinic back the next morning, but they just kept telling us to give him Tylenol. They made me believe it was a normal reaction. He was my first baby. I had nothing to compare it with."

Steven appeared to recover, although he was more irritable and less content than before the shot. He was given his second DPT shot three months later, when he was almost six months old. Again he ran a 104-degree fever and screamed for nearly four days.

Shortly after his second shot, he began pulling constantly at his ears. His nose started to run and he became more and more irritable. At times, he could cry inconsolably. When Jo took him to the clinic, the doctors told her he had "a little fluid in the ear."

One month later, Steven was given his third DPT shot. Again Jo and her husband walked the floor for four days with their feverish, wailing baby. Steven was still pulling at his ears, and his nose was running constantly. Jo took him back to the clinic, where the doctors diagnosed otitis media and prescribed antibiotics.

In the next few months, Steven became very restless. He would rub his forehead with his little hand as if he were trying to wipe pain away. His right eye began to wander off track, and he would often stare into space as if in a trance. Sometimes he would arch his back and scream just as he had after his earlier shots. He also began turning his thumbs into his fists, like a newborn baby. Jo could not understand why her child, who had been so neurologically advanced at birth, was not developing as he should.

Steven did not sit up until he was almost ten months old. At thirteen months, he was still screaming for as long as an hour and a half several times a day. He could not bear to ride in a car and even the sound of a voice could throw him into a tantrum. He did not want to be held and would often crawl into the bathroom and bang his head on the floor or the bathtub.

"By now he was on antibiotics almost all the time for the ear infection and runny nose that wouldn't go away. And he had this crazy cough day and night. But the worse part was that he acted as if his whole body hurt. He couldn't stand to be touched or even talked to at times. I had to put pillows in front of the bathroom and kitchen doors so he couldn't crawl in and bang his head on the floor."

When Steven was almost sixteen months old, his baby brother, Nathan, was born. Steven still could not walk. One day, after his nap, he crumpled up in a little ball on the living-room floor and held his head without moving.

"I took him back to the doctor for what seemed like the hundredth time and told him I thought Steven was having headaches. He said, 'Children that age don't have headaches.' I told him Steven was deliberately hitting his head on the hardest surface he could find and was having uncontrollable screaming fits every day for no reason. He said, 'Don't worry, lots of kids throw tantrums.' I told him Steven was always sick. He said, 'He just has a little respiratory infection and fluid in his ears.' I told him Steven seemed delayed in learning to walk. He said, 'Some babies walk later than others.' He made me feel like I was an hysterical mother who was worrying too much. But I knew there was something wrong with my son."

When Nathan had his DPT shots, Jo and her husband were prepared for the worst. They thought they would have to spend days and nights walking the floor with another screaming baby. But Nathan did not react at all to his DPT shots; there was no fever or screaming. Compared to Nathan, Jo realized how violent Steven's reaction had been.

When Steven was two years old, his father resigned from the Air Force rather than take a one-year assignment in Alaska without his family. Neither he nor Jo felt Steven's problems could be handled by Jo alone.

By the time Steven was three, his knees and legs were frequently covered with bruises from constant falls. He was still screaming several times a day at the least provocation and alternately staring off into space. His nose was still running; he was still coughing; and he continually rubbed his forehead.

"The smallest request was too much for him. If I would so much as suggest we get dressed or eat, he would run screaming through the house like a wild man. When we went to church, we would always be called out of the service to come to the nursery to get Steven because he was screaming. At preschool he would not interact with the other children and at times would scream uncontrollably and I would have to come and get him. At home, when he was playing outside, he would sit and dig in the dirt for hours."

When Steven was three and a half, Jo began feeding him foods recommended in the Feingold diet designed to help control hyperactivity and behavioral problems in children. It helped him cope at home, but he still could not handle any form of outside stress. Jo believes, however, that the Feingold diet saved her son from being placed in an institution for emotionally disturbed children, and he is still on the diet today.

When it became apparent that Steven's behavior, constant cough, and runny nose all became much worse during the spring and fall at the height of the allergy season, Jo had him tested by an allergist, but all the tests came back negative.

Jo was told by teachers at the preschool that Steven should have diagnostic testing. By age four, he was diagnosed as having "significant expressive language delays, significant fine motor and gross motor delays, and visual memory delays." The county diagnostic center recommended physical, occupational, and speech therapy. Jo and her husband decided, however, that they would consult a private psychologist and a neurologist to have their son evaluated.

"I was a physical therapist," said Jo. "I have always relied on traditional medicine to give me the answers for health problems. I had also been taught that you don't question your doctor. A doctor is going to tell you what is wrong with your child. So I kept taking Steven to doctors in search of an answer."

At fifty dollars a session, the psychologist played with Steven three times a week; the neurologist charged the same amount for a ten-minute consultation once a month. At the end of six months, the psychologist diagnosed Steven as "developmentally delayed, possible minimal brain dysfunction" and pronounced him to be "trainable but not educable." He recommended that he be placed in a special preschool for speech- and language-delayed children.

"He also suggested," Jo said, "that because my husband and I had Steven and Nathan so close together, we may have neglected Steven and paid too much attention to Nathan. I couldn't believe it. If there is one thing you cannot do with a child whose needs were as great as Steven's, it is ignore him."

Jo was particularly upset that the psychologist painted such a dark picture of her child's future. "I couldn't believe a psychologist was willing to label my four-year-old son as 'trainable but not educable.' Despite the fact Steven was never well and could not control his behavior, at the age of four he was teaching himself to read and to add numbers. I became convinced that his problems were primarily physical and not intellectual. But I couldn't convince any of the doctors of that."

At four and a half, Steven was enrolled in a special school for speech-and language-delayed children. His parents paid $175 per month for him to attend two and a half hours a day, three days a week.

The school decided Steven needed "anger therapy," and Jo was told that when he was angry, he should be allowed to do whatever he wanted to do. She was apprehensive because she had been trying to teach him to control his behavior, even though she knew it was often beyond his control. She had made a rule that he could only scream in his room, the playroom, or the backyard, and he had tried very hard to adhere to that rule.

"During the time they were trying 'anger therapy' on Steven, he would come home and kick the wall and scream wherever he wanted to scream. One day I found him in his room, smashing and throwing his toys against the wall. I asked him what he was doing. He said, 'I'm angry.' I asked him what he was angry about. He said, 'I'm angry at myself because I am throwing things and I can't stop.' You can't tell a four year old who has worked really hard to gain self-control that self-control doesn't matter. You can't take that away from him and leave him with nothing. It scared me because I realized there could come a time when he would turn that anger on himself."

Jo withdrew Steven from the school and placed him in a church day school. He did well over the winter, but in the spring when the trees began to bloom, she would get calls from the school to come and pick him up. In the background she could hear him screaming.

"It was like picking up an animal. He would just arch his back and scream as if he was in agony. He was inconsolable."

By this time, the neurologist was telling Jo, "I don't know what is wrong with him. Perhaps he will outgrow it," and recommended more psychological testing. Still searching for alternative treatments, Jo took Steven to a dentist specializing in TMJ (temporal mandibular joint) cranial therapy used by osteopathic physicians and dentists to realign bones in the face, jaw, and head. The dentist found that Steven had a TMJ misalignment and helped relieve the pressure on Steven's sinuses that had been contributing to his head pain.

Jo enrolled her son in a private kindergarten. He had not been there for more than a couple of weeks when his nose started to run profusely, and he coughed day and night. Jo was still taking him for TMJ therapy as well as following the Feingold diet. One day the school called her and told her to pick up Steven. She could hear him screaming.

"Steven told me, 'I'm so sick I'm dying.' I kept trying to downplay what he was telling me. But he insisted that he was dying. In a way, I think he was."

Steven spent a whole day just sitting in his room unable to move. Jo took him back to the allergist. This time the tests showed he was slightly allergic to dust and pollens but not allergic enough to need shots or medication other than the over-the-counter variety.

Jo became desperate. After talking to a friend, she decided to take Steven to an orthomolecular physician. The tests he conducted revealed the effects of pertussis vaccine in Steven's body as well as a candida yeast infection probably caused by the antibiotics he had been on throughout his life.

"I was stunned. I had never thought to connect his problems with the vaccines he had been given as a baby. I called my husband and said, 'What are they putting in these vaccines? Do they know what they are doing?' All of a sudden things started falling into place."

After treatment with homeopathic remedies and mycostatin prescribed by the orthomolecular physician, Steven stopped screaming and began acting more like a normal six year old. He did well in first grade with only one phone call from the school. Although he is still more emotional during the spring and fall allergy seasons, he is able to cope with the stresses of school without falling apart emotionally and behaviorally.

"When I saw those severely brain-damaged children on TV in Lea Thompson's documentary on the pertussis vaccine," Jo said, "I turned to my husband and said, 'There but for the grace of God goes Steven.'"

* * * * *

Jo spreads out Steven's medical records on the couch and table. They are piled high in stacks, falling over each other. Steven walks in smiling self-consciously. With his tousled blond hair, wide-set blue eyes, and turned-up nose, he looks like a little gamin.

He tosses off a quick "Hi" and runs over to whisper in his mother's ear. "What is nine multiplied by eleven?" she asks him back. "I don't know. What is it?"

"Ninety-nine," he replies confidently and runs back to finish working in his activity book. At seven and a half, there is no doubt that Steven is bright, almost precocious.

"I look at Steven and think about the basket case he was a year ago and wonder how many thousands of other children are now being affected less or more severely than he was. If I hadn't gotten answers when I did, he would probably be in a school for the emotionally disturbed and learning disabled today," Jo says.

Pointing to the stack of papers comprising Steven's medical records, she continues, "I took him to every kind of doctor I could find. Nobody could tell me what was wrong with him. It is frightening to think about the numbers of parents out there who don't know what happened to their child. My husband and I began to think we were the problem."

Jo looks down at her lap, her voice momentarily falters and her eyes moisten. "We really felt we must have psychologically damaged Steven in some way for him to be so totally out of control. In church, they told us we were letting him watch too many cartoons because he always was pretending to be Superman. If I had been as sick and weak as Steven was, I would have wanted to be as strong and healthy as Superman, too."

Steven and his younger brother, Nathan, enter the room eating gingerbread cookies. Nathan is almost a head taller than Steven, although he is fifteen and a half months younger. Steven watches Nathan bite off the nose of the gingerbread pig and he starts to cry.

"What is the matter, Steven?" asks Jo.

"He is eating the pig's nose," squeals Steven unhappily. "I don't want him to do that."

"You are eating your gingerbread pig and Nathan is eating his. I can make more cookies another day," explains Jo patiently. Steven evidently decides that eventually he is going to have to eat his gingerbread pig's nose, too, and he stops crying.

"Steven is a little touchy right now because it is fall again, and the mold is on the leaves. But his emotional outbursts are nothing compared to what they were during the first six years of his life. A year ago, he would be screaming on the floor instead of just crying a little. He still has a way to go, but it took a while for him to get here.

"I think Steven had a predisposition to allergies when he was born. But whether the increasing severity of his allergies would have manifested itself in emotional disturbances, hyperactivity, and learning problems had he not been given the pertussis vaccine or, perhaps, a combination of the vaccines, I have no way of knowing. The pertussis bacteria is a congestion producer. Have scientists ever really studied what effect injecting pertussis bacteria into a sensitive immune system, such as Steven's, has on that system?"

Remembering Steven's reactions to his DPT shots, Jo believes other parents are not sufficiently aware that high-pitched screaming and a prolonged fever indicate a serious reaction to the DPT shot, and are contraindications to further pertussis vaccine.

"My husband and I both remember the agony Steven was in after his DPT shots. I couldn't even go in and take a shower. I just held him in my arms while he was screaming. I'd call the clinic and say, 'He is really sick,' and all they would tell me was to give him more Tylenol. I am sure that is the response that thousands of other parents are getting too. Just because a child doesn't go into convulsions or collapse doesn't mean he isn't affected neurologically and physically in some way," says Jo.

"I also will never know what Steven would be like if the doctor had paid attention to his first reaction and not given him four DPT shots. I suspect the cumulative effect of the shots contributed to the severity of his condition."

For his booster shot, Steven received only the DT. "My husband said there is no way we will allow Steven to have more pertussis vaccine. We would go to court and take all Steven's medical bills along with us. If they want to make problems, we would take the Department of Health to court."

Asked if she believes in vaccination as a disease prevention tool, Jo answers, "I do believe in the killed polio vaccine because polio is a devastating disease, and I believe that tetanus and diphtheria vaccines are safe and necessary. I am very skeptical about the MMR vaccine for measles, mumps, and rubella, because most children are going to survive those diseases without permanent damage. I would definitely not take another chance on the pertussis vaccine until a safer one is developed."

Jo believes that the pertussis vaccine may be contributing to the increase in learning disabilities, hyperactivity, and emotional disturbances among children. "Doctors and scientists cannot explain in biological or genetic terms why there are steadily increasing numbers of learning disabled and hyperactive children. We give the pertussis vaccine to virtually every child in the United States. It is known to cause neurological damage. Why doesn't someone study the possible correlation between the two, particularly in children with sensitive immune systems?"

Steven and Nathan are playing in the recreation room downstairs. Occasionally Steven can be heard shouting in frustration.

Jo listens and then says, "The brain has miraculous recuperative powers. I don't want to believe that Steven will always be affected to some degree by the damage that was done to him. But only time will tell."

✿   ✿   ✿   ✿   ✿

Steven was re-evaluated in the summer of 1984 by a psychologist who found that, although tests showed Steven now has an I.Q. of 126, he appeared to have episodic losses of consciousness for a few seconds at a time during the testing. Steven's mother is consulting specialists to determine if he has petit mal seizure activity. The psychologist also found that Steven has visual and depth-perception problems that continue to affect his gross and fine motor skills to a marked degree.

9

Do We Know the Extent of the Damage?

There is no question that there is a risk. There is considerable difficulty in defining that risk.

Walter Dowdle, M.D.

"**T**here appears to be a conspiracy of silence about reactions, and there is a failure to communicate all along the line. Babies find it difficult to communicate to anyone. Mothers find it difficult to convince their doctor just what happened. The doctor who does the immunization is often not the same doctor who is called out to see the baby who has a reaction. The doctor observing these reactions is upset in seeing an adverse effect to a procedure which he has recommended and is often loath to blame the procedure. Medical officers of health are in a predicament because they do not want to publish figures of reaction rates which might discourage the acceptance of an immunization procedure which, by and large, they consider worthwhile."

George Dick made this statement in 1967, but he could just as well have made it today. G. S. Wilson, who has written a definitive work on the hazards of vaccination, expressed it this way: "A large number of accidents, I suspect the majority, have never been reported in print, either through fear of compensation claims, or of giving a weapon to the antivaccinationists, or for some other reason."

Miller and Stanton observed in 1954: "It must be admitted that, in the heat of the emotional battle provoked by propaganda for and against prophylactic inoculation, there has been a tendency on the part of the medical profession to turn a blind eye to unfortunate individual

142

complications of procedures which have the indisputable sanction of social value."

Because most physicians have a very hard time accepting the documented fact that a procedure designed to save lives can, in some instances, actually take or ruin lives, there is a tendency to deny that vaccine damage exists. Because physicians have been recommending pertussis vaccine to parents for more than forty years and are afraid they will be sued by former patients should it be shown that the pertussis vaccine causes a wide range of problems, there is a tendency to put the blame for injury on some other cause.

As the West German physician Wolfgang Ehrengut suggested in one of his studies (1980), it may be that doctors have a negative bias against vaccine reactions, an unwillingness to believe, because "what must not be, therefore cannot be." It must not be true because, they think, whatever will we do if it is true?

This negative bias, this denial that vaccines can cause death and injury, has had devastating consequences for mothers and their children. Because many doctors refuse to believe in vaccine reactions and others are confused about the definition and consequences of a severe reaction, mothers have never been told to watch for reactions. Consequently, they do not look for signs indicating their child may be reacting neurologically.

The root of vaccine damage is ignorance on the part of doctors and mothers. The mother is told her baby "may be a little fussy and run a fever for a couple of days." Often, when she calls to report that her baby is screaming in pain or running a 105-degree fever, the doctor tells her, "Don't worry about it. It's a normal reaction." Several days later, when the child begins to have convulsions or other neurological problems, neither doctor nor mother connects the convulsions with the DPT shot. Should the mother suggest such a connection, often the doctor will deny it.

Added to the basic ingredient, ignorance, is the chance that a child may fall between the cracks of the medical bureaucracy. Having had a severe reaction to a DPT shot, he or she may not return for more shots to the doctor who administered the first one. A mother may go to a private pediatrician for the first injection and a public health clinic for the second one. This can increase the risks of vaccine damage because the child may continue to be given pertussis vaccine despite a prior severe reaction.

In a private pediatrician's office, where one doctor may handle twenty to thirty children a day, or in a public health clinic, where that number may be far greater, medical records are not always adequately kept and sometimes may even be lost. Often doctors do not feel there is either time or necessity to give a child a full medical examination or take a medical history before giving the shot. When a reaction does occur and is recognized, doctors are nervous about admitting it or reporting it.

No one wants to take responsibility for injuring a child with the pertussis vaccine. It is not surprising that no one knows the extent of vaccine damage in this country. Without such knowledge, there cannot be a credible analysis of risks.

There has been a terrible breakdown in communication, and the truth about the risks of pertussis vaccine will only be known after careful repair of all the links in the reporting chain—from the baby and parents, whose lives can be ruined, up through the doctors and government health agencies responsible for setting vaccine policy and monitoring adverse reactions.

The Channels of Communication: Infant to Mother

The first breakdown in communication occurs when a baby tries to tell his mother that he is sick after a DPT shot. A mother, who knows her child better than anyone else, usually senses when her baby is not feeling well. But many mothers, like many doctors, do not connect their baby's strange behavior with a recent vaccination. They fail to make the connection until much later when they are informed about vaccine reactions or start checking back through a baby book or medical records as did this parent, who recalled:

"That's when I came home and started going through his baby book. And I looked at when it first happened and went through all his medical records. I looked at what happened before the second time, and it just clicked. There they were—both shots exactly six days before he had begun his symptoms and then both times exactly fourteen days after the shot he was put in the hospital."

"She had just fallen asleep that night," another mother said. "Looking back on it now, I realize she had a very mild seizure lasting about three to four seconds. She opened her eyes wide, opened her mouth and made a short, loud funny noise. It never entered my mind she was having a seizure. I didn't know what seizures were then."

It is easy for parents to miss neurological signs, especially when they have never been told to look for any at all. Many times these reactions go unreported to the doctor. Later, when a mother connects the shot to her child's injury, she suddenly realizes the reaction may have occurred much closer to the day of the shot than she remembers noticing it.

One mother said, "The first head nod he had was within a week of the third shot. I should say that it was the first head nod I noticed because they are easy to miss. They happen so fast. He could have been having them in his crib and because he wasn't sitting up right after the shot, I wouldn't have known."

Yet another mother expressed regret at her lack of knowledge about neurological signs. "When we first came in to the pediatrician, he told us our son was having petit mal seizures every twenty seconds, but he didn't know how long he had been having them. I didn't even know what a petit mal seizure was or that he was having them, they were so quick and slight."

But when parents are asked specifically to observe any change in their baby's behavior or physical condition after a shot, as was done by Barkin and Pichichero in Colorado in 1979, a very high proportion report unusual symptoms. In their study, only 7 percent of the parents reported no reaction at all; 27 percent reported mild reactions; 59 percent reported moderate reactions; and 7 percent reported severe reactions.

They concluded, "This study delineates the high reactogenicity of diphtheria-pertussis-tetanus vaccine in a pediatric population receiving the product in accordance with current recommendations and underlines the necessity to reevaluate current guidelines and vaccine."

It is extremely important that parents be given information about reactions to vaccines so that they can recognize what their baby is trying to tell them and report it to their doctor. At that point, of course, doctors must be knowledgeable enough to recognize the significance of what mothers are telling them.

Private physicians in most states today have no obligation to inform parents about the possible dangers from an adverse reaction before giving the DPT shot. Public Health Service clinics using federally funded vaccines, however, do have such an obligation. Since 1978 they have been required to give the parent an "Important Information" form to read and sign before a vaccination is administered to a child.

This Important Information form (1983 revision) attempts to tell parents about the benefits and risks of vaccination: "Most children will have a slight fever and be irritable within two days after taking the shot. One half of children develop some soreness and swelling in the area where the shot was given." It continues, "Convulsions or episodes of limpness and paleness may each occur after 1 in every 1,750 shots. Unusual high-pitched crying may occur after 1 in every 1,000 shots. Rarely, about once in every 110,000 shots, inflammation of the brain (encephalitis) may occur and permanent brain damage may occur about once in every 310,000 shots."

Although private doctors are not required to inform parents of vaccination reactions and risks, they can always be asked to provide a copy of the product information sheet included in every package of vaccine. Mothers can also ask their pediatrician to explain in greater detail the symptoms of the more severe reactions such as convulsions, collapse, excessive sleepiness, or high fever as well as the steps that should be taken if these symptoms are observed.

Mother to Physician

When a mother senses that her baby is acting strangely, she usually calls the doctor for advice. Again, ignorance and denial can cause a doctor to reassure her that nothing is wrong and everything is going to be just fine. The desperate mother becomes more desperate as she tries to make the doctor believe her:

"The doctor wasn't really concerned about her shaking. I couldn't get anyone to admit there was anything seriously wrong with my child. He kept telling me I was overreacting. I used to try to run to the doctor's office when she would start having her seizures. She might have several a day and then go a few days without one. So I would run to the doctor's office and sit there, hoping the doctor would see one. He wouldn't believe me."

Doctors try to reassure mothers who bring in paralyzed or convulsing children after a DPT shot that their children will "get better." As this mother commented, "These doctors try to pass it off as a transitory thing. My doctor kept saying, 'Oh, she's going to get better.' Now you can't just tell a mother whose daughter is lying there not doing anything that it is okay, she is going to get better."

In their disbelief and denial of DPT vaccine reactions, doctors will even go so far as to suggest that the distraught parent needs psychiatric help. One mother whose doctor refused to believe that her baby was having seizures after a DPT shot said, "My pediatrician told me that I needed psychiatric help because there was nothing wrong with her. I knew something was wrong with her. I am never going to let another doctor tell me anything that I will accept on blind faith. I am going to check it out."

But, even when doctors are willing to admit a baby is acting abnormally, it is difficult for them to accept that the behavior is due to the recent DPT shot. Some do not want to believe it while others may be covering up to protect themselves.

A favorite way to escape the undeniable truth that a child is having neurological problems following a DPT shot is to claim that the problem is due to "other causes." Doctors will try to convince parents that the child had an "underlying seizure disorder," which would have eventually been manifested even without the DPT shot. Or they will try to convince the parents that such convulsions often occur spontaneously, even if the baby reacted within hours of the shot. These and other common justifications of neurological reactions following DPT shots are discussed more fully in Chapter 14.

One mother expressed her frustration at this typical line of reasoning by doctors, saying, "Nobody will listen to us. They keep telling us, 'She must have had an underlying seizure disorder.' I don't believe that, but even if she did have an underlying seizure disorder, I can't believe the shot didn't trigger it into activity. The neurologists I go to laugh at me when I say there is a connection with her DPT shot. I get furious."

Parents who have reason to believe the DPT shot caused their child to become ill often try to get confirmation from a doctor but cannot. One parent said, "None of the doctors will talk to us. Our family doctor won't say, yes or no, it was due to the shot. But since the television publicity about reactions, he agrees that we shouldn't give the vaccine to our other children."

One reason American doctors have difficulty believing that vaccine reactions exist to any great extent is that the DPT shot is mandated by law in forty-one states. They cannot imagine that a medical procedure credited with saving millions of lives by eliminating a disease, which is compulsory, recommended in medical textbooks, and advocated as overwhelmingly safe and harmless by the American Medical Association, American Academy of Pediatrics, and Centers for Disease Control, can cause serious injury and even death.

After the broadcast of "DPT: Vaccine Roulette," WRC-TV in Washington, D.C., received telephone calls from pediatricians who asked if the DPT shot could be so dangerous. The typical comment, according to producer Lea Thompson, was "I really didn't know. I didn't think I had to know because, after all, the thing is mandated."

The physician who finally realizes that the vaccine can do harm lives in fear of malpractice suits, especially if he has ignorantly given more pertussis shots to a child who has reacted severely to a previous one. This can lead to a steady and convincing stream of denials that the vaccine is in any way connected to the child's problems.

When a doctor does have the courage to report a reaction, he will often do it only after a child has been hospitalized. Ehrengut in West Germany criticized the British NCES study of adverse reactions because the doctors conducting it only included children whose seizures lasted more than thirty minutes and were hospitalized, noting that ". . . 20 percent of convulsions following various vaccinations are missed because patients are not admitted to hospitals" (see Chapter 20).

In addition to being afraid of a lawsuit that could damage his professional reputation and economic welfare, a doctor is often worried about the impact of bad publicity on a public health program he supports and believes in. And the knowledge that each child in his practice must routinely be scheduled for many office visits to receive DPT and MMR shots, as well as oral polio vaccine, during the first six years of life reinforces his profound belief in the wisdom of mass vaccination.

Doctors have an enormous incentive to disbelieve and deny vaccine reactions. For all of these reasons, they have developed stock rationalizations for apparent reactions to the vaccine: "spontaneous seizures" occur in unvaccinated populations; mental retardation has many causes; the DPT shot just "precipitated" a medical condition that was inevitable anyway; the mother is "imagining things." While any one of these explanations may be true in a particular case, they are not always true. But doctors are quick to claim that they are. Their denials translate into infrequent recognition of the reality of adverse reactions to the vaccine.

As Janice Cockrell, M.D., a Virginia pediatrician, put it, "Vaccine surveillance is a self-reporting method. . . . In other words, this reporting is dependent on the parents' perception of the severity of illness and whether or not a physician was visited, as well as the motivation of the patient and the individual physician to report the adverse reaction."

So, the breakdown in communication continues. The minimizing of risks continues.

Physician to Manufacturer, State, or CDC

Even if a doctor recognizes and accepts a mother's account of her child's severe reaction to the DPT shot, or has observed the reaction himself, this information is of no statistical value in measuring vaccine risks unless it is reported to an agency which can collect, analyze, and compare the data.

For this reporting system to work properly, doctors must be compelled to report reactions, and some central recordkeeping agency must be ready to receive these reports. Neither requirement exists in the United States. Private physicians, who administer half the DPT shots in this country, are not legally required to report reactions. And there is no single agency where adverse reaction data from all sources are brought together and analyzed.

The American reaction reporting system does not compare with that of Sweden, where for years physicians have been required to fill out annual questionnaires on vaccine reactions. Swedish physician Justus Ström suggests this is why Swedish estimates of pertussis vaccine reactions, death, and permanent damage have always been higher than those of other countries. He has expressed little confidence in a reporting system which relies solely on a sense of obligation on the part of the individual physician, and wrote (1969): "If you rely upon a recording duty for your physician, you will have no reactions."

With all the reasons a doctor has not to report a reaction and no legal requirement to do so, is it any wonder parents doubt the reliability of the federal government's analysis of the risks of pertussis vaccination? The Office of Technology Assessment of the U.S. Congress reported in 1979:

"The Federal Government at present has no effective means by which to compel private sector physicians to report the number and types of vaccinations they administer, let alone the number of adverse reactions to these vaccinations . . . Neither the Bureau of Biologics nor any other Federal agency currently collects data needed to conduct comprehensive postmarketing evaluations of the safety, efficacy, or conditions of use of licensed vaccines . . . Neither the Federal Government nor the pharmaceutical industry systematically surveys vaccines to determine the incidence of adverse reactions to licensed vaccines."

Even if a doctor is determined to report a bad reaction and have it included in national adverse-reaction statistics, he has a variety of places to send the report, instead of to a single recordkeeping institution. First, he can send it to the vaccine manufacturer, who must keep it for one year in a complaint file that can be inspected by the FDA. The manufacturer does not have to report the reaction to the FDA unless the agency asks for it, although recently vaccine manufacturers have been voluntarily providing "summaries."

The doctor may also send a reaction report to his state health department, which is supposed to forward it to the Centers for Disease Control's Monitoring System for Illness Following Immunization (MSIFI); or the doctor may himself send it directly to the CDC.

On the other hand, doctors in public health clinics do not have to decide the best way to report a vaccine reaction because they are required to use the MSIFI set up by the CDC. But this system has repeatedly been attacked, even by the CDC itself, as inadequate for obtaining a comprehensive picture of vaccine reactions.

Here is how the MSIFI is supposed to work: Parents receive an Important Information form on vaccine benefits and risks and are asked to read and sign it. At the bottom of the form is the statement: "If the person who received the vaccine gets sick and visits a doctor, hospital or clinic in the four weeks after vaccination, please report it to. . . ." A blank is left for the local public health clinic to fill out; each clinic is supposed to enter its phone number for the parent to call. When a parent does telephone to report a severe reaction, the clinic is supposed to fill out an official form, "Reporting of Illness Following Vaccination," which is forwarded to the CDC.

What is wrong with this process? First, a mother who brings her child to a public health clinic for a free DPT shot may seek out a private physician or hospital if a severe reaction occurs. In any case, she is not likely to go back to the public health clinic with a child in the midst of a convulsion. A major breakdown in communication has just begun. The public health clinic will never learn about this reaction unless the mother remembers to report it later.

But a distraught mother with a very sick child is unlikely to do that. She and the private physician may not connect the illness to the DPT shot. It is anybody's guess how many reactions are not reported because mothers forget; or lose the Important Information form and do not know whom to call; or do not realize the baby is sick because of the DPT shot recently administered at the clinic.

Secondly, if a mother does report a reaction, clinic personnel have to be conscientious enough to fill out the "Reporting of Illness Following Vaccination" form and send it to the CDC. This is a job rarely handled by a physician and is often left for a health aide or clerk who may not relay to the CDC a precise clinical description of the reaction reported by the parent.

Harrison Stetler, a medical epidemiologist in the CDC, stated at the 17th CDC Immunization Conference (1982), "At present our system provides an accurate number of doses administered for the public sector but an incomplete accounting of the frequency of illness. Our estimates of illness following immunization thus provide only minimal estimates of rates of occurrence even in the public sector."

Stetler went on to lament that reactions reported to the CDC by private physicians via telephone call or letter may never be recorded unless the doctor also submits the official CDC reporting form. He notes that some states will only report reactions resulting in the child being hospitalized, while others report all reactions. Sometimes a reaction is reported twice.

As for providing a comprehensive picture of vaccine reactions in the United States, the CDC's MSIFI is virtually worthless. Though half of vaccinations each year are given in public health clinics and half are given in private practitioners' offices, less than 10 percent of MSIFI data comes from reports by private physicians.

The U.S. Office of Technology, confirming that the CDC adverse-reaction reporting system has no way of analyzing vaccine risks, wrote, "because it relies on voluntarily submitted case reports, CDC's system will not generate data needed to calculate the incidence of severe adverse reactions to particular vaccines." Janice Cockrell echoed this view when she concluded in 1982, "The CDC monitoring system represents a grossly inadequate picture of the incidence of reactions to DPT vaccinations."

A doctor may also send adverse reaction information to the Quality Assurance Branch of the FDA, which has been keeping a data bank since 1973. In the years 1978 to 1982, when approximately ninety million doses of DPT vaccine were distributed in the United States, the FDA and the CDC together received reports of seven cases of permanent vaccine damage due to the DPT shot. In the first five years of operation, the CDC's MSIFI received reports of forty-four deaths occurring within four weeks of DPT vaccination, only one of which was attributed by CDC officials to the DPT shot itself. In the early 1980s the CDC was receiving from one to three reports every year of "acute encephalopathy" associated with DPT shots given in the public sector.

Kevin Geraghty, M.D., a California pediatrician and clinical immunologist in private practice, is a critic of MSIFI. He studied the incidence of SIDS deaths in Contra Costa County (San Francisco Bay Area) and found that ten deaths had been diagnosed as SIDS during the first half of 1983. Of these, five occurred within eight days of a DPT shot, but only one of the five was in the state records—and, therefore, in the federal records—even though all are supposed to be reported to the state and the CDC. (Interestingly, although the shot had been given in a public health clinic, the reaction report was filed by the baby's private physician.)

Geraghty also found that the five so-called SIDS deaths temporally related to the DPT shot which he pinpointed in Contra Costa County during the first six months of 1983 were more than all of the deaths temporally related to the DPT shot reported to MSIFI for the whole United States in 1981 (four). He said, "My criticism of MSIFI is based not only on its failure during our clustering in Contra Costa County during the first half of 1983 but also retrospectively on its performance based on data reported previously. . . ." Geraghty's Contra Costa study is discussed further in Chapter 20, where a provisional benefit/risk analysis of the pertussis vaccine is presented.

Obviously the government's adverse-reaction reporting system is grossly deficient. By extension, so is its analysis of vaccine risks. Certainly, without an honest and accurate study and measurement of adverse reactions and the resulting death and permanent injury, no credible benefit/risk analysis of the pertussis vaccine is possible.

10

Profile:
Surviving Whooping Cough

> And by his health, sickness
> Is driven away
> From our immortal day.
> *William Blake*

A few days after giving birth to her second daughter, Deborah began to cough. "I didn't feel sick at all until the day after Sarah was born," she recalled. "I started having a short dry cough, and I thought it was my allergies acting up because I wasn't running a fever and didn't have a sore throat."

Like most mothers who have just given birth, Deborah was drained with fatigue trying to breastfeed and tend to her newborn daughter, Sarah, while her husband, Jim, helped her care for two-and-a-half-year-old Miriam. Happily, Sarah was thriving on her mother's milk and was a sweet-natured baby.

"By four weeks old, Sarah was a chubby little tub. She was a good eater and sleeper, but by that time, my cough had really gotten bad. Every time I coughed, I felt like my insides were going to fall out. I couldn't believe how hard I was coughing. I would cough and then gasp for air because it felt like I couldn't catch my breath. Each cough took so much energy that sometimes I was exhausted."

Even though Sarah appeared to be thriving when she was a month old, Deborah noticed that she too was starting to cough a little. Deborah took her to their family doctor for a routine checkup and the doctor told Deborah that Sarah was a healthy baby. In the next seven days,

154

however, Sarah began sleeping almost continuously. She did not want to nurse as often as before, and when she did nurse, she would spit up her feedings within thirty minutes.

"At five and a half weeks old, Sarah's cough was like mine," Deborah said. "When she coughed, her face got red. She coughed day and night. She wasn't nursing very often. In fact, we were using a diaper service, and I suddenly realized that she was only using thirty diapers a week. At four weeks old, she had been using over one hundred diapers a week. I started changing her whenever she got the least bit damp. I suppose I was trying to reassure myself that she was still breast-feeding enough."

Deborah took Sarah back to her family doctor again. Sarah was not running a fever, and the doctor reassured Deborah that her baby only had "a little flu bug." But in the next few day, Sarah's cough worsened to the point where she often turned blue and gasped for breath. Deborah and Jim were careful to make certain that Sarah was lying on her stomach when they put her down to sleep because they were afraid she might choke on mucus while she was coughing. She was still sleeping almost continuously and vomiting up her feedings.

Understandably frightened, Deborah made an appointment with a pediatrician to get a second opinion on Sarah's condition. The pediatrician was puzzled.

"He didn't know what she had," Deborah said. "She wasn't running a fever and she didn't have a runny nose. He sent us to get a chest X-ray for her, and the next day he called us at home. He told us to get Sarah to the medical center immediately. In fact, he said, 'Don't stop for anything—GO!' "

Deborah and Jim rushed Sarah and Miriam into the car and started racing for the medical center. On the way, Sarah went into a fit of coughing that would not stop. Her face turned red, her eyes bulged, she stared straight ahead and coughed. As she tried to catch her breath and couldn't, she turned blue.

"I thought she wasn't going to make it," Deborah recalled. "I thought she was going to die. Somehow she managed to start breathing again. We finally arrived at the hospital, and we ran into the emergency room. As they were checking Sarah and trying to get an I.V. in her, she stopped breathing and they had to revive her."

The doctors suspected that Sarah and Deborah both had whooping cough. To confirm their suspicions, they took a swab and inserted it deep into Sarah's nose; they did the same to Deborah. Both swabs were sent to the laboratory where cultures were grown for pertussis confirmation.

Sarah was admitted to Intensive Care and placed on oxygen and intravenous ampicillin. The doctors felt that in addition to whooping cough, Sarah also had bronchitis as a secondary complication. The antibiotic ampicillin was prescribed to treat the bronchitis. Since there is no medicine or "cure" for whooping cough, there was nothing else the doctors could do except treat Sarah's symptoms. Deborah was also placed on an antibiotic to lessen her chances of further infecting others.

While Sarah was in the Intensive Care Unit (I.C.U.), she continued to have from fifteen to twenty-five paroxyms of coughing and cyanosis (turning blue) each day. The nurses would suction her to make sure she continued breathing.

"Because she was in Intensive Care," Deborah said, "I couldn't sleep beside her. I had to sleep in the waiting room, and the nurses would wake me so I could nurse Sarah when she woke up. We were really lucky that, even though she was so sick, she continued to breastfeed. I was still coughing hard and was totally exhausted from that as well as the strain of wondering whether or not my baby was going to survive."

After three days, the doctors decided that Sarah could be removed from Intensive Care and placed in an isolation room. She was still coughing but had not stopped breathing during her three-day stay in I.C.U.

"We definitely thought she was getting better," Deborah said. "They put her in an isolation room and hooked her up to a monitor that would sound an alarm if she stopped breathing. Since she was out of I.C.U., they allowed me to sleep beside her. The third night she was in her new room, the monitor went off. I looked at the monitor, and her breath measurement was zero and her heart rate was near zero. The nurses came running in, grabbed her, and ran out of the room. I prepared for the worst. I thought she wouldn't make it this time."

But the medical team did revive Sarah. "They started her breathing again by putting this little black bag over her mouth and nose and suctioning her with tubes. When they brought her back into her room, I held her the rest of the night and nursed her whenever she woke up."

Deborah sat beside her baby for several more nights, praying for her recovery. "I don't think I have ever been so frightened or completely drained in my whole life. I stayed beside her day and night, listening to her cough and gasp for air, coughing myself, and wondering if it would ever end. I couldn't really sleep because the monitor kept going off, sometimes due to a problem with the monitor being too sensitive and sometimes because Sarah really did need to be suctioned. I prayed a lot. I tried to mentally prepare myself in case she died."

Now Sarah's sister Miriam also started coughing, although her cough was much milder than Sarah's. The doctors at the medical center immediately took a pertussis culture from Miriam.

"Miriam's cough was nothing like mine or Sarah's. You couldn't really tell Miriam was sick. She was eating, sleeping, running around. She didn't have any fever or vomiting," Deborah recalled.

Sarah was discharged after a ten-day stay in the hospital. The pertussis cultures came back positive for Sarah and Miriam but negative for their mother, Deborah. The doctors theorized that Deborah was the first member of the family to come down with whooping cough, but by the time the culture was taken, she had had the disease too long to obtain a reliable culture reading.

"The doctors agreed to discharge Sarah and let us take her home because I had taken CPR training, and they felt I was an alert mother who could handle suctioning Sarah," said Deborah. "They gave me a refresher course on infant CPR. So we left the hospital, still worried but more confident that we could help her if she needed assistance breathing."

After Deborah and Jim returned home with Sarah, they watched her every minute and never left her alone. They kept her in their bed so they could monitor her all night long. She continued to cough for six more weeks, but she began to nurse more frequently and to gain weight. Gradually, she had fewer and fewer episodes of coughing.

From the time Sarah started coughing to the day she was discharged from the hospital, she dropped in weight from ten pounds, four ounces to nine pounds, six ounces. Even though her baby lost almost a pound during her bout with whooping cough and almost died several times, Deborah believes Sarah may have survived because she continued to breastfeed.

"I was lucky that Sarah continued to nurse. I feel she received antibodies from me and had an easier time keeping her food down. Breastfeeding also let her remain physically, emotionally, and psychologically connected to me while she was so ill. There was a little baby girl who was the same age as Sarah in an isolation room on another floor of the hospital. The doctors thought she had whooping cough, too. She was unconscious most of the time and was being fed intravenously because her mother was not breastfeeding. She couldn't keep anything in her stomach, and she was still there when we were discharged. She was so weak. I don't know what happened to her."

At four weeks of age, Sarah was too young to have received a DPT shot. At two years of age, Miriam had received four DPT shots. At thirty-one years of age, Deborah had received five DPT shots. At thirty-one years of age, Jim had had whooping cough as a child and had never received a DPT shot. Although his wife and children caught whooping cough, he did not. Most probably he was naturally immune to the disease.

* * * * *

Sarah wiggles as she sits on her mother's lap, laughing and crinkling up her big brown eyes. Now two years old, she looks and acts like any other two year old. Deborah is proud of the fact that Sarah has already begun to recognize letters and numbers.

"I know we were lucky that Sarah pulled through because she was so very tiny when she got whooping cough. I know how terrible it felt to have whooping cough as an adult with that mucus clogging my fully developed air passages. I can't imagine what it must have been like for her with those little four-week-old air passages."

Deborah smiles as Sarah scampers away to play with Miriam. She admits that the experience of almost losing her made her especially protective of Sarah for a while.

Nobody knows where Deborah caught the whooping cough that she eventually gave to both her daughters. "I suppose someone in church or at the store had whooping cough and coughed near me. I know that adults and even children, like Miriam, can have mild cases of whooping cough and not know it. Of course, just because they don't have overt symptoms doesn't diminish their ability to infect others. I am sure I could have infected others besides my daughters because I coughed for weeks after Sarah was born before I knew I had whooping cough, and I was going to church, grocery stores, shopping malls, everywhere."

Deborah finds it interesting that she had been given all her DPT shots and that Miriam had received four DPT shots, yet both of them came down with whooping cough. "It makes me wonder just how effective the shots are when it comes right down to it. I mean, maybe you could explain away my case by theorizing that my protection had worn off after some twenty-five years. But Miriam received all her DPT shots on time, and it had only been a year since her last one. Perhaps that is why she had such a mild case. Still, it makes me wonder how many fully vaccinated adults and kids are walking around with whooping cough and spreading it to others without knowing it, especially if they have mild cases like Miriam had."

Sarah runs up to her mother and complains loudly that Miriam has just taken her favorite doll away and won't give it back. Deborah leaves to arbitrate the dispute and, when she returns, discusses her feelings about the pertussis vaccine.

"I am sure most people would assume that, because I almost lost my daughter to whooping cough, I would be wholeheartedly in favor of the pertussis vaccine. It isn't true. After we had whooping cough, I began studying the disease and the vaccine, and I really believe that I would rather take my chances with the disease than with the vaccine. With what I know about the pertussis vaccine now, I could not in all good conscience deliberately subject my child to the risk of vaccine brain damage. I would rather risk fate and the disease. Of course I don't have to worry about Miriam and Sarah now. They will never have to have pertussis vaccine again because they both have had whooping cough."

After a moment of thought, she adds, "Sometimes I wonder if we know what we are doing when we allow our children to be injected with so many different kinds of vaccines. Sarah had a bad reaction to her MMR shot. Supposedly, she now is protected against measles, mumps, and rubella. I had measles when I was a child, and so I am immune to it for life, just as Jim is apparently immune to whooping cough because he had it as a child. But I have read that some kids who have been vaccinated with MMR are getting these diseases as adolescents after the vaccine wears off and are becoming very sick and occasionally permanently injured because the diseases are so much more serious when people are older. Then there are other children who become brain damaged from the vaccines. To tell you the truth, I think scientists should rethink the question of disease cure and prevention and come up with a whole new concept that is safer and more effective than vaccines or else make better vaccines."

Sarah and Miriam bounce into the room, wearing cowboy hats. They are chasing each other, running in circles and squealing with delight.

Seeing that their mother is not doing anything exciting, they retreat to another room.

"I suppose a doctor who really believes in the pertussis vaccine could say to me, 'Oh, you just say you would rather take your chances on whooping cough because your child was lucky enough not to die or be brain damaged afterward.' It's true, Sarah is perfectly fine today, and she certainly couldn't have been much younger when she caught it. Am I lucky or is that the outcome for most babies who get whooping cough in America today?"

Sarah comes running back into the room and jumps on her mother's lap and gives her a big hug. Deborah cuddles her.

"One thing I know for certain. I was very fortunate to be in a large medical center that provided such excellent care. I think she pulled through because of a combination of reasons, because of the good medical care and the fact she was fat and healthy when she got sick. I'm positive that breastfeeding made a difference. She didn't have a fever or go into convulsions, and they gave her antibiotics to fight the bronchitis. American medicine has come a long way since the 1920s when so many children were dying from whooping cough. That has to be a big reason why she made it. I just thank God she is alive and healthy today."

11

Whooping Cough Today

> I thought it of particular interest to show what a significant
> effect a rising social standard can have on the character of these
> ordinary infectious diseases [whooping cough, measles, scarlet
> fever]. Not only does mortality diminish, but the entire spec-
> trum of the diseases shifts towards increasingly mild, abortive
> forms with a corresponding reduction of the severer, clinically
> typical cases. There is reason to dwell upon this point since
> proposals have been made within socially advanced countries
> for all kinds of universal vaccination. The demands on the
> vaccines, their efficiency and freedom from risk, must be all the
> greater the less the importance of the disease to be combated.
> *Justus Ström, M.D.*

Evidence from around the world indicates that whooping cough
has become a milder disease in developed nations with good
nutrition, medical care, and sanitation. It is no longer the "hundred-day
fever" and no longer kills or injures the numbers of people it did in
former times.

In the United States there was a steady drop in whooping cough cases
and deaths from the end of the nineteenth century until the early
1950s, when doctors began giving pertussis vaccine on a mass scale.
In 1926, for example, there were more than 200,000 cases of whooping
cough with 9,000 deaths. In 1934, which was another high-water mark,
there were more than 265,000 cases, but the deaths had declined to
7,500. These figures are in stark contrast to the less than 2,000 cases of
whooping cough and only nine deaths reported in 1981. In recent years
the number of whooping cough deaths reported in the United States
has varied between ten and twenty annually (see Chapter 20).

Since the rate of decline was steeper after the early 1950s, when the vaccine began to be used on a mass basis, the vaccine appeared to deserve most or all of the credit. But according to Edward K. Mortimer, M.D., and Paul K. Jones, M.D., of the Case Western Reserve University Medical School, "It is not possible to attribute this salutary trend to pertussis vaccine with any degree of certainty."

D. L. Miller, of the University of London, Middlesex Hospital Medical School, wrote in 1982, "If mortality rates from, say, diphtheria or poliomyelitis are compared for the periods before and after the introduction of immunization against each disease, the impact of immunization is both obvious and immediate. Immunization against pertussis, which was introduced at a time when mortality from the disease had been falling steeply for seventy years, made a much less convincing impact."

Nevertheless, few experts have questioned the vaccine's ability to prevent or lessen the severity of whooping cough. Even one of its most prominent critics, Gordon Stewart, M.D., of the University of Glasgow, stated in 1980, "I have never doubted the partial and temporary protective effect of pertussis vaccine, because it obviously has immunizing potency."

There is also evidence that the disease is milder in vaccinated children, and as a German physician reminded the medical community at the 1978 Brussels International Symposium on Immunization, "As physicians we have responsibility to decrease the incidence of misery as well as mortality."

A Decline in Vaccination and Whooping Cough Returns

The pertussis vaccine's ability to prevent whooping cough is evident in countries that have stopped using it. In Britain, where vaccination has never been mandatory, coverage declined from 80 percent to about 30 percent (and to as low as 10 percent in some parts of the country) after a television program on vaccine damage was aired in 1974. Clinically reported cases of whooping cough then rose from 9,000 in 1975 to 66,000 in 1978 and 65,000 in 1982. (At the same time, according to A. H. Griffith, claims under the national vaccine damage compensation system "virtually dried up," indicating that a drop in the vaccination rate brought a dramatic decline in cases of neurological damage attributed to the vaccine.)

The same happened when Japan's population stopped using the pertussis vaccine in 1975 following publicity about two pertussis vaccine-related deaths. Coverage rates dropped from 70 percent in 1974 to between 20 and 40 percent in the following years. As a result, whooping cough cases shot up—from 393 cases and no deaths in 1974 to more than 13,000 cases and 41 deaths in 1979.

In West Germany, the Federal Department of Health ended the mass pertussis vaccination program in 1976. According to Ehrengut, rates among infants dropped from 58 percent in 1970 to less than 10 percent in 1978. With that drop in coverage, there was a rise in whooping cough cases.

The Swedish government withdrew its support from the pertussis vaccine in 1979, because authorities were beginning to doubt its effectiveness in controlling whooping cough and were worried about the large number of serious reactions. According to a 1982 letter from Ström, "The vaccine had been changed, the toxicity was lowered. The experts carried on their attempts to make the vaccine less risky. At the same time the vaccine got more and more ineffective, and because of that and the fact that reactions continued to occur, the vaccination was suspended in 1979." Thereafter the incidence of whooping cough rose almost to the prevaccination levels.

Still, Iceland is the only Western European country to require the pertussis vaccine. The communist countries in Eastern Europe continue to require pertussis vaccination, but Western European doctors, scientists, and parents evidently share the view expressed in 1979 by two associates of the Vienna Institute for Specific Prophylaxis and Tropical Medicine, who concluded that in Austria, "vaccination against whooping cough has lost its justification."

It may be that the public in Western Europe listened to the rational appeal voiced a quarter of a century ago by Ström, in his 1960 *British Medical Journal* article, "Is Universal Vaccination Against Pertussis Always Justified?" "Pertussis is still a great child-killer in many countries," he wrote. "Effective vaccines are now available but are not devoid of risks, especially of a neurological nature. In some countries— for example, Sweden—the illness has assumed increasingly mild forms and the mortality is now very low. Thus, the situation may arise when we must weigh up the relative advantages and disadvantages of vaccination."

A Cyclical Disease

What are the reasons for this general abandonment of pertussis vaccination programs in Western Europe? Why are these countries not concerned about the increase of whooping cough in their populations?

First, health authorities recognize that whooping cough is a cyclical disease with a natural rise in cases every three or four years, even in a vaccinated population. Despite high levels of immunization, there were increases in whooping cough in England in 1963 and again in 1967. (The same increase in whooping cough was seen in the U.S. in those years, despite mass vaccination.) Even if England, Sweden, and West Germany had continued their programs, a definite increase in whooping cough would still be registered in peak years. At least some of the recent increases in whooping cough cases, which have been blamed on epidemics caused by a drop in vaccination rates, can be attributed to the cyclical pattern of the disease.

Second, physicians have a stake in vaccination programs. There is a natural tendency to underreport whooping cough when it occurs in a vaccinated population, and to overreport it when it appears to be occurring in an unvaccinated population. Some of the supposed increase in whooping cough cases in countries which have declining vaccination rates may, in fact, be due to increased reporting.

In the United States, where more than 95 percent of the children have been vaccinated, it is estimated that only 5 to 10 percent of whooping cough cases are reported to the Centers for Disease Control. The same is true in Japan. Translated into numerical figures, this means that instead of the 1,000 to 3,000 cases of whooping cough reported to the CDC annually, there may actually be as many as 30,000 to 40,000 cases of whooping cough in the U.S. every year.

Underreporting and Overreporting: Is It an Epidemic?

A British physician asked his colleagues in 1963 if they routinely reported pertussis cases, and the answers were (1) "I did not know it was notifiable"; (2) "I never notify measles or pertussis because I don't like the health authorities coming around to see my patients; it upsets them"; (3) "It is difficult to be sure nowadays, because some of the cases are so mild."

After these replies were received, the doctor commented, "I did not trouble to ask any further."

Stewart believes there is a reluctance among physicians to report the disease. He said, "In some practices whooping cough is never notified in a vaccinated child." In a vaccinated population, physicians tend to underreport cases of whooping cough.

By the same token, when vaccination rates decline, physicians tend to diagnose pertussis "every time a baby clears his throat," to quote Robert Mendelsohn, M.D. As George Dick put it (1978), many doctors think pertussis is "a disease with a cough which takes longer to clear up than the 'usual' type of respiratory infection of infants and children, which often occurs at night, and is sometimes associated with vomiting."

The state and federal government health agencies do not hesitate to reinforce this misinformation. Within a few months after "DPT: Vaccine Roulette" was shown on WRC-TV in Washington and on NBC-affiliated stations throughout the country in April 1982, the states of Maryland and Wisconsin reported whooping cough "epidemics." Health officials from the Maryland State Health Department implied that this rise in cases was due to parents having watched the pertussis vaccine TV documentary and no longer having their children inoculated.

Timothy Johnson, M.D., devoted one of his 1982 *Healthbeat* syndicated television shows to this very possibility. In a program that attempted to discredit "DPT: Vaccine Roulette," Johnson announced that there was an outbreak of whooping cough in the state of Maryland and compared it to the rise in whooping cough in England. He said, "The pattern seems to be the same. Negative reports on the risks of the vaccine frighten parents into not having their children immunized against pertussis. Such concerns have prompted officials in Maryland to look back on the impact of the WRC program."

Johnson interviewed Robert Longenecker, of the Maryland Health Department, who said, "The controversy that existed at that time about the adverse effects of the vaccine had an impact on the parents. It pretty much undermined their confidence in the use of pertussis vaccine."

By autumn of 1982, forty-one cases of whooping cough had been reported in Maryland, and the press release issued by the Maryland Department of Health was picked up by the local and national media. But when these cases were analyzed by J. Anthony Morris, Ph.D., who is an expert on bacterial and viral diseases, he found that in only five cases was there a definite laboratory diagnosis of whooping cough; and that all five of these children had been vaccinated: three (aged two to three months) had received their first DPT shot; one (aged ten months) had received two shots; and one (aged four years) had received four shots. The "epidemic" was much smaller than was announced by the state health authorities and, such as it was, was occurring in a largely vaccinated population.

Later that same year, the Wisconsin Health Department announced a similar "epidemic" of forty-three cases. Morris again analyzed the data and found that the diagnosis was confirmed by laboratory data in only sixteen of the forty-three cases. And fourteen of the sixteen had had one or more shots, according to the vaccination schedule recommended by the Public Health Service and the American Academy of Pediatrics. So, again, the "epidemic" was minuscule in size and occurred almost entirely among vaccinated children.

The state health departments and even the CDC merely take the physician's word, without verifying the accuracy of the diagnosis. An officer of the CDC stated in 1982 at the FDA Symposium: "We accept any diagnosis of pertussis made by a physician and a form filled out and submitted to the CDC. On the form there are places where you can specify the clinical features . . . the presence or absence of a whoop, the apnea, pneumonia, seizures, encephalopathy. Then separately we specify the laboratory results. But we don't make the stipulation that a case must have a whoop and a positive laboratory result."

In any case, an epidemic cannot begin within a few weeks or even months after a drop-off in vaccine acceptance. It takes years for herd immunity to wear off. This fact was substantiated by John Robbins of the FDA in 1982: "In the U.K. the increase in whooping cough which occurred was observed two to three years after the decline in the acceptance rate of pertussis vaccine." The Maryland and Wisconsin whooping cough epidemics are discussed further in Chapter 14.

While the British whooping cough epidemic of 1982 did count 65,785 cases of pertussis with fourteen deaths, one of the physicians intimately involved in caring for patients, Herbert Barrie, M.D., of London's Charing Cross Hospital, formally protested the "campaign of terror" being waged over the pertussis vaccine in a 1983 issue of the *American Journal of the Diseases of Children*. He asked, "Why all the fuss about a dozen possibly mismanaged whooping cough deaths when we have an annual toll of 1,500 cot deaths, 2,000 child deaths from accidents, and 2,500 avoidable perinatal deaths?"

Barrie found it hard to justify the "stream of statements, bulletins, and memoranda" which "poured forth through television, radio, post and press." He described the British government's media blitz:

"Hardly a day passed without the latest whooping cough returns appearing somewhere. 'Pertussis Peaks Again,' 'Epidemic Claims Another Victim,' or 'Killer Disease Strikes Again' . . . were typical headlines. A recorded message phone-in service encouraging parents to have their children vaccinated was set up. Terrified parents were greeted with a hair-raising series of paroxysms from a child close to expiry, followed by a diatribe on the imminent dangers of death, brain damage, and lasting lung disease. The message ended, in the tradition of such commercials, with the urgently voiced hysteria-toned exhortation: 'If your child has not been vaccinated, do not delay. There is an epidemic. Get your child vaccinated now!' More coughing. The campaign of terror was on."

Barrie concluded that pertussis vaccination was being heavily stressed by the National Health Service because "promoting it costs next to nothing since the Child Health Centres, their physicians, and health visitors already exist, unlike the massive investment needed for research into cot deaths, accident prevention, and neonatal intensive care. In the eyes of the Health Department, what hath no need of gold glitters."

What is more, Barrie questioned the statistics of the 1982 epidemic. In a 1984 interview he stated, "There is no question but that the pertussis incidence in 1982 was overreported. British physicians tend to overreport supposed pertussis incidence cases in an epidemic year and underreport them at other times. And the cases were very mild. I doubt if more than a small percentage were hospitalized. In the Charing Cross Hospital, which serves twenty-five thousand children, we had only six hospital admissions, which were all mild cases and home again within two weeks. The problem with diagnosis of whooping cough is that serologic or bacteriologic tests are done in only about 50 percent of the hospital cases and virtually never if the infant is not hospitalized. So how can you be certain that what you are seeing is pertussis?"

There is also question about the fourteen deaths attributed to whooping cough in the 1982 pertussis statistics in Britain. Stewart, who has analyzed them, asserted in a personal communication that about half the deaths may not have been due to whooping cough at all but to other diseases. He said, "About half the deaths were in children who already had complications like cerebral palsy or some other handicap. There were only about four or five out of the fourteen that were straight whooping cough deaths."

One point that has become obvious as a result of the debate about the pertussis vaccine is the general fuzziness of the statistics. Even Jeffrey Koplan, M.D., who undertook a benefit/risk analysis of the vaccine for the United States under the auspices of the Centers for Disease Control and the Harvard Medical School, concluded in 1979, "Our analysis . . . suggests the need for prospective collection of reliable data on vaccine complications in a large population [and] close observation of the epidemiology of pertussis in the United kingdom and the United States. . . ."

But four years later, in May 1983, Harrison Stetler of the CDC told the Eighteenth Immunization Conference in Atlanta, Georgia, "Although rates of common reactions such as fever or local reactions can be defined, the occurrence and frequency of the rare but more serious illnesses that might be due to the vaccine cannot be determined. . . . Improvements are needed in the quantity and quality of the data obtained by [the MSIFI] surveillance system if meaningful results are to be obtained." Benefits and risks are discussed further in Chapter 20.

Diagnosis of Whooping Cough: Who Knows?

The true extent of a whooping cough "epidemic" is difficult to evaluate, in part because of the defects in the laboratory tests used to diagnose whooping cough. As Morris's analyses of the mini-epidemics in Maryland and Wisconsin showed, most cases are diagnosed from the symptoms of the patient, with all the inaccuracies this involves.

Dr. Walter Dowdle, then director of the Center for Infectious Diseases at the CDC, testified before the U.S. Senate Committee on Labor and Human Resources in July 1983 that "Current diagnostic tests are technically difficult or have an unacceptably high frequency of error. Most cases are diagnosed on clinical grounds alone."

At present, two laboratory tests are used to confirm that a person has pertussis—one a culture, the other a blood test.

The bacterial culture test involves collecting a sample of the patient's sputum or mucus in an attempt to grow B. pertussis bacteria in a medium. It is thought to be the most conclusive way of confirming whooping cough, but unfortunately the pertussis bacteria are plentiful only during the initial stages of the disease when the patient appears to be suffering from nothing more than a cold. In the violent stage of coughing, which occurs later, the bacteria have usually disappeared.

As Alan Hinman of the CDC stated (1983), "Often by the time the diagnosis is suspected, it may not be possible to recover the organism and culture it."

Various studies have shown that the bacteria can only be recovered about half the time—because the disease has reached the coughing stage, because the patient is taking antibiotics, or because the laboratory simply does not have the skill and experience to perform the culture correctly.

Philip Brunell, M.D., a prominent member and later chairman of the AAP's Red Book Committee, which recommends vaccine policy for America's pediatricians, alluded to this "misdiagnosis" problem at the 1982 FDA Symposium on New Pertussis Vaccines when he said, "The other problem with that is the poor laboratory diagnosis, both in terms of culture and FA. And I suspect that many clinicians are really terribly naive in terms of how poor this is. I can give you a number of anecdotes about reliability in laboratories. . . ."

The second commonly used diagnostic laboratory test for pertussis, known as the "fluorescent antibody" (FA) test, involves examining a specimen of the patient's blood for antibodies to the pertussis micro-organism. Several types of this serologic test exist, but according to the Swedish scientist Marta Granstroem, of the National Bacteriological Laboratory in Stockholm (1982), "None has been found to be quite satisfactory."

Sometimes the patient can have a negative bacterial culture and positive FA. Different laboratory technicians may interpret the same slide differently. In one study, three readers of the test agreed only half the time in interpreting immunofluorescence smears, and it is thought that FA tests can give "false positive" (meaning an incorrect finding of antibodies in the blood) results from 6.7 percent to 40 percent of the time.

Claire V. Broome of the CDC pointed out in 1978 that "although direct immunofluorescence may be useful for rapid presumptive diagnosis, it would be hazardous to use it alone as a diagnostic method without confirmatory cultures."

When J. Anthony Morris asked the FDA in 1983 about the reliability of the FA test, the response was that "some workers do not consider previously developed serologic assays, such as the immunofluorescence assay . . . to be totally satisfactory to serve as a laboratory verification of [pertussis] infection." Morris commented, "It is generally accepted that a demonstration of fluorescent antibody by itself, in the absence of an antibody demonstrated by another technique, is of limited value. . . ."

And yet it is these two tests that are most widely applied to "prove" that a whooping cough epidemic exists. In truth, probably the most precise way of diagnosing whooping cough is when a doctor recognizes the classic "whoop" and both the bacterial culture and the FA tests come back positive. This confirmation, however, may be hard to obtain if a doctor gives a patient antibiotics prior to obtaining a mucus sample for testing, because the laboratory tests can then come back negative. In fact, no causative agent can be found in from 10 to 50 percent of the cases that are clinically diagnosed as pertussis.

Broome in her 1978 article stated, "The sensitivity of culture for identification of B. pertussis is affected by the amount of time between disease onset and obtaining the culture and the prior use of antibiotics known to eradicate B. pertussis from the nasopharynx. Other factors which may result in variation in culture results include the age and immunization status of the patient."

It is known that although antibiotics cannot "cure" or lessen the severity of whooping cough once a person has it, they can help prevent the spread of the disease to others as well as lessen the chance of developing such complicating secondary infections as bronchitis, pneumonia, and otitis media. Medicine has never found a medication or any other therapy to treat whooping cough itself.

Is It Whooping Cough or Chlamydia?

The whooping cough picture is further clouded by the fact that other diseases mimic whooping cough. As medical students have been told over the years, "All that whoops is not whooping cough, and all whooping cough does not whoop." A number of other bacteria such as B.

parapertussis, B. bronchoseptica (usually but not always limited to animals), Chlamydia, Mycoplasma pneumoniae, and various adeno-viruses cause symptoms similar to whooping cough.

Stewart commented in 1978, "What we call whooping cough is a syndrome; the symptoms of whooping cough that lead to a case being identified as whooping cough and reported as whooping cough can arise from a variety of causes, if by causes we mean the isolation of particular pathogens."

Brunell added in 1982, "It is clear that other agents can mimic this disease. We are also told that at different ages the disease may have varying clinical manifestations. It makes the clinical diagnosis very, very difficult."

Particularly when the child is unvaccinated, physicians may diagnose whooping cough when actually the disease is allergic bronchitis, influenza, or atypical viral pneumonia.

But the vaccine only protects against whooping cough caused by B. pertussis. This confusion about what is really whooping cough can have major repercussions on clinical trials of new pertussis vaccines. In 1982, Brunell expressed concern about this confusion: "Unless we can precisely identify cases of pertussis, we are going to make our instrument extremely dull in terms of defining efficacy. And the worst thing that could happen is that we go in and make a clinical diagnosis of pertussis and start a vaccine trial on that basis, and it turns out to be Chlamydia."

On the other hand, whooping cough caused by B. pertussis can take a variety of different forms resembling other diseases. In babies, the characteristic whoop can be absent. Sometimes vomiting, especially at the end of the coughing spell, is a more reliable diagnostic indication. If the child has been vaccinated, the disease may take an atypical, milder form which is also very difficult to recognize. The same is true for adults who catch whooping cough after their pertussis vaccination has worn off.

All of these factors, together with the inexperience of most doctors with actual cases of whooping cough, mean there is little accurate diagnosis of the disease. Most younger physicians will have seen one, maybe two, cases of whooping cough throughout their whole period of medical studies and are not equipped to diagnose it instantaneously. Therefore, there is no reliable yardstick with which to measure the true incidence of the disease in modern industrialized societies and the ability of the pertussis vaccine to prevent it.

Has the Sting Gone Out of Whooping Cough?

One of the major difficulties in diagnosing whooping cough is its increasing mildness in industrialized countries. As Stewart has said, "The sting went out of the disease." And Ström pointed out as long ago as 1967 that pertussis is shifting toward "increasingly mild, abortive forms with a corresponding reduction of the severer, clinically typical cases." In a 1982 personal communication he wrote:

"Pertussis was very rare in Sweden in the 1960s. About 90 percent of all infants were vaccinated at that time. In the first years of the 1970s, whooping cough returned and since the middle of that decade the disease is again endemic. A few smaller local outbreaks have occurred. The number of cases is, however, relatively modest. In the years 1977–81, between 2,100 and 5,200 bacteriologically verified cases were reported to the National Bacteriological Laboratory in Stockholm. Of course, these figures represent only a smaller proportion of all cases. In general, the disease has been mild even in infants. No deaths and no cases of brain damage caused by the disease have been seen."

John Taranger of the Vastra Frolunda Hospital in Sweden confirmed Ström's report of modern-day whooping cough in Sweden. In a 1982 letter to *The Lancet*, he wrote, "Due to the ineffective vaccine and the present mild clinical course of pertussis in Sweden the vaccination was stopped in 1979. . . . Despite the fact that since the mid-1970s pertussis has again become endemic in Sweden and now has reached incidence rates approaching those of the pre-vaccination era, no child has died of pertussis since 1970. The clinical course in Sweden has become milder." Taranger noted that there had been 19,000 cases in the years 1977 to 1979 without a single death.

Ehrengut has reported a similar experience with generally milder cases of whooping cough in West Germany, another country which stopped mass pertussis vaccination in the 1970s. "Though vaccinations had been performed on a low level (about 10 percent, later 20 percent, in infants in the period 1979 to 1981), the fatalities due to pertussis had the lowest level ever recorded; 1979: seven cases; 1980: eight cases in West Germany. . . . In the last two to three years we had an increase in pertussis cases but [they were] of mild nature."

In a 1982 letter Stewart wrote, "We have outbreaks about every four years. The last one in 1978/79 was more widespread, but the death rate was the lowest on record. In this city of over one million people

[Glasgow], with less than 50 percent of children vaccinated, there have been no deaths since 1971 and we have no evidence of more severe or persistent complications due to pertussis. We do, on the other hand, have very clear evidence of some children having been hopelessly incapacitated following vaccination and of at least one unexplained death."

Robinson and his colleagues in Manchester, England, reported in 1981 on 127 hospitalized cases of whooping cough. There were no deaths and no permanent damage. Robinson also observed that the disease takes a much milder course today.

This shows that while many doctors have noticed that the disease is milder in vaccinated children, it is also milder in unvaccinated children. In 1976, Stewart studied 252 hospitalized cases of whooping cough in the United Kingdom and concluded, "There was no significant difference between immunized and nonimmunized cases in the duration of illness, complications, level of lymphocytosis, presence of whoop, and isolation of B. pertussis of serotype 1,3." Ehrengut reported a similar conclusion after studying whooping cough cases in West Germany. This leads to the question of the effectiveness of the pertussis vaccine.

How Effective Is the Pertussis Vaccine?

Some of the earlier pertussis vaccines used in England were judged to be only 20-percent effective (protecting only one child in five), while the best were only 60-percent effective. The British vaccine was subsequently made more potent and is now thought to be 80-percent effective.

America's pertussis vaccine is judged by William H. Foege, former director of the CDC, to be from 63- to 94-percent effective. In the remaining 6 to 37 percent of children, the vaccine does not "take," and these children can and do catch whooping cough. The CDC estimates that there are about 34,000 cases of whooping cough annually in the United States today, even with over 95-percent vaccination of children (see Chapter 20). Severe cases of whooping cough can occur in vaccinated children just as they can occur in unvaccinated children. But this 6 to 37 percent of children, in whom the vaccination does not produce immunity, still run the risk of a serious reaction to the vaccine.

A final factor in evaluating the benefits of pertussis vaccination is that the effect wears off after a few years, although nobody appears to be quite certain how long this takes to happen. A person who has recovered from whooping cough has usually acquired either lifelong immunity or many years of immunity to the disease. But since the U.S. adult population is basically a vaccinated population that has only a temporary immunity and is no longer being periodically reexposed to whooping cough, it cannot periodically reinforce its immunity.

The possibility remains that many adults are highly susceptible to whooping cough. A 1972 article in *The New York Times* reported two outbreaks of whooping cough among the staff of the University of Colorado Medical Center and pointed out "a paradoxical situation in which doctors are diagnosing cases of the childhood disease among a small but growing number of adolescents and adults."

The article goes on to state that "though the vaccine is highly effective in preventing the disease among children, its immunity begins to wane after a decade. And because whooping cough vaccine can cause serious reactions when injected into adults—not children—the Public Health Service does not recommend booster doses after the age of 6 years." Today 6.5 percent of whooping cough cases occur in persons older than fifteen; in the late 1940s this figure was 1.2 percent.

Whether there are whooping cough "carriers" in a vaccinated population, who innocently infect others, especially vulnerable infants, is an issue that scientists and physicians have been unable to resolve. Claire Broome reported in 1981 that it is often hard to identify the source of whooping cough infection because of "atypical clinical presentation or the failure of physicians to consider the possibility of pertussis in adults."

This problem of possible "carriers" is especially relevant in view of the increased number of cases of whooping cough in babies under one year of age. CDC figures presented at a 1982 FDA symposium indicate that 60 percent of modern cases are in babies less than one year of age, with more than three quarters of these cases in those younger than six months. In the 1940s, less than 10 percent of whooping cough cases were in such young babies.

J. D. Nelson pointed out in a 1978 article that adults may well serve as the source of infection for young children, especially if the adult's symptoms are atypical due to previous vaccination.

Few today would follow the example of the American doctor in the 1940s who revaccinated all children every three years up to the age of twelve, but the problem of the short-lived nature of whooping cough immunity remains. The 1979 FDA Bacterial Vaccines Panel alluded to the possibility that "the need to immunize adults, as well as children, may have to be considered in the future."

There is every indication that pertussis in modern industrialized countries has gone the way of tuberculosis and other disease epidemics of the past. In 1980 Mortimer said, "The possibility that changes in the nature of B. pertussis occurred has its precedents, as attested to by experience with tuberculosis over the centuries and with streptococcal infections since the end of the nineteenth century, as well as with measles and diphtheria more recently."

Any infectious disease is the outcome of an interaction between the cause and the host. It appears that in industrially advanced countries the superior nutritional status of the populations and their better environmental circumstances are strengthening the hosts and thus helping to tame the formerly lethal cause of whooping cough. Finally, antibiotics and other forms of therapy are capable of controlling secondary complications of the disease, such as pneumonia, which used to claim as many children as the disease itself.

Ström observed in 1967: "In that way the morbidity in clinically typical diseases can be said to be a manifestation of social conditions. . . . The persons attacked have an increasingly improved resistance. . . . The general social, economic, and hygienic development, and the preventive care of mothers and children, have resulted in an extremely satisfactory state of child health."

Or, as the British physician John L. Emery, M.D., of the Children's Hospital in Sheffield, asked in the *British Medical Journal* (1981), "Are we now in danger of advocating a program based on a concept of the efficiency of vaccination in reducing the general level of infection? A factor which was valid perhaps thirty years ago, when we had many nutritionally substandard children, is not valid today."

The Third World and Whooping Cough

Although the risks of pertussis vaccination may prove to outweigh the benefits in America and Europe, this may not be the case in the Third World for many generations to come. High vaccine risks may well be offset by the much more prevalent death and damage suffered by Third World children who catch whooping cough where there is virtually no sanitation to inhibit its spread or medical care to prevent secondary complications.

The World Health Organization (WHO) has estimated that 1.5 million children die from whooping cough in the Third World each year. According to WHO Director-General Halfdan Mahler, it is the fourth leading cause of death in these poorer underdeveloped countries (after diarrhea, pneumonia, and measles). The case fatality rates in these countries can be as high as 15 percent. This is, for example, in sharp contrast to the 1977–79 outbreak in England which had 26 deaths out of 102,500 cases for a case fatality rate of .025 percent, or the 1982 epidemic where the rate was .02 percent.

A 1960 investigation of the West Indian island of Antigua concluded that, in the hundred years between 1860 and 1960, whooping cough was responsible for 10 percent of all the deaths of infants between the ages of twenty-nine days and twelve months. A 1962 report from Senegal estimated that half the children in that country develop whooping cough before the age of one.

A 1966 publication by D. Morley, of the Wesley Guild Hospital in the Nigerian town of Ilesha, observed that "The picture in West Africa is compared to that seen in England in the past," with a case fatality rate in the Ilesha Hospital of 15.5 percent. Morley observed that the violent coughing starts at the end of the second week of the disease, and "the paroxysms become longer and more intense. The rapid spasmodic cough is at this stage generally associated with choking and vomiting, with the production of sticky, stringy sputum. . . . A proportion of small infants may die of a 'suffocating' bronchospasm with their lungs full of tenacious viscid secretion without developing a characteristic cough."

In a quarter of all Nigerian pertussis cases, the cough persists for as long as ten weeks. Sometimes the coughing spasms cause convulsions and death. Many of the children lose weight and take weeks, even months, to regain it. In some cases this leads to permanent digestive disorders and protein caloric deficiency. Some develop pneumonia during convalescence because of collapsed lungs; others have permanent neurological complications.

But the pertussis vaccine has sharply reduced the incidence and mortality of whooping cough in the Third World. Morley reported: "The introduction of whooping cough vaccination has almost completely removed the infection from the village."

In 1978, John Cameron noted that the Third World continued to need the pertussis vaccine. He said, "I think those of us today who are indulging in the luxury of this argument about reactions vs efficacy ought to appreciate that the argument is wholly irrelevant in developing countries. When you have had the experience, as I have, of finding that the dose [of vaccine] has been reduced by half to prevent reactions when people were dealing with a disease with a 25-percent mortality rate, you realize the heavy responsibility that lies on our shoulders to see that this kind of misinformation does not get into areas where it can be so badly and dangerously misinterpreted."

There seems to be little doubt of the benefits of whooping cough vaccination in Third World countries. But whether these benefits necessarily apply to the industrially developed countries is a question that should be debated by Americans with full disclosure of all the information available.

12

Profile: For Love of a Son

> . . . a man's reach should exceed his grasp,
> Or what's a heaven for?
> *Robert Browning*

Maryl and Bill were struggling to help Bill finish graduate school when their first child, Samuel, was born. He weighed in at eight pounds and was a robust, contented baby from birth. When he was six months old, Maryl took him to his pediatrician for his regular checkup and his third DPT shot. It was his third DPT shot in three months.

"I remember the doctor telling me that Sammy was in perfect health and neurologically fine. There was no discussion about reactions to DPT shots in those days. I had been told nothing except that our baby might be fussy and run a fever after the shots. I was a new mother and I trusted my pediatrician to tell me everything," recalled Maryl.

Soon after Maryl returned home with Sam, he began to cry. "It was a shrill cry. It sounded strange, several octaves higher than normal. He had never cried like that before. He also ran a fever but I can't remember how high it was. After all, this was fifteen years ago. I remember I wasn't particularly worried because my pediatrician had told me that Sammy might be fussy and run a fever."

Sam's high-pitched screaming subsided later that night. It was not until ten days after his third DPT shot that Maryl realized something was seriously wrong with her son.

"When Sammy woke up that morning, he did not babble as he usually did. He just lay quietly in his crib. I picked him up, and his body became

178

rigid and he cried shrilly just like he had when we first got home after his DPT shot. He was stiff and held his head to one side in an odd way."

Sam continued to act strangely for the rest of the day. He screamed almost constantly. The next morning, Maryl found him lying in his crib. He did not move the right side of his body or respond to the sound of her voice or to her touch. He was paralyzed on his right side, and he could not raise or turn his head. He was having difficulty breathing. Maryl and her husband, Bill, took him to the best children's hospital in the city.

"Sammy was admitted to the hospital, where he stayed for ten days. All the tests came back negative, and no reason could be found for the paralysis. With each passing day, he was able to move more of his body. First, he moved his legs, and by the tenth day, he could raise his head. The paralysis disappeared, and we thought he was going to be fine. But three weeks later, I found him lying in his crib, this time paralyzed on the left side of his body. We took him to a university research hospital. Again the doctors were unable to find a cause. This went on for months, his paralysis alternating between the left and right sides of his body. Each time it went away, we thought it wouldn't come back," said Maryl.

Maryl and Bill took Sam to more specialists for more tests at different hospitals, including the Mayo Clinic. A pediatric neurologist diagnosed Sam as having akinetic seizures and alternating hemiparesis. By this time, he had stopped developing altogether.

"For the next three years, Sammy could not do anything, could not feel anything in his body. His eyes could not focus. He did not react to pain. He had no reflexes. When they took blood from him, he did not move or cry out. He did not respond to sound or touch. At one point, we thought he was totally deaf. Feeding was a task that required at least one hour per meal. Sammy would hold baby cereal in his mouth sometimes for as long as an hour without swallowing. He could not sit, stand, creep, or crawl," said Maryl.

During those years, Bill and Maryl took their son to countless pediatric neurologists and hospitals in search of a cause for his condition. They tried all the prescribed drugs to help control his seizures. No doctor could find a cause for his condition or a way to treat it. Even with Sam's serious brain dysfunction, his EEGs came back normal, as they do to this day.

"When it first happened," said Bill, "I kept thinking it was just a temporary condition. Sammy's paralysis would come and go, and each time it went I wanted to believe that it was gone forever. Basically, we had this fantastic sense of hope that one day we would wake up and it would all be a bad dream and everything would be fine. But instead we woke up one day and realized that what Sam would become would be the result of what we helped him become. And rather than concentrate on what caused his condition, which no doctor could explain, we decided to find a way to help Sammy achieve as much as he could."

Bill and Maryl were referred to the Institutes for the Achievement of Human Potential in Philadelphia, where parents are taught to retrain the brains of their handicapped children.

"It wasn't until we got to the Institutes that we found a way to help Sammy begin to develop," said Maryl. "We retrained his brain through an intensive therapy program, repeating a rigorous series of exercises every day for as many as twelve hours a day. We started out with the most rudimentary skills, such as trying to help him increase his intake of oxygen through better breathing. We progressed from there to trying to develop every area of his body and brain that could be developed."

Maryl and Bill and hundreds of volunteers worked intensively with Sam day and night for six years, and watched him eventually sit up, creep, crawl, stand, and speak using single words and short phrases. He did not take steps by himself until he was eight years old. Now sixteen, he can only walk with great difficulty. His movements are very similar to those of people with severe cases of cerebral palsy. He frequently goes limp for periods of twenty to thirty minutes during the day when he loses the strength in his body and cannot move and can barely speak. He is on medication, which is supposed to control the grand mal seizures he has once or twice a year.

"As Sam gets older," said Bill, "it gets easier in some ways but in other ways it gets harder. We used to be able to take him to a department store or playground or museum, and when he went limp, we could pick him up easily and carry him. Now, when he goes limp, he is dead weight. I can barely lift him myself and Maryl hasn't got a chance because he is both heavier and taller than she is now."

But, as profoundly physically and neurologically handicapped as Sam is, he is able to speak, read, spell, count. His intellectual capabilities are remarkable considering the severe brain damage that he sustained.

"Sam has been a frustrated kid," said Maryl. "He knows so much and he understands and remembers things we have all forgotten. But he has learned to do so many things intellectually rather than automatically that if he talks while he walks, he usually falls. Mentally he feels he can do everything that he wants to do. He has a beautiful body and a wonderful mind and spirit trapped by a damaged brain. But he never stops surprising us with what he can do and his determination to do it."

In all the years that Maryl and Bill were searching for the reason why their healthy baby had suddenly become profoundly neurologically damaged, no doctor ever made the connection with Sam's third DPT shot. Neither did Maryl or Bill until they saw the television documentary "DPT: Vaccine Roulette" in April 1982.

"When we watched the program," said Maryl, "we were stunned. We have taken Sam to various kinds of special schools and programs, but the only time we have ever seen a collection of children who looked and behaved like Sam was when we saw 'Vaccine Roulette.' There is just a general aura about DPT kids that is different from children who have Down's syndrome or cerebral palsy or other kinds of neurological damage. I believe that kids who have been hurt by the pertussis vaccine are very different and that schools for the physically and mentally handicapped are not equipped to handle them."

Bill added, "We had stopped thinking about what had caused Sam's condition, and that television program was like a bolt out of the blue fourteen years after the fact. Now that I know how he was hurt, I think I feel better. Of course, that does not take away from the fact that the pertussis vaccine is an inherently neurotoxic vaccine and parents haven't known it."

The television documentary also had a tremendous impact on Maryl. "What affected me most about the program was that parents continue to bring wonderfully healthy, strong babies to be vaccinated, and some of them end up severely handicapped with futures that cannot even be imagined. I would do anything to help prevent that from happening to other children," Maryl said. "Primarily because I know what it means to raise a neurologically damaged child. And what it means for that child. I am just overwhelmed with sadness for Sam, for the thought of how he is going to have to live the rest of his life."

❀   ❀   ❀   ❀   ❀

Sam lurches through the kitchen doorway holding onto the sides of the walls with both hands. His legs are bent at the knees, and his high-top brown leather shoes do not prevent his feet from bending inward so that he rests his weight on his collapsed ankles. Each step requires extraordinary effort. That he walks at all is a miracle.

He is dressed in corduroys, a white shirt, and a bright red sweatshirt with white letters that read "Cornell University." The colors complement his light olive skin and wavy chestnut-brown hair. Big hazel eyes are the most beautiful feature of his face, which is as masculine and strong-boned as the rest of his body. It is easy to picture him on a baseball field hitting a home run or taking a girl to the junior prom.

"Come and read this magazine with me," says Bill.

Sam has only two more steps to take before he reaches the couch where his father sits. He totters precariously, his weight shifting to one leg that threatens to give out under him. Somehow he manages to lunge toward the couch and fall into a sitting position next to his father.

"Look at that," Sam drawls slowly, pointing to a picture in the wild-life magazine that Bill is sharing with him.

Sam speaks haltingly in almost a monotone. He can enunciate quite clearly, but sometimes he slurs his words together or drops the volume of his speech to an unintelligible level. His mother and father can interpret what he is saying, no matter how he speaks.

"That is a lungfish," Bill replies.

"Is. . . it. . . dangerous? What does. . . it. . . do, Bill?" Sam asks slowly. (Usually he calls his father "Bill" unless he is particularly upset and resorts to "Dad" or "Father," a habit he has had since he was a little boy.)

"I think it eats other little fishes in the rivers in Africa," says Bill as he turns the page. "What is this?"

"A. . . kang. . .a. . .roo," answers Sam matter-of-factly, putting emphasis on the sound "roo." He is resting his head on his father's shoulder.

"That's right," agrees Bill. "What is this?"

Sam lowers his head and studies the open magazine intently. "A. . . bear. A. . . polar . . . bear," he decides.

"That's right. Where does the polar bear live?" asks Bill.

"In the. . . Arctic. . . where it. . . is cold. At the. . . North Pole," replies Sam, dragging out the answer as if it requires a tremendous mental effort to translate each thought into words.

"That's right. Who does this look like, Sam?" asks Bill pointing to a picture of a balding man with spectacles.

Sam inspects the picture for a moment and then, in his usual monotone, says confidently, "He. . . looks like. . . Ben Franklin. He discovered. . . electricity."

Sam sees another picture and asks his father if the buildings in it were built in "the old days." He identifies South America on a map. He announces that the first President of the United States was George Washington and that Christopher Columbus discovered America in 1492. He sings a song with his father, finishing the phrases his father does not.

When it is time for lunch, Sam tries to stand up. He leans over the arm of the couch and attempts to use his arms to raise his body into an upright position. But he cannot make his arms do what his mind is telling them to do. He ends up falling to the ground and hitting his head on the side of the couch. He cries out briefly, lying on the floor holding his head.

His father gets down on his knees, leans over, and gives him a big bear hug. "Did you hurt the couch, Sam? I'm not worried about that hard head of yours, but is the couch okay?" he teases.

Sam stops crying and starts laughing as his father wrestles with him on the floor.

For lunch, Sam has two hot dogs on a special kind of bread that he loves. He cannot drink milk or eat any dairy products because they may cause him to have seizures as well as further reduce his ability to function. Although Sam has never been diagnosed as having any other allergies, he constantly has a runny nose. Maryl's family has a history of allergies, particularly those which result in wheezing, respiratory ailments, and sinus conditions.

"Sam has been in a full-time residential school for the mentally retarded for the past year," says Maryl. "They are always careful not to give him dairy products, and he knows what he shouldn't eat. He refuses those foods that aren't good for him."

Bill and Maryl placed Sam in the residential school when their county public school system could not develop an appropriate special-education program for him. Although they are happy that Sam has developed social skills he never had before he entered his new school, they are less satisfied with the educational program.

"When I think about Sam's school, it reminds me of our working in a foreign country for the Peace Corps," says Bill. "Nothing is automatic. Everything takes extraordinary effort. The most frustrating aspect of our experience as Sam's parents is that the schools and special education teachers are not able to provide programs that are effective for kids with unique handicaps.

"There is very little innovative, individualized programming for a child, such as Sam, who falls between the cracks and does not fit into preexisting programs. For example, Sam has never been able to print or write, and no equipment is used to this day to enable him to communicate in a written form, despite the fact we have been requesting it on his IEP (Individualized Education Program) for the last four years. Then, frequently, teachers complain that Sam disrupts the class by speaking out loud!

"I have told them," he continues, "that if they don't challenge Sam more and provide opportunities for him to learn new things, as we have done for all his life, they will have a rebellion on their hands. Sam has the intuitive grace of a toreador in terms of finding your button and pushing it if he is not challenged. Although Sam requires twenty-four-hour supervision, custodial care is not what he needs. The quality of life for him and the other kids can be vastly improved by setting higher standards and enabling them to reach and push themselves to achieve. What they finally grasp will be much more than if they had never reached it in the first place."

Maryl is particularly concerned about the battle she and Bill have fought with many doctors over the years: trying to keep the amounts of medication prescribed for Sam at low enough levels so Sam can function.

"I have battled the doctors for years about not increasing the dosage of Sam's anticonvulsant medication. Every time they change or increase it, which they do at every opportunity, Sam loses his balance, falls down more often, and eventually has to crawl to get where he wants to go. For a five-foot-tall sixteen year old, that is a terrible situation. The increased medication also dulls his mental faculties to the point where he responds at a pitifully slow rate, which makes him unbearably frustrated and often triggers very disruptive behavior."

Maryl gives a poignant example of why she fights doctors about increasing Sam's medication. "Sam has a major seizure about once a year, and when it is over he sleeps. One year he had his annual seizure at school and was taken to the emergency room where doctors gave him an extraordinarily high dosage of Valium. By the time I got there, Sam was resting as he usually does after his seizures, and I took him home over the objections of doctors at the hospital. A week later, I received a letter from the county officially charging me with child neglect. I got charged with child neglect in the same year we were spending ten thousand dollars for physical therapists, special tutors, pediatric neurologists, occupational therapists, and special programs for Sam," says Maryl.

The county required Maryl to take Sam to a pediatric neurologist who gave Sam a new drug to control his seizures. "That year was the worst we ever had," said Maryl. "Sam stopped learning, and his behavior deteriorated to a point where the school personnel were pushed to their limits. After six months of living hell for Sam and us, the doctor finally admitted that Sam reacted negatively to the drug, and we were allowed to take him off of it. Then the county was satisfied and the doctors were satisfied we had done what they wanted. The only loser was Sam. He had to endure an entire school year of frustration and punishment for bad behavior."

Maryl concludes that if doctors would listen to parents, children would not have to suffer with treatments that don't work or do more harm than good. "Doctors see lots of kids every day. Parents see one child all the time. Doctors know a lot about many conditions and medications. A parent knows a lot about one child's condition, and the effects of different medications on him. It doesn't make sense for doctors to discount parents' observations about the effects of medications on their child."

Since Sam has been home for Thanksgiving vacation, Bill and Maryl have been encouraging him to walk, even though his legs have been further weakened because the school puts Sam into a wheelchair much of the time. Maryl and Bill refuse to allow Sam to lose the thirteen long years of muscle building and hard work he put in to becoming all that he could be.

After lunch. Sam sits on the couch with a Speak 'n' Spell computer toy on his lap. It beeps a computer sound.

"Would you like a drink, Sam?" asks his mother.

"No. . . thank you," he says as he listens to the toy rattle on. Suddenly he looks up and announces, "I am. . . thinking about. . . something sticky."

"What are you thinking about?" Maryl questions as she walks back into the kitchen.

"Something. . . sticky. The no-cavities. . . sticker," Sam says in a loud voice so Maryl can hear him in the next room.

"Who gives you that?" Maryl asks.

"The. . . dentist," he replies.

The Speak 'n' Spell squawks again. Sam tries to lift the toy, but it slips from his hand. The color drains from his face, and his body loses all muscle tone as he slumps against the couch. He fights the loss of control, trying to move. He takes a big breath.

"Maryl. . . MOM!" he yells loudly, unable to move.

"Yes, Sam," says Maryl calmly, walking back into the living room.

"Mom. . . I feel. . . kind of. . . floppy," Sam says weakly. By the time he gets to the word "floppy," his voice is almost inaudible and his face is chalky white.

"How about if I get you some pineapple juice?" she offers and walks quickly back into the kitchen.

"I. . . feel. . . floppy," he repeats without moving.

Maryl returns with a small glass of pineapple juice and puts it down on the coffee table beside the couch. "How are you going to get strong?" she asks kindly in a way that suggests she has asked him this question many times before.

"Rest," he whispers.

"Okay. When you get stronger, you can have some juice." She pushes back the hair from his forehead.

Sam stares at the ceiling, still motionless. "I. . . am. . . weak," he says softly.

"I know you are," agrees Maryl as she sits down beside him. Sam's head is like a rag doll's and it rests heavily on his right shoulder. She cups her hand under the right side of his face and gently lifts his head. "Can you push up?"

"I can't," he says simply.

"What are you going to do?" she asks. "Push harder. A little more."

Sam appears to try to lift his head, but there is only the tiniest movement in the muscles of his neck, and his head remains heavily resting against his mother's open hand. "I. . . am. . . very. . . floppy," he repeats in despair.

Maryl holds the glass of pineapple juice up to his lips with one hand as she continues to support his head with the other. He slurps the juice noisily and then coughs.

"I think you can push your head up, Sam. Come on. Try again," she encourages, placing her face directly in front of his and looking straight into his eyes.

Sam groans and appears to try to regain strength in his neck but fails again.

"Push. Push *up!*" Maryl coaches, breaking into a broad smile.

A smile begins to appear on Sam's face, too, and their eyes lock in what has been a lifetime of shared frustration and determination.

Sam leans limply against her, still pale.

"I. . . don't. . . like to. . . be. . . weak," he finishes sadly, staring away from his mother.

"I know you don't like to be weak," says Maryl, trying to keep the momentary desperation that is on her face out of her voice.

"I. . . want. . . to be. . . a. . . bad walker," says Sam.

Maryl laughs, and Sam smiles when he hears her laughing. "A bad walker! Well, you know what that calls for," she replies. "Here, push up. Push your head up."

"I can't," says Sam.

"Can you lift either arm, Sam? Which arm can you lift?" she asks.

Sam apparently tries to raise his left arm but manages only to briefly flick the fingertips on his left hand. "I. . . am. . . still. . . weak," he concludes.

There is a long silence. Maryl cradles his head, the pain in her eyes spilling out into the room and floating above them both.

"This is a very heavy head! There must be a lot of stuff in there," she says almost gaily, determined that Sam will not know how she feels.

"I. . . am. . . weak," repeats Sam tonelessly.

"Is it hard to think when you are weak?" she asks.

"Yes," answers Sam.

"How do you do it?" she asks.

"I. . . stop. . . thinking," he says.

"What? I NEVER saw you stop thinking!" Maryl laughs. She pauses. "Do you think I am going to sit here all day and hold up your head?"

"I think. . . you had. . . better. . . carry. . . me," Sam grins.

"I couldn't possibly carry YOU! You are going to have to start carrying me. You are bigger than me. Isn't that the deal? The bigger one carries?" Maryl teases.

"I. . . can't. . . carry you. . . Mom," Sam states. "It. . . is. . . hard. . . to. . . walk."

"But you've been walking since you came home this vacation!" Maryl says.

"Are. . . you. . . proud. . . of. . . me?" Sam asks his mother, knowing what her answer will be.

"I AM proud of you!" she exclaims with enthusiasm, taking her hand away from his face and embracing him.

Sam smiles, and the color starts to return to his skin. Just as suddenly as his paralysis came upon him, it seems to be dissipating. Gradually he sits up and maintains control of his head.

"Sam is a special kid, a bundle of contradictions," his father says. "Raising him has been an unbelievable challenge, but it has also been fun because Maryl and I really get a kick out of Sam. He has made our relationship much stronger over the years, and he has made me a better person."

"Sam is a wonderful story," his mother says. "To go from a child who was essentially a vegetable to an individual who can walk and talk and read and spell and think is a remarkable achievement. We have achieved it together with the help of lots of special people, who spent enormous amounts of time trying different approaches and developing relationships with Sam that enabled him to develop and grow. We have done it with a kid who is highly motivated in a society that doesn't understand what it means to be brain damaged."

Sam's first act, after he regains his strength, is to try to get up from the couch and walk. He manages to stand up and take three steps before he crashes into the wall. If only he had wings so he could fly as high as his spirit would surely take him.

❖　❖　❖　❖　❖

In summer 1984, the directors of the full-time residential school that Sam had been attending notified Bill and Maryl that Sam could no longer attend the school. The county sent a letter confirming this fact and told Sam's parents that there was no appropriate school in the state, private or public, which could accommodate Sam's needs. Sam is once again at home, and Maryl and Bill, who both hold full-time jobs in order to raise the money that will be needed to provide decent care for Sam for the rest of his life, are again searching for ways to help Sam find his place in the world.

13

Contraindications

Who shall decide when doctors disagree?
Alexander Pope

A contraindication is a condition which precludes the further administration of a drug or vaccine. Contraindications should be observed to screen out children who are most likely to react to the pertussis vaccine.

Yet the lack of scientific knowledge about the precise effects of the pertussis vaccine, together with the pursuit of nationwide, 100-percent vaccination coverage, has led to a serious underestimation of the importance of identifying high-risk children and observing contraindications. In a time when getting a DPT shot is as routine for an American child as a dental checkup, the definition and observance of contraindications has become the orphan discipline of immunology.

Confused Contraindications = Confused Doctors

Today a doctor or parent interested in learning exactly what does and does not constitute a contraindication to giving the pertussis vaccine is confronted with a number of contradictory guidelines and opinions. The three entities responsible for informing doctors about when and when not to vaccinate—the vaccine manufacturers, the American Academy of Pediatrics (AAP), and the U.S. Public Health Service—do not agree with each other about contraindications.

Three private drug manufacturers have been the principal distributors of DPT vaccine in the United States during the past decade— Wyeth Laboratories, the Lederle Laboratories Division of American

190

Cyanamid Company, and Connaught Laboratories. Each has included a list of severe reactions and contraindications in product information inserts which accompany the packages of vaccine distributed to private physicians and public health clinics. (Wyeth Laboratories announced in June 1984 that it would no longer manufacture the pertussis component of the DPT shot. All references herein to the product inserts of the three principal manufacturers are to the editions in effect in 1984 prior to Wyeth's withdrawal from the market.)

The Committee on Infectious Diseases of the AAP periodically publishes a report known as the *Red Book.* It is used primarily by private pediatricians and contains information on what the AAP considers to be severe reactions and contraindications to vaccines.

The U.S. Public Health Service's Advisory Committee on Immunization Practices (ACIP) devises recommendations on the use of vaccines, including contraindications, and the Centers for Disease Control (CDC) publishes them in the Morbidity and Mortality Weekly Report. These guidelines are used by physicians in public health clinics.

Other sources for information about contraindications are the findings and recommendations of vaccine researchers published in the scientific and medical literature. It is safe to say that nobody agrees on what does and does not qualify as a bona fide contraindication to the pertussis vaccine.

Take the question, "How high a fever must a child run after a DPT shot before it is considered a contraindication to further pertussis vaccine?" Page 11 of the AAP's 1977 *Red Book* says 103 F. and page 205 says 105 F. The Wyeth Laboratories DPT vaccine product insert stated 103 F. in one section and 105 F. in another. Connaught Laboratories and Lederle Laboratories state 103 F. The 1982 AAP *Red Book* dropped the 103 F. and retained the 105 F., adding only that infants who run a 105 F. fever "probably should not receive additional doses of pertussis vaccine, although these phenomena are of unknown significance." The 1984 ACIP recommendations call a 105 F. fever, "usually within forty-eight hours" of immunization, a "definitive" contraindication.

The vaccine manufacturers, the AAP, and the ACIP are in agreement on the significance of such neurological reactions as convulsions, encephalitis, collapse/shock, or focal neurologic signs; they list them as absolute contraindications to further pertussis vaccine. But high-pitched screaming is listed as an absolute contraindication by the ACIP and the vaccine manufacturers while the 1982 AAP *Red Book* states only that its significance is "unknown" and that the child "probably" should not receive more pertussis vaccine.

Yet another neurological sign—excessive somnolence (sleepiness)—is regarded as an absolute contraindication by Lederle and Connaught, while the 1982 AAP *Red Book* states that its significance is "unknown" and that the child "probably" should not receive further shots. The ACIP guidelines do not mention somnolence at all, although they do mention "severe alterations of consciousness" as a contraindication.

A 1982 article in the *Journal of the American Medical Association* quotes Leonard P. Rome, M.D., chairman of the AAP's Chapter Chairman's Committee, as commenting that "excessive somnolence" following a DPT shot is "a state of sleep from which the infant cannot be aroused; a drowsy child who wakes up to eat is not experiencing this reaction." The article goes on, however, to say, "When a worrisome reaction occurs that does not actually contraindicate further pertussis immunization—for example, considerable drowsiness from which the child can be aroused, with moderate fever persisting for two days—some pediatricians prefer to include only half the normal dose of pertussis vaccine in the next immunization. If the reaction recurs, they administer DT from then on." (See the discussion of half doses of the vaccine in Chapter 16.)

In addition, the time period in which a reaction must occur to be considered causally connected to the DPT shot has, until very recently, not been spelled out in any of the guidelines. Because most doctors have been taught in medical school that vaccines are safe, they may recognize severe reactions only if they occur within minutes or hours of an inoculation, if they identify them at all.

The 1982 *Red Book* states that reactions such as fever and malaise "occur within several hours of immunization" but indicates nothing about the time period for convulsions, collapse, or encephalitis. Connaught and Lederle offer different advice, stating that more severe reactions "almost always occur within 24 to 48 hours after injection but have been thought to appear after an interval as long as seven days." Formerly, the ACIP recommendations referred to the seven-day period established in England by the National Childhood Encephalopathy Study but appeared to discount the results by adding, "However, pertussis vaccine could account for only a small proportion of cases of serious neurologic disorders in the population studied." The 1984 ACIP recommendations state that reactions occur "usually within forty-eight hours."

How many American pediatricians or family practitioners know that Britain's 1981 National Childhood Encephalopathy Study, designed to evaluate the pertussis vaccine, found that "there were statistically significant associations between the onset of the various neurological disorders notified and immunization with DPT vaccine within the previous seven days"? How many doctors know that in 1983 the AAP agreed that convulsions occurring within seven days after a DPT shot could be considered related to the shot and therefore eligible for compensation under the proposed National Childhood Vaccine Injury Compensation Act?

What is the average doctor supposed to do with these ill-defined and conflicting contraindication guidelines? What is he to do with the AAP's caveat, "Probably should not receive additional doses of pertussis vaccine although these phenomena are of unknown significance," or the *Red Book* admonition, "Frequently only a temporal association is noted between reaction and vaccine administration with no proof that pertussis vaccine caused the reaction"?

In most states pertussis vaccination is required by law. The doctor knows a child must have a certain number of DPT shots in order to attend school. Probably, the doctor has been taught very little in medical school about reactions, contraindications, or the permanent neurological damage that can be caused by the pertussis vaccine. Probably, he will give more pertussis vaccine even after a mother reports that her child ran a high fever or cried strangely or slept excessively after a previous DPT shot. If vaccine authorities themselves cannot agree which reactions are important, it is easy to understand why many doctors do not consider these same reactions to be contraindications.

Janice Cockrell, M.D., surveyed ten pediatric practices in Richmond, Virginia, in 1982 to "determine the local incidence and management of reactions." What she discovered was that "the definitions of mild and severe reactions to DPT are not clear in the minds of many well-trained pediatricians. This is disturbing in that the average pediatrician in our survey administered *at least* one immunization per day. This lack of criteria for defining reactions is probably not only due to the confusion existing in the 1977 edition of the *Red Book*, but to a failure of residency programs to deal with this matter adequately."

Children in the Hands of Uninformed Doctors

Cockrell's statement that severe reactions are "not clear" in the minds of pediatricians is a medical understatement. Not only was the doctor in the following case not clear about pertussis vaccine reactions and contraindications, he did not recognize a convulsion.

Within fifteen hours of her first DPT shot at six weeks of age, Theresa started high-pitched screaming and running a 102-degree temperature. (Theresa's case was described briefly in Chapter 7.) For two weeks after her shot, she alternately screamed, turned blue, and went into a state of collapse. When her mother called the doctor, he blamed the whole thing on Theresa's birth.

"I kept calling my doctor," she said, "and he told me that, because Theresa had been delivered by cesarean section, she was screaming. He told me it was because I had been put to sleep to have the C-section."

By the time Theresa was due for the second shot two months later, she had stopped her screaming spells and was starting to sit up. Within twenty-four hours of the second shot, she again ran a 102-degree temperature and alternately screamed and went into a state of collapse. But this time, she started jerking her head, then dropping it down to her chest.

Her mother again called the doctor: "I didn't know what the head jerking meant, so I went back to my doctor, and he told me 'A lot of babies do it. It's muscle spasms. She will outgrow it.' I was still worried though, because when she would jerk her head, she would get a real dazed look. You could talk to her, and she wouldn't respond. At first it only lasted a few seconds, and then it got worse where she did them more often and they lasted longer. And she wouldn't sleep at night. I'd be up all night long with her screaming."

The doctor proceeded to give her a third DPT shot. Within twenty-four hours, she ran a 102-degree fever and had severe collapse episodes.

"After her third shot, she would go in and out of seizures all day long," her mother said. "We couldn't even talk to her and have her look at us. She would turn blue and get so still that you couldn't even tell she was breathing. One time she definitely stopped breathing because we couldn't get a pulse on her or a breath out of her. I picked her up and started running with her because I didn't have a car to get to the doctor. My mother took me to the doctor's office, and when we got there,

Theresa was still coming in and out of seizures. The nurses told me that my running with her probably jarred her back into breathing."

The nurses at the doctor's office saw Theresa collapse. "They told the doctor they thought Theresa was having seizures. He looked at her and told me she might have a brain tumor and referred me to a neurologist. The neurologist told me that all her tests were negative and that some kids just jerk their heads and no one knows why they do it. I felt the shot had something to do with her problem, but they kept telling me it didn't. See, after every shot she had she would be real sick and then would get better. The head jerking would get less and less, and then when she would get another shot, she would be so sick again."

Even with all these neurological signs occurring within twenty-four hours of three separate DPT shots, the doctors still insisted that Theresa receive more pertussis vaccine. "They are trying to make me bring her to get her fourth DPT shot. They tell me I can't get her into school without it. I have tried pediatrician after pediatrician, and they all tell me to get the shot. I have asked them if they will leave out the pertussis, and they won't do it."

Is it any wonder that more and more physicians are finding themselves targets of malpractice suits for repeatedly giving pertussis vaccine to babies who have had obvious neurological reactions to previous DPT shots? Even though the AAP, CDC, and vaccine manufacturers have not come up with a comprehensible set of guidelines for physicians to follow, there are numerous reports in the scientific literature by independent vaccine researchers who have warned physicians about contraindications.

Four Decades of Warnings

As early as the 1940s, when physicians and researchers became aware of adverse DPT reactions, they reported them in the literature and often recommended that health practitioners look for warning signs indicating a child at high risk of reacting to the pertussis vaccine.

In 1947, Matthew Brody was one of the first doctors to suspect that if a child reacts with neurological symptoms to a previous shot of pertussis vaccine, he should not receive another dose. He came to this conclusion after observing two babies who were repeatedly injected with pertussis vaccine despite a variety of neurological signs that appeared after each injection.

In the *Brooklyn Hospital Journal*, Brody described the mental deterioration and eventual death of a five-month-old boy who had a questionable neurological history even before vaccination and displayed increasingly severe neurological signs two weeks after his first pertussis shot, one week after his second shot, three days after his third shot, and within twenty-five minutes after his fourth shot. He became completely paralyzed and died seven weeks later at the age of three.

Brody concluded, "The appearance of somnolence, convulsions or other neurologic complications within two weeks of inoculation with pertussis vaccine should be considered a contraindication to further such inoculations," and warned about "giving these inoculations in the presence of an undiagnosed disease of the central nervous system."

In 1949, John A. Toomey collected data on thirty-eight cases of severe reactions to the pertussis vaccine and warned physicians in the *Journal of the American Medical Association* that "no child should receive injections of pertussis vaccine in large amounts who has (a) any family history of convulsions (b) a present history of convulsions or (c) illness of any kind, especially if it pertains in any way to the central nervous system."

In 1953, W. C. Cockburn, reviewing whooping cough and pertussis vaccination in *The Practitioner*, warned physicians that "children with a personal or family history of organic nervous disease should not be inoculated" and that "vaccination should not be attempted before the age of six months and should be carried out after diphtheria immunization, which is the more important."

In that same year, Karl-Axel Melin wrote in the *Journal of Pediatrics* that it is appropriate for physicians "to follow the children carefully during the immunization and to interrupt the procedure at any signs of complication, especially if a convulsion occurs in connection with the immunization."

The large field trials conducted by Britain's Medical Research Council to assess the efficacy of pertussis vaccine in children from six to eighteen months old excluded any child "with a personal or family history of convulsions, epilepsy, hydrocephalus, mental defect, or similar conditions," as well as any child who had recently been sick with "measles, mumps, influenza, chicken-pox and similar diseases." This is a good indication that the physicians conducting these trials believed that children with these preexisting conditions were at risk of reacting and perhaps being damaged by the pertussis vaccine.

In 1958, J. M. Berg analyzed 107 cases of pertussis vaccine damage reported in the literature up to that point and told physicians in the *British Medical Journal*, "Any suggestion of a neurological reaction to a pertussis inoculation should be an *absolute* contraindication to further inoculation."

In 1960, Ström noted in the *British Medical Journal* that "continued vaccination is absolutely contraindicated in any suggestion of a neurological reaction to a previous pertussis inoculation."

In 1961, J. M. H. Hopper wrote in *The Medical Officer*, "In this study, some of the children were given further doses of vaccine when illness had followed the previous injection. In many cases, illness of a similar severity recurred. . . . Certainly all are agreed that, following the more severe manifestations of illness following pertussis vaccination, no further pertussis vaccine must be administered."

In 1967, Ström again warned physicians in the *British Medical Journal* about neurological reactions to the pertussis vaccine, stating that "the great majority of reactions occurred after the first injection. Repeated injections appeared to produce the same reaction."

In 1969, Hannik told physicians at the International Symposium on Pertussis that "once a major reaction has occurred, further vaccination with DPT-polio vaccine is contraindicated."

In 1974, Kulenkampff, with others, published a study of pertussis vaccine brain-damaged children in the *Archives of Disease in Childhood* and told physicians that "in as many as a third of our patients there were contraindications to inoculation with pertussis vaccine, in that there was a previous history of fits, or family history of seizures in a first-degree relative; reaction to previous inoculation; recent intercurrent infection; or presumed neurodevelopmental defect." They recommended that pertussis vaccine be withheld from this high-risk group of infants and postponed in those recently ill.

In 1979, Stewart published an article in the *Journal of Epidemiology and Community Health* informing physicians about the "Toxicity of pertussis vaccine: frequency and probability of reactions." He noted that out of 197 cases of pertussis vaccine brain-damaged children, 129 were given a first shot of pertussis vaccine despite contraindications and 25 more were given more pertussis vaccine despite reactions to a previous injection or injections.

In 1981 the UCLA-FDA study (published in *Pediatrics*) informed physicians that 1 in 1,750 immunizations of DPT results in a shock reaction, and 1 in 1,750 immunizations results in a convulsion (i.e. 1 in 875 DPT shots results in either a convulsion or collapse). The authors advised that children who reacted with convulsions, collapse, or prolonged or peculiar crying should be given only DT in future vaccinations.

In 1981, the National Childhood Encephalopathy Study conducted in Britain found a significant correlation between serious neurological illness and pertussis vaccine and gave the following contraindications to pertussis vaccination: "a personal or family history of epilepsy or other neurological disorders, a history of convulsions or cerebral irritation in the neonatal period, evidence of developmental neurological defects, and the presence of a febrile illness at the time of the proposed vaccination."

These references in the medical literature over a period of nearly four decades are only a small proportion of what is available for American physicians to read on the subject of pertussis vaccine reactions and contraindications. Yet despite a convincing number of studies pointing out severe reactions and intelligent contraindications, in 1980 Ronald Illingworth, a prominent British physician specializing in immunization, wrote that no epidemiological or pathological evidence existed for considering "general or local reactions to a preceding dose" as a contraindication to the pertussis vaccine.

Physicians taught to believe that vaccine reactions and histories of convulsions are unimportant will not recognize a severe reaction or consider a child's medical history carefully before deciding whether or not to give more pertussis vaccine. As late as 1982, the AAP's guidelines stated, "Convulsions that are infrequent, occurred months or years ago, or are well controlled do not contraindicate pertussis vaccine." Yet consider the following case:

Dylan was born without any problems and developed like any other healthy newborn. He was given his first DPT shot by a general practitioner at exactly two months of age. Four weeks later, he was hospitalized with a grand mal seizure that lasted for eight hours. All tests came back negative, and no cause could be found for the convulsion. He was placed on Phenobarbital.

One month after this eight-hour grand mal convulsion, Dylan was given another DPT shot at a public health clinic. This time the convulsion occurred ten days after the shot. Again no cause could be found, and his dosage of Phenobarbital was increased.

Despite his history of two grand mal convulsions and despite being on anticonvulsant medication, Dylan was given a third DPT shot seven months later. Within a few hours, he had a third grand mal convulsion, and from that point on they became frequent and uncontrollable. At age eight, he was severely retarded.

Dylan has a family history of febrile seizures. He has asthma and his brother also has asthma plus a severe allergy to milk.

His mother said, "Some of Dylan's seizures are so violent, he has had cardiac arrest with them. He is in a special class for severe and profoundly retarded children. My pediatric neurologist said he didn't know much about the vaccine, but it was his understanding that only seizures taking place within twenty-four hours after the shot were due to the vaccine. He said he didn't think Dylan's problems were due to the vaccine, but he couldn't say definitely not, because Dylan's condition runs so closely along the lines of pertussis vaccine seizures."

Dylan's parents cannot get supplemental social security income for their son, and as a result, his medical bills have already put them into bankruptcy once. Now the state school system is pressuring them to have Dylan's brother injected with more pertussis vaccine.

"My youngest son is five years old, and I don't want him to receive his booster DPT shot because I am afraid he might react with seizures," said Dylan's mother. "But the school system is insisting I give him the booster before he goes to school."

❖ ❖ ❖ ❖ ❖

In the summer of 1984, Dylan developed leukemia, went into status epilepticus, suffered cardiac arrest, and died.

Which Children Are At High Risk?

As soon as researchers perceived that pertussis vaccine had serious side effects, they realized that many of the babies damaged were in poor physical or neurological condition or had family histories of certain medical conditions.

In 1969, Johannes Melchior observed: "It appears reasonable, as has been done previously, to recommend that great care be exercised with every form of vaccination both as regards ordinary contraindications such as acute infections or poor general conditions and also the more particular contraindications such as information concerning possible cerebral damage (family predisposition, difficult deliveries, neonatal neurological symptoms, developmental deviations)."

Physicians who conduct research on the pertussis vaccine will often eliminate what they consider to be high-risk children from their studies, even though these same categories of high-risk children in the general population are routinely given pertussis vaccine. At the 1982 FDA Symposium Philip Brunell, M.D., chairman of the AAP's Red Book Committee, described one study he conducted on the pertussis vaccine at the 1982 FDA Symposium: "The children included in this study were all healthy. There were no premature infants with any CNS [central nervous system] problems. . . . Before children were enrolled in the study they had a physical examination to exclude any underlying problems that might perhaps put them at additional risk."

As with other kinds of diseases and traumas, the extent of vaccine damage is determined by an interaction between an external cause (the pertussis vaccine) and the condition of the host (the child). If a child is congenitally vulnerable to the pertussis vaccine, has had a difficult birth, or had poor health in early life, that child could be a likely candidate for vaccine damage.

The first indication that a child may be at risk of reacting is contained in the personal and family medical history. Mothers should ask the physician or nurse to take a medical history of the child and his family before giving the first shot. The following information should be included: a history of convulsions or neurologic disease in the child or in the immediate family; a history of previous cerebral irritation; a strong history of severe allergies in the child or the immediate family; prematurity or low birth weight; chronic illness or a recent severe illness; a brother, sister, mother, or father who had a severe reaction to the DPT shot; or a severe reaction by the child himself to a previous DPT shot.

History of Convulsions or Neurological Disease

Vaccine policymaking groups in England, Sweden, The Netherlands, and other countries have considered a history of convulsions or neurologic disease in the child or immediate family (brother, sister, mother, or father) to be a contraindication to the pertussis vaccine. West Germany, East Germany, and Japan have considered a history of convulsions in the child to be a contraindication. Generally, however, the vaccine policymakers in the AAP and the U.S. government have not recognized a history of convulsions—even in the child—to be a contraindication.

In 1977, the Department of Health and Social Security in England stated that children should not be given pertussis vaccine if they have either of the following: "history of seizures, convulsions, or cerebral irritation in the neonatal period. A history or family history of epilepsy or other diseases of the central nervous system."

In 1975, a WHO-sponsored international meeting of pertussis vaccine experts recommended that "children from families with a history of neurological disorders should not be vaccinated."

But vaccine policymakers in the AAP and the government do not agree with the rest of the world, and U.S. vaccine manufacturers are divided on the subject. Lederle Laboratories states, "Routine immunization with this product should not be attempted if the child has a personal or family history of central nervous system disease or convulsions." Connaught Laboratories states, "The benefit/risk ratio of routine immunization with this product should be carefully considered by the responsible physician if the child has a personal or family history of central nervous system disease or convulsions."

But the Wyeth Laboratories insert did not mention a personal or family history of convulsions or neurologic disease and only stated, "The presence of an evolving or changing neurologic disorder is a contraindication to use." Wyeth's recommendation agreed with the Public Health Service 1981 recommendations, which read, "The presence of an evolving neurologic disorder contraindicates use of pertussis vaccine. A family history of neurologic disease or a static neurologic condition like cerebral palsy is not a contraindication. . . ."

The 1982 *Red Book* stated, "Most frequently, questions arise about children with convulsive disorders with or without other neurologic abnormalities. Convulsions that are infrequent, occurred months or years ago, or are well controlled do not contraindicate pertussis vaccine. Similarly, nonprogressive neurologic conditions such as cerebral palsy and most instances of developmental retardation are not contraindications. . . . A family history of convulsions or other neurologic disease is not a contraindication."

Ultimately, the 1982 *Red Book* advised against vaccination only in the presence of "progressive or evolving neurologic disease (such as progressive encephalomyelopathy)," and then "if only because confusion might occur regarding the relationship of the vaccine to disease progression."

The *Red Book* justified its position with a statement that touches on the belief of many doctors that the danger of whooping cough is far greater to a child with neurological disorders. It stated, "the risk of the disease and its complications must be weighed against risks from the vaccine. The current local prevalence of the disease should be considered, and it should be remembered that the disease itself is associated with severe central nervous system complications at a greater rate than is the vaccine."

What the AAP was saying as late as 1982 was that a doctor should weigh the danger of whooping cough against that of a pertussis vaccine in a child who has a history of convulsions or other kinds of neurological problems. With over 95 percent of the U.S. population vaccinated against pertussis, why was there so little questioning of the wisdom of vaccinating a high-risk child with convulsions and neurological problems?

In 1983, the Interagency Group to Monitor Vaccine Development, Production and Usage, as well as the ACIP and the AAP, began discussing the possibility of adopting the view held by a majority of the world that a child who has a history of convulsions or neurologic disease should not receive pertussis vaccine. They also discussed the possibility that a family history of reactions to the pertussis vaccine might be considered a contraindication.

But in April 1984, the ACIP announced, "For infants and children with stable neurologic conditions, including well-controlled seizures, the benefits of pertussis immunization outweigh the risks, and such children may be vaccinated." The government went on to recommend that a child with an "evolving neurological disorder" expressed in the form of continuing convulsions should have the DPT shot delayed for a few months. If, by that time, the disorder has stopped evolving or is "well controlled" (with Phenobarbital or other drugs), the ACIP suggests that vaccination may be carried out. In August 1984 the AAP modified its recommendations to conform with those of the ACIP.

Whatever future changes are made in pertussis vaccine policy will not affect Caroline. It is too late for her. She was a very bright baby, sitting at four months and crawling at six months. After her first DPT shot, she ran a fever of 102 degrees and was a little fussy. One month later, she had her first grand mal convulsion.

Despite this history, she was given a second DPT shot, and she again ran a fever of 102 degrees and was cranky. Two weeks later, she had her second grand mal convulsion.

Her pediatrician still did not consider her history of seizures to be a contraindication to further vaccination. He gave her a third DPT shot. Within twelve hours, Caroline had a one-and-a-half-hour grand mal convulsion.

"She had her shot in late morning or early afternoon," her mother said. "And she was real jerky all evening. I could feel her jerk in my arms every so often. I didn't realize it was seizure activity. During the night, she had a grand mal for one and a half hours."

The hospital could find no infection or reason for Caroline's seizure, although she was again running a fever of 102 degrees. "The doctors told us she had a low fever threshold. My husband's brother had had a few febrile seizures as a child."

But in the following months, Caroline began having seizures without a fever. She has been diagnosed as having idiopathic epilepsy. Over the past five years, Caroline's seizures have become more frequent, and she has been on a long list of anticonvulsants that do not work. She sometimes has a grand mal convulsion once a day.

"We have learned to live with the seizures," her mother said, "but the learning disabilities are really difficult to overcome and they are getting worse. Tests show her I.Q. is dropping."

There will never be any way of knowing whether Caroline's seizures would have become as frequent and uncontrollable as they are today if the pediatrician had removed the pertussis vaccine from her second and, particularly, her third shot. But her case, and many similar ones, suggest that children with a history of seizures are at high risk of developing more serious seizure conditions when given further injections of pertussis vaccine.

History of Previous Cerebral Irritation

In the first few days of life, some babies may experience signs of cerebral irritation due to complications of pregnancy or difficulty in delivery. Such signs may include encephalitic screaming, opisthotonic posturing (the baby bends his head and heels backwards and arches his back), or unusually restless and irritable behavior. Whatever the cause, such signs should be reported to a physician.

England considers a history of "cerebral irritation in the neonatal period" to be a contraindication. Reports from parents of vaccine-damaged children seem to support this. The mother of Linda, whose reaction is detailed in Chapter 5, recalls how her daughter reacted with high-pitched screaming, collapse, and excessive sleepiness within one hour of her first DPT shot and describes her difficult pregnancy.

"I had not menstruated for five months before I became pregnant with her. I had a thyroid condition and was throwing up all the time while I was pregnant, and they had to put me on medication. But I had a very easy delivery."

She remembers that before her daughter got the shot at six weeks of age, she was very restless and irritable.

"She was very restless from the day she was born. She never slept for more than two hours at a time. Most babies, when you lay them down on a bed, would lie still for at least a moment or two. But she would flop about and squirm and not lay her head down. She would constantly flop and wiggle like she was a fish out of water. Then when she got her first DPT shot at six weeks old, within one hour she screamed very strangely. It was a horrible scream that I had never heard before. Then she passed out and went to sleep for twenty-four hours and I couldn't wake her at all."

Linda continued to "pass out" hundreds of times for the next several years, and is now hyperactive with an emotional disorder and an attention-span deficit.

History of Severe Allergies

The question of whether a history of severe allergies in the child or the immediate family puts him at high risk of reacting to the pertussis vaccine is another source of controversy. In England in past decades, a personal or family history of allergy was regarded as a contraindication, while today it is not a contraindication in either Britain or America. However, East Germany warns that "persons with manifest allergic disease symptoms" should not be given a DPT shot less than four weeks following recovery.

No manufacturer or official body today mentions a history of asthma as a contraindication, although the 1979 *Bacterial Vaccines Report* revealed that the Dow Chemical Company's DPT product insert in the 1960s stated: "fractional doses are recommended in infants with cerebral injury, asthma, a strong family history of allergy. . . ."

In the early days of pertussis immunization there was more discussion of allergies and asthma. As discussed in Chapter 7, Köng in 1953 described a child who had an "asthma-like condition during the hay-fever season" and who reacted violently to a DPT shot (tonic-clonic convulsions). He urged that infants with "allergic diseases" or a family history of allergy not receive the vaccine.

Halpern and Halpern in 1955 observed that some physicians were calling for fractional doses in asthmatic and allergic children. One mentioned that his "own daughter had a severe asthma attack and angio-neurotic edema one-half hour after a booster alum-precipitated pertussis vaccine," and added, "I have had three children in my practice develop angio-neurotic edema and/or asthma within one hour after a booster dose or a dose other than the first one of the combined diphtheria, pertussis, tetanus alum-precipitated vaccine." A third physician "knew of an infant who developed asthma following the second and third injections of DPT. None of these children had a personal or family history of allergy."

In 1961, Hopper found that, in a group of babies who reacted violently to the pertussis vaccine, there was twice as common an incidence of eczema, asthma, hay fever, and allergic skin rashes in the child, its siblings, parents, and grandparents as there was in a control group of the same size.

In 1969, Hannik found a positive family history of allergies in a significant proportion of infants who reacted with high-pitched screaming, shock, and convulsions.

These observations were reinforced by Lawrence Steinman, who published a study in 1982 concluding that genetic predisposition may play a role in susceptibility to pertussis vaccine reactions. His work with mice suggests that a personal or family history of allergies, particularly milk allergies, may be a warning sign. (See Chapter 7.)

It is no news to Lisa and her mother that a severe personal and family history of allergies puts a child at high risk of reacting to the DPT shot. Now a young mathematician, Lisa was born with exceptionally severe allergies and an exceptionally high I.Q.

Her mother said, "Lisa has always had severe allergies. She was born with eczema covering her from head to toe. My mother, myself, and Lisa are very allergic to milk. Lisa had a lot of colic and had to be put on soybean formula, like all of my children because they are all allergic. I have eczema and food allergies. Lisa is so highly allergic to peanuts that one peanut butter cookie almost killed her. Her father had severe asthma, and Lisa has asthma."

She was a very special baby because she started talking at five months and was speaking in sentences at seven months. She became the subject of a study at a major university and researchers continued to followed her progress as she grew older. Lisa reacted to her first three DPT shots with a high fever, high-pitched screaming, and a large, hot, red lump at the site of the injection.

Her mother said, "Her fevers after the first three shots were quite high. I had to give her tepid baths. Her crying was more like screaming with severe colic or pain. And the lump was about the size of an egg, hot and red."

But it was Lisa's fourth shot at the age of six that brought on petit mal convulsions. She received the shot in the morning and returned to school. Within four hours, her teacher found her pale, drooling, and staring unresponsively with dilated eyes. It was her first petit mal seizure.

She was immediately admitted to a hospital, where the doctors could find no reason for her seizure. One week later, she had another petit mal seizure. She was placed on anticonvulsant medication until the age of eleven; she was then seizure-free until seventeen. She had just arrived at college, when she had her first grand mal convulsion. From that point on, her grand mals were uncontrollable despite medication.

Lisa said, "To this day, I can't drink milk, or I will break out in hives. And if I get anywhere near peanut oil, I could die. Everybody in my family has severe allergies, but mine are the worst. No doctor has ever been able to find a lesion in my brain. My diagnosis is 'seizure disorder: cause unknown.' "

Lisa and her mother both know the devastating effect that Lisa's seizure condition has had on her life. Her mother said, "Lisa was and is an exceptionally gifted individual. Before that fourth shot, her only health problems were severe allergies. Now she must cope with the fear of whether or not she is going to have a grand mal at her job or in a store or at a party. People don't really understand what seizures are.

There is still a lot of discrimination and ostracism of people with epilepsy."

Lisa speaks firsthand of her fears. "I am on six tablets of Tegretol a day, and I never know from one day to the next if I will go into a grand mal and lose ten minutes to an hour and a half of my life. It could happen anywhere at anytime—at work or home or out on the street. It is terrifying to come out of it and not know what I have said or done."

Jackie is another child who has a strong personal and family history of milk allergy. She reacted within ten hours of her second DPT shot with a seizure and has uncontrollable seizures today. She has never been able to drink milk. Her mother said, "She spit up a lot and had constipation from birth when she was on milk formula. We switched her to soybean formula and she stopped being constipated and spitting up. She is still on soybean, even though she is eighteen months old, because every time I try to switch her to skim milk she spits up."

Jackie's father was highly allergic to cow's milk as a baby. "My mother-in-law told me that he was so allergic to milk he almost died. He had violent projectile vomiting and lost so much weight in his first few weeks of life they were afraid he would die. They switched him to soybean formula and he was fine," her mother said.

Jackie's uncle could not drink milk as a child, and both his sons also had to be put on soybean formula. "His son was found blue and not breathing within five hours of his first DPT shot. He was given mouth-to-mouth resuscitation and put on a heart monitor for a year," said Jackie's mother.

Jackie did not react to her first DPT shot, but on the day of her second shot, her mother found her in the middle of a convulsion. "She was holding her arm really stiff, and she was quivering. Then she made gurgling sounds in her throat. The seizure lasted about forty-five minutes."

Today she has three to four convulsions a month, despite medication. Her mother said, "She started walking at fifteen months, but she doesn't really talk. It is hard to get her attention. She falls a lot and seems delayed. She is also prone to ear infections. She didn't have an ear infection until that second shot at four months old, but she must have had ten ear infections since then."

Although doctors told Jackie's parents that her first seizure was a DPT reaction, they now deny it. "After the first seizure," her mother reports, "they said it was a reaction to the DPT shot, but then, when her seizures continued, they denied it was a reaction to the shot. What really makes me mad is that I was worried about Jackie getting the shot because of what had happened to my husband's brother's son. But my doctor told me it was an isolated, rare incident and it would never happen again."

Many other parents of vaccine-damaged children have reported that their babies spit up their milk, screamed with colic, had constipation or diarrhea, and were eventually determined, or suspected, to have a milk allergy. A significant proportion of parents of vaccine-damaged children have reported a strong family history of allergies to other foods, medications, pollens, and grasses (see Chapters 5 and 7).

In 1946, Sauer cautioned physicians against vaccinating infants with "feeding problems." Many times a colicky baby will also spit up his milk, and both these symptoms can point to a milk allergy. Although the cause of colic has never been scientifically defined, it may have an allergic basis. William J. Cates, M.D., an allergist in Rockville, Maryland, maintains: "I have never seen a case of colic that wasn't due to allergies."

The Steinman study, together with the numbers of parents who are reporting milk allergies in their children who have reacted violently to the vaccine, raises the question of whether or not "colic" or milk allergy should be considered a contraindication to the pertussis vaccine. Approximately 25 percent of all the children in the United States are believed to have severe allergies, with perhaps as many as 10 percent having milk allergies and 5 percent having asthma.

Certainly the question of whether a personal or family history of allergies puts a child at high risk of reacting to the pertussis vaccine deserves further serious investigation.

Prematurity and Low Birth Weight

Babies with low birth weight are often difficult to distinguish from those who are truly premature. But both cases raise the possibility that the infant's neurological and respiratory systems have not developed sufficiently to withstand the shock of early vaccination.

Research on low-birth-weight infants during the past two decades has revealed the relationship between low birth weight and lower-than-normal mental and neurological development. The nervous system and brain develop most in the last three months of pregnancy, and can be harmed by a premature delivery.

Many low-birth-weight babies originally thought to be premature have been found to be actually full-term babies who had been under-nourished in the uterus because the mother herself was eating poorly. In the 1950s and 1960s, when doctors were encouraging mothers to gain a minimum number of pounds during pregnancy (as few as fifteen to eighteen pounds in some cases), there was a large crop of under-sized babies combined with an increase in perinatal mortality, congenital neurological disease, cerebral palsy, blindness, deafness, and mental retardation.

In the 1960s, the NIH studied more than 50,000 babies born between 1959 and 1966 and found that those who weighed more at birth had significantly less morbidity and mortality. One of the directors of the study, Kenneth Niswander, commented that "abandonment of the traditional obstetric practice of keeping weight gain during pregnancy to a minimum might significantly reduce the incidence of prematurity and its attendant mortality and morbidity."

Like Cindy and Heather, whose reactions were described in Chapter 5, Katie was born prematurely, weighing just over three pounds. She weighed only eight pounds when given her first DPT shot at two and a half months of age. An adopted child, she appeared to be a contented and cheerful baby when her parents took her home for the first time, but her behavior changed after the DPT shot.

"We picked her up on Friday, and that whole weekend she was very happy when she was awake and slept peacefully. She got the DPT shot on Monday. After the shot she didn't sleep and was very fussy while she was awake. Then I noticed that she wasn't breathing very well. I told my husband and he timed her and we found she was only breathing every twelve seconds or so."

Katie was put on a monitor and supplied with oxygen, and her mother noticed that "as soon as she was put on oxygen four days after the shot, she was well and happy again. That is why our pediatrician thinks her periodic breathing was brought on by the pertussis vaccine."

Katie was kept on the monitor for eight months. She was eventually taken off it but continued to have occasional periodic breathing. At fourteen months, she only weighed twenty-four pounds, but the doctors encouraged her mother to have Katie vaccinated with another DPT shot. She said:

"We really don't want to give her more pertussis vaccine. One doctor wanted to keep her on a monitor and give her three DPT shots in close succession. Another specialist wants her to get more pertussis vaccine because he says that, with her breathing problem, she could have a hard time with whooping cough if she caught it. But the doctors say there is no guarantee that, if we put her back on the monitor and give her another DPT shot, that she won't react or die of SIDS the day after we take her off the monitor."

Katie is at high risk of being damaged or dying from whooping cough as well as at risk of reacting to the pertussis vaccine. Unfortunately, the dimensions of both these risks in America today are unknown. Just how great a risk premature or low-birth-weight infants are taking when they receive the pertussis vaccine is a subject that should be more thoroughly investigated by scientists and physicians.

Chronic Illness or Recent Severe Illness

Often a child has a cold, a runny nose, or a slight fever at vaccination time, or has just recovered from a mild case of the flu or diarrhea. Other children may recently have been sick with something more serious, such as meningitis. The doctor who has looked to the AAP or the CDC for guidance about whether or not to vaccinate under these circumstances has not gotten a clear answer.

Although British authorities have urged postponing vaccination in the presence of "any febrile illness, particularly respiratory, until the patient has fully recovered," such a suggestion was not made by the 1982 *Red Book*. The 1981 ACIP recommendations stated, "A severe febrile illness is reason to defer routine vaccination. Minor illness without fever, such as a mild upper respiratory infection, should not be cause for postponing vaccination."

The manufacturers have not spoken with one voice on this subject either. Wyeth stated, "A febrile acute respiratory infection or other active infection is reason for deferring administration." Lederle advises against vaccination during "any acute illness," but Connaught states, "A minor illness not associated with fever such as upper respiratory tract infection need not preclude vaccination."

Harry Jennison, executive director of the AAP, recommends that children who have recently had a "bad cold" should defer DPT vaccination. In response to a question in 1983 by television reporter Lea Thompson concerning how ill a child must be to defer the shot, Jennison said, "A bad cold, or if he has a fever and obviously any other more debilitating illness. If a child had a cold last week but is better now, Mom says, that is probably enough to say, 'Let's take our time.'"

But Robert Ancona, M.D., who sits on the Maryland Medical Society Committee on Infectious Diseases, stated on a 1983 television program, "In my practice and in most of my colleagues' . . . for very minor illnesses . . . child has had a runny nose for a week and a half and is now getting better but may still have a little runny nose, that sort of thing, they would not feel . . . that they should delay the shot on that behalf."

Alan Hinman, M.D., of the CDC, made the following statement in a March 1983 meeting with representatives from Dissatisfied Parents Together: "I don't think there would be general agreement in the U.S. medical community that a full exam is necessary prior to vaccination. Is the child sick now? is the question that is enough in most cases. Besides, it is common practice to give a child immunizations at a well-child exam. If a physician had to give a physical exam to every child before a child received a vaccination at a public health clinic, it would either dismantle the public health system or increase your taxes to the point that you wouldn't tolerate it."

Hinman went on to state that "you can't have nurses or other personnel give the child a physical exam because that would mean they were practicing medicine and that is prohibited because they aren't medical doctors."

Cases of vaccine damage reported in the medical literature indicate that a recent or present infection may put a child at high risk of reacting to the pertussis vaccine. In 1968, Hannik suggested the possibility of a "subclinical infection triggered by the vaccination." In 1978, she urged that an effort always be made to diagnose the presence of coinciding latent virus infections which might be triggered by the vaccine.

In 1953, John M. Sutherland mentioned that vaccination "might activate a previously latent neurotropic virus," while Ehrengut agreed with the concept of the vaccine "triggering" a latent virus into activity. In England, there were several cases of "provocation poliomyelitis" in the 1940s and 1950s, caused by vaccination with diphtheria and pertussis vaccines. The Connaught and Lederle product inserts advise against vaccinating during an outbreak of poliomyelitis, although Wyeth's did not.

In 1974, Archie Kalokerinos, M.D., published *Every Second Child*, describing his experiences treating aboriginal babies in Australia. He maintained that a portion of Sudden Infant Death Syndrome is caused by acute vitamin C deficiency triggered by vaccination.

"A health team would sweep into an area, line up all the aboriginal babies and infants and immunize them," wrote Kalokerinos. "There would be no examination, no taking of case histories, no checking on dietary deficiencies. Most infants would have colds. No wonder they died. Some would die within hours from acute vitamin C deficiency precipitated by the immunization. Others would suffer immunological insults and die later from 'pneumonia,' 'gastroenteritis,' or 'malnutrition.' If some babies and infants survived, they would be lined up again within a month for another immunization. If some managed to survive even this, they would be lined up again. Then there would be booster shots, shots for measles, polio and even T.B. Little wonder they died. The wonder is that any survived. . . . We were actually killing infants through lack of understanding."

It is known that a vaccination can deplete the body's reserve of vitamin C, just as an infection lowers the body's vitamin C levels. Kalokerinos asserts that in an infant who is fighting a cold or other viral or bacterial infection, the already subnormal vitamin C levels can plunge to a fatally low level after vaccination. Infants with poor immune systems who are prone to constant infections or allergies would be at special risk.

His book describes several cases of children who went into shock after vaccination and would have died if he had not injected them with a large dose of vitamin C. Recovery sometimes took place within thirty minutes. Kalokerinos's theories are controversial, and he has been criticized by colleagues for his stand on the importance of vitamin C just as Linus Pauling was criticized. Whether he is right or wrong, it seems reasonable to recognize the wisdom of his argument that the best time to vaccinate is when a child has been healthy for a significant period of time.

In 1974, Kulenkampff noted that some of the damaged children in her study were vaccinated during "recurring intercurrent infection." In 1981, Cavanaugh described three cases of infants infected with a virus at the time of DPT vaccination who ended up with paralysis, seizures, mental retardation, and blindness. He concluded: "Although it is impossible in retrospect to determine the etiological role of each of the infective agents in causing severe encephalopathic illness, nevertheless it is possible that the severity of the illness in these children was compounded by the coincident presence of antigens of B. pertussis either occurring as a result of natural infection or as a component of the vaccine." Cavanaugh went on to recommend: "In administering vaccines of any kind, care should be taken to exclude the likelihood of infection in the child, his family or other close contacts."

A particular danger exists when a child is vaccinated with pertussis vaccine and is coming down with whooping cough or is recovering from it. The problem is particularly difficult when the disease is atypical and the child does not have the characteristic whoop. Ehrengut noted in a 1974 article that inoculating children with pertussis vaccine when the disease is in the incubation stage can increase the chance of an adverse reaction and brain damage. In 1947, Brody reported a case in which an infant may have been vaccinated while sick with an atypical case of whooping cough. He suffered a severe neurological reaction to the vaccination and eventually died after several more injections of the vaccine.

Leigh came down with viral meningitis at the age of two months and was sent home after a five-day hospitalization. Even though she did not have bacterial meningitis, the doctors had placed her on antibiotics. She then began to have diarrhea.

"The doctors said her diarrhea was from the antibiotics she got in the hospital," her mother said. "And she also came down with two colds in the month following her hospitalization. But we were really happy because she wasn't damaged in any way from the meningitis. She was starting to reach for the side pads on her changing table, and she would lie on her back and swing her arms back and forth and giggle."

Barely three and a half weeks after Leigh's bout with meningitis, her doctor administered the first DPT shot. Leigh's mother was worried about it because Leigh had caught a cold four days earlier and still was occasionally having diarrhea.

"I knew of a little girl who had been retarded by the vaccine, and I told my doctor that while I didn't want Leigh to have another horrendous disease, I was worried about the shot. I told him she had just come down with a cold. He asked me if she still had a fever, and I said no. He said, 'Well, I don't think it will be any problem then.' He added that kids who are in danger of reacting to the shot are those with prior neurological problems.

"I asked him if he didn't think her meningitis counted as a neurological problem. But he said, 'The kind of problem I am talking about is a permanent one. They have something going on with them neurologically, and the shot just makes them worse. Leigh certainly seems fine to me, so we don't have to worry about it.' "

Leigh's mother remembers what happened after they got home. "A little more than an hour after Leigh had the shot, she started crying hard. Then she had violent explosions of gas. At the same time, the site of her injection swelled up. It was a huge, swollen area. Then she started screaming.

"She screamed for sixteen hours nonstop. Her scream sounded so painful, I thought she had meningitis again. She finally got a little sleep the next morning, but she literally cried for sixteen hours without stopping. After she woke up, she cried on and off for two more days and nights."

Within the next few days, Leigh began clenching her fists, bending her elbows, and turning her arms inward to her body. She was no longer able to stretch her arms out in front of her or over to her side. She did not sit until she was twelve months old or try to crawl until she was fourteen months old. Now she is almost three and cannot talk. She has been diagnosed as mentally retarded.

"A neurologist told me that, unless she had a grand mal seizure within twenty-four to forty-eight hours of the shot, they don't consider it a causal relationship. Since Leigh was due for her second DPT shot, I called my pediatrician in a panic. He just laughed at what the neurologist said and told me that Leigh would only get the DT from then on."

Would Leigh be mentally retarded today if she had not received her DPT shot while she had a cold and diarrhea, and had recovered from viral meningitis only three and a half weeks before?

A Family Member Who Has Reacted to the DPT Shot

In 1983, the Interagency Group to Monitor Vaccine Development, Production and Usage echoed Steinman's view: "The possibility that adverse reactions to routine immunization may be under genetic control seems novel." This attitude is puzzling in view of the impressive number of statements made by vaccine researchers for decades that

DPT reactions are "idiosyncratic" responses, in that they are under genetic control.

As mentioned previously, in 1946 Werne and Garrow reported the deaths of identical twins within twenty-four hours of their second diphtheria-pertussis shot. The same outcome in identical twins is strong evidence of a genetic predisposition. And not only has the possibility of such genetic or constitutional predisposition been mentioned frequently in the literature, it has also been evidenced in reports of several vaccine-damaged children in a single family.

After analyzing a group of infants who became ill after pertussis vaccination, Hopper noted, "This evidence suggests that the cause of this illness following pertussis vaccination is handed down from the preceding generations, just as many other traits are." Halpern and Halpern mentioned "constitutional peculiarities of the patients themselves" as causal factors.

Ström referred to a "certain individual predisposition." Kulenkampff reported a case of reactions in identical twins, where one became temporarily blind and then mentally retarded while the other died in status epilepticus. She suggested that the reactions may be due to an "idiosyncratic response." Ehrengut also mentioned reactions by identical twins, indicating "genetic predisposition."

In 1982, Linthicum and his coworkers used B. pertussis to deliberately cause acute autoimmune encephalomyelitis. They found that strains of mice can be inbred to resist the capacity of B. pertussis to cause encephalomyelitis, suggesting that this feature is under genetic control.

As Sutherland wrote in 1953, "A constitutional tendency or an individual susceptibility is sometimes postulated. This view is not at variance with the widely held belief that an allergic or pathergic state of the nervous system is responsible. Such a state may be an expression of previous specific or non-specific sensitization."

Pittman wrote in 1970, "There remains the likelihood that pertussis vaccine does cause on rare occasions a neurological reaction in a child with an individual predisposition. The nature of the reactive factor is unknown." And the 1979 Bacterial Vaccines Panel reported, "Some reactions are intrinsic to the process of human immunization and range from psychic trauma to fatal idiosyncratic reactions that are extremely rare and are an unavoidable hazard of introducing foreign substances into humans."

The important problem of how to screen children for genetic pre-disposition is being worked on in England where researchers are trying to find a genetic marker in children who develop complications from the pertussis vaccine. Steinman is also further investigating the question of genetic predisposition.

Obviously, many factors must come together to predispose an infant to react violently to the DPT shot. In a child without genetic predisposition, even poor health may not lead to a severe reaction. If such a child is in good health with a well-developed neurological system, even the presence of a milk allergy may not tip the scales and trigger a pronounced reaction. But some combination of prematurity, low birth weight, underdeveloped neurological system, a personal or family history of convulsions, neurological disease, severe allergies, a recent or present infection plus the pertussis vaccine, may be sufficient to bring on early death or a lifetime of uncontrollable seizures, paraplegia, and mental retardation.

The reason why the Interagency Group regards the concept of genetic predisposition as "novel" may be because the idea is unwelcome. Louis Cooper, M.D., professor of pediatrics at Columbia University and chairman of the New York chapter of the AAP, stated on *The MacNeil-Lehrer Report* in 1983, "One of the problems that all of us face is that we don't know what the real indicators of risk are."

No technique yet exists for pinpointing which babies have such a genetic predisposition. This means that, for the present at least, a certain number of children may be condemned to death or permanent damage by the pertussis vaccine because of an inherent and as yet undiscoverable predisposition.

This is an idea that doctors find unpalatable. It could constitute a serious block to any program of compulsory mass vaccination. It is far more acceptable to government health officials to trace "hot lots" of vaccine than to search for the unknown numbers of babies who might be genetically vulnerable to a vaccine that is safe for so many others. And even if the key is someday found, these babies may never be saved because identifying the genetic marker may prove too costly and unwieldy to be used for screening the more than three million babies vaccinated each year.

If vaccine researchers had discovered a genetic marker twenty years ago, five members in one family might not have been affected by the vaccine. Eleven-year-old Ken is one of four children. His father had reacted severely to the DPT shot as a child. His mother's brother had his first seizure within forty-eight hours of a DPT shot and is in a mental institution with uncontrollable seizures. Ken and his three brothers and sisters ran very high fevers for days after their DPT shots, and all projectile vomited their milk formulas until they were a year old.

Ken vomited his formula the most and also had the most severe reaction to his three DPT shots. "He ran a 104-degree fever for four days in a row after his first shot and cried constantly," said his mother. "He was really sick. My mother-in-law stayed up with me the second or third night because I just didn't get any sleep. Ken was up the entire four days and nights. He had the same high fever for days after his second and third shots."

Ken has an above-average I.Q. but is learning-disabled. "He skips words and letters when he reads. When he writes, he runs all the words together so there is no spacing between words. One teacher said that he had written a report, and she couldn't read a word of it. She had him read it in class, and he read through it really fast and knew exactly what he had written. Ken enjoys sports but he is not coordinated like the other kids. He is being seen by a man who works with children who have visual perception problems."

Two of Ken's sisters, who also had high fevers for several days after their DPT shots, are also in learning disability classes, but their visual perception problems are less severe than Ken's. His youngest sister was given only one DPT shot, and she has no learning disabilities at all.

When Ken's father reacted severely to a DPT shot as a baby, his mother made a notation in his baby book about how sick he was. "My mother-in-law wrote down that he cried a lot and was very sick," Ken's mother said. "What is interesting is that he had trouble in school with reading and writing. He still has horrible handwriting."

Ken's uncle is twenty-two years old and in a mental institution. His first seizure came within forty-eight hours of a DPT shot, and they are now uncontrollable.

"They have to keep changing his medication to try and control them," Ken's mother said. "They have done all kinds of tests on my brother, and everything comes back negative. My mother talked to the administrator at the institution he is in, and he said it looked like the shot is what caused his seizures and retardation."

Ken's mother has recently changed doctors, and her new doctor agrees that the family's medical history of severe reactions to the pertussis vaccine should have exempted her other three children from being given the vaccine.

"My new doctor said that Ken should never have been given any more pertussis vaccine after the first shot when he had a 104 fever for four days. I had no trouble convincing him to not give any more pertussis vaccine to my baby. In fact, he said my baby should never have been given even one dose of pertussis vaccine because of our family history of reactions."

Ken and his sisters all had colic and projectile vomiting after drinking milk formula. Ken's was the worst.

"I tried to breastfeed him, but my nerves didn't last. All of them were on milk formula most of their infancy. They all vomited so bad that I remember deciding there was no sense in cleaning our carpets until they were older. When Ken threw up, it must have gone a foot or two across the room. If we would go to church and I would hold him on my shoulder, he would throw up on the person behind me.

"If we could prevent just one family from going through what we have gone through, we want to do it. Our whole family has been affected. What happened to my brother hurts me the most. And the fact that what happened to him could have happened to my children because we gave them the pertussis vaccine is frightening."

There are other families in America who have several pertussis vaccine-damaged children. One of the most tragic stories may be that of a family in the South who watched one son die from an adverse reaction to a DPT shot and are now watching their second son die in the same way.

"My first son, Brandon, died at nineteen months for the same reason that my son Tom is now dying. Both of my boys had fevers after the shots and then developed convulsions. Within a week of his first DPT shot, Tom began staring and making irregular movements with his hands. He would twitch and throw his hands around in ways he had never done before. Just like Brandon's were, Tom's convulsions are so bad that he keeps aspirating saliva down into his lungs, which causes pneumonia."

When Tom began having seizures after the first DPT shot, a doctor told his mother that there was a DPT connection. "The doctor said he thought Tom's problems were caused by his shot, and then he pulled out Brandon's records and said it could very well be that Brandon was damaged by the same thing. He said they both reacted the same way."

Brandon's convulsions were uncontrollable, and so are Tom's. Tom is taking three different anticonvulsants three times a day.

"Brandon died because he got so weak. He was having so many seizures he couldn't relax or eat. He finally developed chronic pneumonia, and went downhill and died at nineteen months old. Now I am watching Tom do the same thing," his mother said. "He was eight years old yesterday, and the doctors have just put a tube down his throat so we can feed him. He just lies there on the couch. He can't walk or talk or feed himself. He hardly ever cries except when he has an earache. He has a lot of ear infections. He has had seven seizures today. The last two times he has been in the hospital, they have been having to do cutdowns for I.V.'s, because his veins are so weak they can't get an I.V. in him."

Tom's mother cares for her dying son around the clock. She says she does not know how she has the strength to watch a second son die as the first one did. "Every time the doctors tell you something bad, you break down and cry all your tears out. Then you dry them and start in again with the business of living through it. When they told me I was going to have to feed him through the tube this week, I thought, I can't stand this again. I remember how I fed Brandon through a tube, too, for a while before he died. It is for Tom's benefit. You can't just let him lay there and starve to death. So you just do it."

She is afraid for her two-year-old daughter, afraid what will happen when the state insists that she be vaccinated for school. "I don't know if they can make me give it to her when she goes to school. I don't want her to get it. My oldest boy has had all his shots. He had a fever but no brain damage. Just Brandon and Tom were not able to survive the shot. But I can't take a chance on my little girl."

How many more families in America have made the sacrifice that this mother has? How many more families with several children experiencing uncontrollable seizures, learning disabilities, or physical handicaps can trace their health problems to the DPT shot?

A Child Seven Years of Age or Older

When is a child too old to be given the pertussis vaccine? The latest recommendations of the AAP, the ACIP, and vaccine manufacturers agree that a child seven years old or older should not get it. Wyeth's product insert stated, "This product should be used for the age group between two months and the seventh birthday," and the AAP as well as the government make the same recommendation in their guidelines. However, at least one doctor ignored these recommendations.

Tony was a bright, active, and alert child. Just one month shy of his eighth birthday, he was scratched by a stray cat.

"Because there is always the danger of tetanus, I called our doctor and asked him if he felt Tony needed a tetanus booster. He made an appointment for the following afternoon to have Tony receive a tetanus booster," his mother said.

Tony had reacted to his state-mandated series of DPT shots. "He always had a high fever and crying. I remember nursing his leg because it had such a big lump in it. And his crying was different than at other times. I remember being desperate when he got his shots because he didn't want me to hold him or anything. He would just scream and be so sick," recalled his mother. "I was always terrified to give him his DPT shots because of our family history of reactions. I talked to the doctors over and over again about whether or not he should have them. They always reassured me and told me that the vaccines today are not like those of years ago, that reactions are rare and I had nothing to worry about."

Tony's paternal uncle had reacted to a DPT shot with convulsions and is now severely retarded. Tony's maternal grandmother was desperately ill following a DPT shot, and nearly died.

"Under no circumstances would I have allowed my doctor to give Tony more pertussis vaccine. He knew our family history. I had talked to him on many occasions about my fear of the DPT shots. But when I took Tony that afternoon for what I thought was a tetanus booster, the doctor gave him a DPT shot without my permission. He didn't even tell me. I went home thinking Tony had been given a tetanus shot."

In the days following the shot, Tony's arm developed a pronounced red, swollen lump, and he became increasingly listless, complaining of a headache. "He began to see double and would knock over things he reached for and walk into walls or furniture. His headache got worse, and he started falling asleep at strange times, even when he was playing outside in the autumn leaves. His eyes drifted to the opposite sides of his head. When we rushed him to the doctor's office, he had to be carried. The doctor took one look at him and said he was reacting to the pertussis vaccine he had given him. He told us to get him to the hospital immediately."

Tony almost died. The myelin in his brain deteriorated. Like a stroke victim, he was totally paralyzed and unconscious for days and in Intensive Care. Fed through his nose, catheterized, and on respiratory and convulsion alert, Tony continued to worsen until steroid treatment was started. In what may have been a medical miracle, he not only lived but regained his ability to walk and speak.

Recovery was slow. He wore a patch on his eye to control double vision for nearly a year and a half. He was unable to walk unassisted for months. For several years, the damage done to the area of his brain that governs emotions caused him to laugh or cry uncontrollably at inappropriate times, and he could not control his feelings of rage.

"He was diagnosed as manic-depressive," said his mother, "and put on Lithium to control his unpredictable behavior. But the Lithium had to be discontinued because it caused liver damage. Psychomotor seizures were diagnosed as an explanation for his spaciness and inability to process information. He was on anticonvulsant medications for two years, but they destroyed his white blood cells so we had to take him off those drugs, too."

Today Tony has been diagnosed as having an auditory-processing deficit and multiple learning disabilities requiring special educational strategies. His continuing medical expenses caused his family to lose many of their assets. The threat of foreclosure and bankruptcy is always present as collection agencies harass his parents. An out-of-court settlement was negotiated with the doctor's insurance company, but because the doctor was insufficiently insured, there was little left for Tony after the legal and medical expenses.

"Tony is brain-injured from a vaccine that he should never have received," his mother said. "The child that was is no longer. His self-confidence has been damaged. He bears permanent scars, and so do we from the nightmare we have been put through and continue to live."

Because of their state's mandatory vaccination law, the family has been told that Tony's three younger siblings must have the pertussis vaccine. "My other children are not going to receive that vaccine, "said Tony's mother. "We are prepared to fight it in court. We will not allow it to happen again."

A Previous Severe Reaction to a DPT Shot

In every pediatrician's office, there should be a sign proclaiming, "DO NOT GIVE MORE PERTUSSIS VACCINE TO A CHILD WHO HAS HAD A SERIOUS REACTION TO A PREVIOUS DPT SHOT." This, above all, is the contraindication that can most easily prevent vaccine damage. Of course, it would help if doctors and manufacturers could reach agreement on the definition of a reaction and on contraindications. In addition, it would be useful if there was more emphasis in medical schools upon educating future physicians about reactions and contraindications to the DPT vaccine.

❁   ❁   ❁   ❁   ❁

If Kurt's doctors and his mother had known about the pertussis vaccine, Kurt would not be brain damaged today.

When he had the first DPT shot at four months of age, he was a normal, healthy baby, but within seven hours of the shot, he was in a grand mal convulsion. Despite medication, he continued to have seizures. He was given two more DPT shots in the second year of his life and continued to have from ten to fifteen grand mals a year.

The year after his fourth DPT shot, he had forty-four seizures. Still he continued to develop. He learned his ABCs, knew colors, and could count. A month before turning five, he had a seizure at preschool and fell down and cut his cheek. He was taken to the emergency room of the local hospital.

"The doctor was going to give him a tetanus booster, but then asked me if Kurt had had his last DPT booster. I told him no, and he gave the DPT shot to him," his mother said. "You see, all these years we had questioned the doctors about the DPT shot being connected to his original seizure but they kept telling us there was no connection. We trusted them. And yet, now that I have Kurt's medical records, I see that one of those doctors suggested he get only a half dose of DPT. But we were never told that."

In the next twenty-four hours, Kurt had ten grand mal convulsions. From that point on, his seizures were completely out of control. "I am just so grateful that Kurt learned what he did prior to that fifth DPT shot because his brain stopped developing at that point. His seizures are so violent now that his whole body goes into contortions, and his lungs are squeezed to the point where he makes loud grunting noises. His knees and legs are covered with scars where he has hurt himself.

He wears a helmet with a face guard to protect his teeth. But even so, he has already chipped one of his new front teeth. He drools really badly, and the saliva backs up into his lungs. He was just hospitalized with a strep throat."

For Kurt's mother his behavior problems can be more difficult to cope with on a day-to-day basis than his seizures. "The longer he goes without a seizure, the worse his behavior gets. It's like steam building up in the pot. When the lid blows off and he has a seizure, he calms down again. Before he has the seizure, it is like he is so mean and nasty that he will pinch or bite or kick or yell something loudly. Yet he can be the sweetest and kindest child. He is like two different people. Sometimes we pray for him to have a seizure just so he can stop being so mean. Then, when the seizures come often, we pray they will stop. It is a Catch-22."

Kurt's mother tries not to be angry or bitter toward the doctors who gave Kurt more pertussis vaccine, particularly the fifth shot. "When Kurt has had a really bad day and has hurt himself, all I can think of is 'those damn doctors, look what they have done to my son.' But I have a very strong belief in the Bible. I trust in God. We will just do the best we can with what has happened to Kurt. I have to continue to hope and believe in life, not only for Kurt but for my other children."

14

Political Immunology

> But man, proud man,
> Drest in a little brief authority,
> Most ignorant of what he's most assured,
> His glassy essence, like an angry ape,
> Plays such fantastic tricks before high heaven
> As make the angels weep.
> *William Shakespeare*

The fire that rages around the pertussis vaccine controversy has illuminated a new line of medical thought which may be called "political immunology." It is the practice of applying pressure through the press and other media for political ends, sometimes with incomplete and distorted versions of medical facts.

Since the American medical establishment long ago committed its prestige and reputation to mass vaccination programs, criticism of any vaccine stimulates strong counterattacks. The Public Health Service, American Academy of Pediatrics, and American Medical Association have money and well-organized press networks available to counter any criticism of their programs. These networks extend not only to the national press but also to practicing physicians throughout the United States.

The reaction in 1982 to the WRC-TV documentary "DPT: Vaccine Roulette" was typical of the medical establishment's rapid and effective deployment of forces to counteract bad publicity about pertussis vaccine reactions. The lead man was Timothy Johnson, M.D., who hosts a national television show and who appeared on *Good Morning America* several days after the DPT documentary. Johnson assured the parents of America that his own children had been vaccinated and so there was nothing to worry about.

Meanwhile, the Centers for Disease Control (CDC) and the AAP were preparing press releases for the national media as well as communiques for physicians throughout the country extolling the pertussis vaccine and painting a cataclysmic picture of whooping cough epidemics should parents take the television show too seriously. Information packets were sent out by the AAP to its members for presentation to their local press and community groups. In letters to radio and TV stations, it urged a "more balanced" and responsible presentation of the problem.

The FDA put out a "Talk Paper" (1982) to guide its personnel "in responding with consistency and accuracy to questions from the public" on the vaccine. *Medical World News* (1982) introduced a "new feature" entitled "Medicine and the Media." The first installment of this new feature was "Did DPT Vaccine Get Smeared on National Television?"

In December 1982, Johnson devoted his one-hour syndicated TV program, *Healthbeat*, to an attack on "DPT: Vaccine Roulette." It began with an uncharacteristically somber warning to the viewing audience: "Our program this month is very different from any we have ever done before, and from any we are likely to do in the near future," and went on to present the establishment view without even a suggestion that disagreement was possible.

Another big gun was a forty-four-page unsigned analysis of "DPT: Vaccine Roulette" issued by the FDA's Division of Bacterial Products (1982). It accused the program of "inaccuracies and imbalance" with a "potential for serious harm" and charged, "It seems likely that parents' confidence may not only have been shaken about pertussis vaccine but also about vaccination programs in general."

The defensive counterattack mounted by the vaccine establishment succeeded in blunting the impact of the vaccine documentary. The NBC network chose not to air the show nationally in prime time. WRC-TV distributed copies to NBC affiliates throughout the country, but some states have never had the documentary shown in its entirety anywhere within their borders.

Press releases issued to the national print media, and warnings of impending whooping cough epidemics should parents be further alarmed about pertussis vaccine reactions, have successfully kept the news about reactions out of magazines and newspapers. Asked in December 1983 why she thought the story had not been picked up by more of the U.S. media, Lea Thompson, the producer of "DPT: Vaccine Roulette," replied:

"I feel the American press has not picked up on this story more in the print media because doctors have squelched it. There is no question in my mind that is what has happened. The AAP put out the word the day we did our story that the story was inaccurate and not to worry. When a reporter calls a local doctor or hospital or medical center, he speaks to doctors who have been told by the AAP and AMA not to worry. To my knowledge, pediatricians in this country have heard absolutely nothing from the AAP on DPT since then."

Discrediting Vaccine Critics

A favorite strategy of political immunology is name-calling of individuals who point out vaccine risks. This is what happened to Lea Thompson. In the desire to cast doubt upon the validity of her report on vaccine risks, doctors and health officials attacked her professional credentials.

The diatribe unleashed against her by members of the medical establishment approached libel and slander. The *Journal of the American Medical Association* in July 1982 stated, "Officially acknowledged experts on pertussis and DPT describe the NBC presentation as 'the most frightening bit of show business journalism I've ever seen,' 'biased, histrionic and inaccurate,' and even 'amoral and psychopathic.'"

William H. Foege, director of the CDC, testified at Senate hearings called by Senator Paula Hawkins (1982), "If journalistic malpractice were a recognized entity, I think the program would qualify." He called it "distorted, verging on the irresponsible. . . . it appears that attempts are being made to provoke a major controversy where one does not currently exist."

Vincent Fulginiti, M.D., chairman of the AAP Red Book Committee, testified at the same hearing on funding of childhood vaccinations. He devoted five out of seven pages of his statement to criticizing "DPT: Vaccine Roulette" and charged the program with an "unbalanced view —bias, in my view—and inaccuracies to carry its destructive message. . . . not an example of responsible journalism."

The FDA's own in-house critique of the show said that the program was "characterized by misinformation and reliance upon the opinions of 'experts' with exaggerated credentials who do not reflect the consensus of health officials in the United States or the rest of the world."

Another tactic of political immunologists is discrediting individuals who question the safety of the vaccine because they are not M.D.'s or Ph.D.'s. "You aren't a doctor," they say, implying that only a bona fide physician or scientist has the intellectual ability and requisite knowledge to understand the complexities of the pertussis vaccine issue. Laymen, they suggest, should not be interfering.

Timothy Johnson implied that Lea Thompson had not done her homework on the issue, was not qualified to discuss it, and was acting irresponsibly when she dared bring the matter to public attention. He told her on the television show, *Panorama*: "I do not attempt to react to the wire copy coming off the news room. I'll get calls from our news room in Boston saying there's a story coming in over the wire. 'Would you please come in and comment on it?' I'll say, 'No way I can do it until I've had a chance to study it, find out all of the background and details.' A day or two later I may be prepared to do so. But I think it's very dangerous, when you're giving advice that can affect people's lives, to react in a very instant sort of off-the-cuff or immediate way. I'll leave that up to brave reporters, but I prefer to wait until we can assimilate the information."

Lea Thompson responded that she and her staff had worked forty hours a week for more than a year on the documentary, and added, "I don't know that, really, health matters are so much different from other journalistic endeavors." Johnson answered, "Ideally, they shouldn't be, but in practical ways they do work out often to be, because of their profound effects on life and death."

The implication is that doctors have the sole right to deal with matters of life and death and that those not possessing a medical degree should not interfere. This tactic is usually employed to deflect attention from an area in which the medical establishment has bodies buried. But, no matter how hard the AAP, FDA, AMA, CDC, and the state health departments tried to prevent the public from being further informed about the pertussis vaccine, they could not stop parents from coming forward with their vaccine-damaged children.

Dissatisfied Parents Together (DPT)

Within a matter of days after "DPT: Vaccine Roulette" was broadcast in Washington, a group of parents in that city banded together to form Dissatisfied Parents Together (DPT) with the goals of gathering information about pertussis and the pertussis vaccine, getting that information out to parents, and finding ways to lessen pertussis vaccine damage. The parent group worked with Congressman Dan Mica (D-Fla.) and Senator Paula Hawkins (R-Fla.) to force the Department of Health and Human Services (HHS) to conduct a study of the pertussis vaccine.

The study, which HHS submitted to the Senate Labor and Human Resources Committee at a July 22, 1983, hearing, was criticized by DPT president Jeff Schwartz as "subtly, but perniciously slanted" to maximize the benefit of the vaccine and minimize its risks. He added, "HHS is clearly just trying to buy time and hopes the issue goes away." He did note later on the *MacNeil-Lehrer Report*, however, that "What's right with it is that it, for the first time, puts the Health and Human Services Department on record as acknowledging that there's a problem with the vaccine."

After networking with thousands of parents across the nation who wrote to the organization for more information, many of whom reported cases of vaccine damage, DPT met with the AAP to develop recommendations for a compensation bill that would provide financial support for the unknown numbers of American vaccine-damaged children and their parents. After eight months of difficult and sometimes heated discussions, the wording of a bill was made final and Senator Hawkins introduced the National Childhood Vaccine-Injury Compensation Act (S-2117) in November 1983.

During discussions with the AAP, DPT representatives described cases of vaccine damage reported to them by parents across the country. At one meeting, at which doctors sitting on the vaccine policy-making Red Book Committee were present, there was an argument about the definition of a vaccine reaction. A frequent statement made by the doctors present was that the vaccine damage cases reported by the parent group were merely "anecdotal."

Philip Brunell, M.D., chairman of the Red Book Committee, said, "You just can't keep citing anecdotal cases of what you believe to be pertussis vaccine damage and state with any certainty that they were in fact due to the pertussis vaccine. You just can't do that. . . . There has to be hard, scientific data backing up the cases. The data you have collected is history, it is not science. There is no way you can prove that a child was damaged by the vaccine. There may have been other factors which caused the damage."

An officer of DPT countered, "I would think that common sense and intelligence would prevail, that anyone with common sense and intelligence could see there is cause and effect here." NIH neurologist Karin Nelson, M.D., replied, "That's not true. You have to have a controlled study, a prospective study." But Georges Peter, M.D., did note with perception and humor, "When DPT presents case histories it is called anecdotal data but when doctors do it, it is called clinical observation."

A Tyranny of Biostatisticians

Today, describing what happens to a child after he receives a DPT shot is generally considered "bad science." "Good science" is defined in terms of "prospective" or "retrospective" studies which abstract the numbers of vaccine-damaged children into statistical analyses.

Kevin Geraghty, M.D., calls this "a tyranny of biostatisticians prematurely making decisions as to rights and wrongs." Although the study of individual case histories has been the cornerstone of medicine for hundreds of years, the practice is currently out of fashion. What a piece of luck for vaccine researchers who can in all good conscience abstract away the descriptions of death and suffering that parents tell and retell in wrenching detail about their children's reactions to the DPT shot.

As Timothy Johnson pointed out, "The hallmark of science vs. nonscience is that it deals with broad statistical analyses rather than individual case reports, what we call anecdotal evidence. . . . We have to do a broad-scale study, a so-called double blind study . . . draw the inferences and give advice based on statistical studies."

Yet "double-blind" and "randomized" studies with "control groups" cannot be conducted unless the researcher first knows and defines the subjects to be studied in all their dimensions. F. S. C. Northrop, of Yale University, one of the twentieth century's leading philosophers of science, has written that the first stage of any scientific investigation must be the collection and description of the facts to be analyzed. If this stage is skipped over, "the result inevitably is immature, half-baked, dogmatic, and for the most part worthless theory." The facts in this instance are nothing more than the case histories of children who have become ill following a DPT shot, and this stage of clinical investigation has been virtually omitted in connection with the pertussis vaccine.

Political immunology does not appear to have room for the "shoe-leather epidemiology" advocated by Gordon Stewart, which requires medical researchers to get out into the population and talk one to one with parents of vaccine-injured children. It is an uncomfortable task for doctors to interview parents whose children have been injured by a procedure recommended for almost half a century. Nevertheless, there seems to be a lack of interest and failure to explore such case histories which reveals an unsophisticated understanding of scientific method.

Are parents really to believe in large-scale statistical studies when they know that those conducting the study failed to explore the details of each case? Are parents to stop worrying about their children dying or becoming brain damaged after a DPT shot because, upon the basis of "double-blind" and "controlled" studies, doctors proclaim the benefits of the pertussis vaccine clearly outweigh the risks? Will parents continue to be pacified by doctors who dismiss as "anecdotal" their descriptions of the devastating injuries their once-normal children sustained shortly after receiving a DPT shot?

Another tactic used by doctors determined to defend the pertussis vaccine is to ask, "So what else is new?" Timothy Johnson hastened to reassure mothers that "immunization experts and physicians have long been aware that the pertussis component of the DPT shot is not perfect. It does cause minor side reactions in quite a few children and occasionally causes a serious side reaction." The *Journal of the American Medical Association* (1982) assured the nation that "to health professionals, of course, the dangers of DPT are nothing new. . . . The whole cell 'P' component, consisting of four units of protective pertussis antigen per 0.5 ml. of DTP, is universally acknowledged to be relatively crude and toxic."

It is not clear why anyone should be comforted by the knowledge that the medical establishment has long known about the vaccine's dangers without doing anything about it. But all of these standard arguments, which have become synonymous with political immunology, are being used on the American public. When they fail to impress, more serious ones are advanced.

Coincidental Death or Convulsion?

The first establishment argument is what Geraghty calls the "Well, it could have been 'coincidental' routine." Is someone claiming that the pertussis vaccine causes convulsions? Political immunologists answer that convulsions occur all the time in unvaccinated children; there is no proof the DPT shot caused the convulsion, there is only a "temporal" (time-related) association with the shot.

A report by the Interagency Group to Monitor Vaccine Production, Development and Usage stated in 1983, "Many medical conditions which occur spontaneously in infants may occur in association with pertussis vaccination by chance alone. Nearly 5 percent of all children will have a seizure before reaching the seventh birthday. Thus the highest incidence of febrile and nonfebrile seizures coincides with the period during which pertussis vaccine is administered."

A press release issued by the AAP to pediatricians and the news media after "DPT: Vaccine Roulette" was broadcast said, "Frequently only a temporal association is noted between reaction and vaccine administration, with no proof that pertussis vaccine caused the reaction." And D. L. Miller and E. M. Ross stated (1982), "An association of the two events in time cannot be accepted as evidence of a causal relationship without adequate clinical information and control data. . . ."

CDC director William H. Foege asserted (1982) that the same is true for brain damage: "Encephalopathy occurs in young children without any identifiable precipitating factor, and the fact that an event follows vaccination does not prove that it was caused by the vaccination."

The argument that these relationships are only "temporal" and not causal is vulnerable for two reasons.

In the first place, it cannot be demonstrated that so-called "spontaneous" convulsions occur as frequently in large groups of unvaccinated American children as in vaccinated children since, for the past twenty years, almost every child in the U.S. has been vaccinated. Under these circumstances, there is no group to study in order to prove that convulsions and brain damage occur in large unvaccinated groups of American children as frequently as in vaccinated groups. At present, therefore, scientists have no way of knowing what role the pertussis vaccine plays in the background incidence of convulsions in American children.

At a February 1983 meeting with representatives from Dissatisfied Parents Together, Alan Hinman, director of Immunization Services for the CDC, admitted that it is impossible to estimate the incidence of "spontaneous" convulsions in the United States. He was asked, "How can you say that convulsions occur spontaneously in the U.S. population in the first six months of life, when for the past twenty years, the acceptance rate for DPT vaccine has been more than 90 percent?" Dr. Hinman replied, after a long pause: "I suppose that is true. We would have to go over to a Third World country, a country where there was a virgin population and make a comparison."

Technically, even this is not true. The unvaccinated population in a Third World country would not have the standard of living, nutrition, or medical care prevalent in the United States. This would affect the general health of newborns and influence the incidence of "spontaneous convulsions."

The second reason why the "temporal relationship" argument is vulnerable is that truly "spontaneous" convulsions or other neurological symptoms will occur randomly throughout a given time period and will not be clustered in the hours or days immediately following the DPT shot. Wolfgang Ehrengut (1974) has shown that in Hamburg, West Germany, this clustering effect was 2.5 times more frequent than would be expected if the seizures were purely spontaneous. Ehrengut has also observed that the same child often reacts with a seizure to each successive DPT shot. When the same baby reacts to two or more shots in succession, the probability of these reactions being "spontaneous" shrinks to one in several million, according to Gordon Stewart (1978).

The argument that seizures are not caused by the vaccine, but only happen to occur at a time when the vaccine is given, does not stand up. But political immunology has a fall-back position: the vaccine does not actually "cause" seizures, but only "triggers" them. Since a certain number of babies born each year are doomed to have convulsions and brain damage anyway, the DPT vaccine only brings on the inevitable. This argument is put forth in an attempt to explain the clustering of seizures after the DPT shot.

A. H. Griffith, M.D., who works for a large British pertussis vaccine manufacturer, summarized this way of thinking in 1982: "What happened was that the act of vaccination brought forward in the first week what would have occurred during the second, third, and fourth week. Instead of having a straight-line background incidence, you brought forward by vaccination a clustering. . . ."

Griffith continued, "The children who have a history, who are prone, who are likely to have neurological effects . . . are the ones that are liable to be precipitated into neurological consequences earlier than they would otherwise. . . . That child is susceptible to convulsions, which he is inevitably going to get in any case, but which the vaccine has brought forward. . . . it is the child who is susceptible and not the vaccine actually causing it."

Bellman, Ross, and Miller made the same argument in connection with infantile spasms (1983): they found a clustering of infantile spasms within a week of vaccination, a higher incidence than would have normally been expected, and concluded that these children were "destined" to have infantile spasms, that the vaccine only "triggered" an earlier onset.

This is an example of how intelligent and well-intentioned physicians and scientists can be misled into ignoring facts; for if the vaccine can precipitate a seizure in a susceptible child, then it is causing that seizure. There is no way of proving that a child who has a seizure after a DPT shot would have had that seizure without receiving the shot.

The "it could have been coincidental" routine is carried to an extreme in connection with Sudden Infant Death Syndrome (SIDS). D. L. Miller and Euan M. Ross, of the University of London, Middlesex Hospital Medical School, wrote in 1982 to the *British Medical Journal*, "A few infant deaths can be expected to occur purely by chance after a procedure as common as immunization. It could be shown, for instance, that on a plausible set of assumptions, seven sudden infant deaths might be expected to occur each year within a week of an event such as a child's christening."

And the CDC stated (1981): "In countries where immunizations with pertussis antigen-containing vaccines are started at six months of age, the age distribution of SIDS is the same as that reported in the United States." The statement implies that the U.S. policy of vaccinating babies at two and four months of age does not increase SIDS deaths at those ages; but upon what scientific evidence is this statement based?

An inquiry to the CDC prompted the reply that this widely quoted statement relies on one study done in Northern Ireland in 1970, involving 148 cases and 148 matched controls.

It might be thought that this study was an investigation of the effect of vaccination on SIDS. In fact, while examining many other factors thought to contribute to sudden infant death, the study did not even look at the vaccination histories of these 296 infants.

A check of the vaccination recommendations in force in 1970 in Northern Ireland reveals that they specified "The earliest age at which the first dose should be given is three months, but a better general immunological response can be expected if the first dose is delayed to six months of age." Since this factor was not investigated, no information is available on when these infants were actually vaccinated. All that can be said is that they were presumably being vaccinated at between three and six months of age, not exclusively at six months of age. The SIDS incidence in Northern Ireland, therefore, could very well have been influenced by the pertussis vaccine.

Furthermore, the authors found "an absence of epidemicity as measured by temporal and space-time clustering methods," which contrasts with Torch's conclusion that, in his own study, "SIDS frequencies peaked at age 2 months in the non-DPT group, and had a biphasic peak occurrence at 2 and 4 months in the DPT group."

What does all of this mean for the CDC's statement about SIDS? Is it an example of deception or simply mishandling of the facts? What is needed is an estimate of the incidence of infant deaths in an unvaccinated population in America. This is not known.

Convulsions and unexplained infant deaths have been occurring in children for hundreds of years. They long preceded the introduction of the pertussis vaccine. Obviously, no one suggests that all convulsions and sudden deaths in infants are due to the pertussis vaccine. It is being suggested, however, that *some* convulsions and sudden deaths are due to the vaccine. The important issue still unresolved is whether or not the "relatively crude and toxic" pertussis vaccine adds to the existing background incidence of "spontaneous convulsions" and sudden unexplained infant deaths.

One way to obtain this information would be to start vaccinating American babies at seven months of age or later. (After 1975, the Japanese did not vaccinate their children with pertussis vaccine until two years of age.) This would give medical researchers a way to compare the incidence of sudden infant deaths and infant seizures in millions of babies in years when they were vaccinated at two, four, and six months of age versus years when they were vaccinated at seven months of age or later. This change in the age of vaccination would generate data to help clarify the broad statistical relationship between the DPT shot and unexplained infant deaths, convulsions, and brain damage.

Bad Logic, Bad Science, Bad Medicine

One reason why physicians and scientists can deny a connection between the pertussis vaccine and death, illness, or injury is because medicine has not pathologically defined vaccine damage. As R. J. Robinson, M.D., explained (1981), "There is no specific syndrome which follows pertussis immunization and which does not occur in unimmunized children. Without figures on the background incidence of acute neurological disorders in childhood, it is therefore impossible to be certain whether an apparent connection with immunization is genuinely causal or merely coincidental."

T. M. Pollack and Jean Morris agreed and stated (1982), "The neurological disorders reported . . . as reactions to DPT were too widely divergent to suggest a common etiological agent. Taken individually, since such disorders are known to occur in unvaccinated children, none could with any confidence be attributed to the vaccine."

The lack of a specific test or recognized pathological profile to prove the relationship between vaccination and damage suffered by certain babies provides much room in political immunology for maneuvering and self-protection. If it is asserted that the vaccine does produce a definable range of negative effects, a "pertussis vaccine syndrome," then vaccine promoters say this cannot be demonstrated with pathological evidence. Yet they turn around and rely on pathological evidence to demonstrate that the vaccine did not cause the injury a child sustained after a DPT shot. For instance, John Robbins of the FDA stated in 1982: "Many cases of encephalopathy that were ascribed to pertussis vaccine were not, in fact; when careful pathologic examination was done, [it was] shown that the cause was another definable cause of central nervous system damage."

This is bad logic, bad science, and bad medicine. If the vaccine works on the body in ways science and medicine admit they have not been able to determine, then physicians cannot rule out a connection between a given illness and the vaccine. If pathological alterations are found on autopsy, there is no way to demonstrate that the vaccine did not cause them or contribute to them. This is especially true of SIDS deaths, where political immunology again takes on Alice-in-Wonderland dimensions.

The cause of SIDS is unknown. If the cause is unknown, then how can doctors rule out the possibility that vaccination was either the direct cause or at least a contributing cause in cases where the only common denominator was death? And yet Alan Hinman was quoted in the *Journal of the American Medical Association* (1982) as stating: "We have received reports of 44 deaths occurring within four weeks of DPT immunization. Thirty-two of the deaths were SIDS. Of the other twelve, in only one was there autopsy or clinical information that would indicate that this was a neurologic or encephalopathic response to DPT."

The Abuse of Statistics and SIDS in Tennessee

Another important technique of political immunology is the abuse of statistics. Modern medicine makes extensive use of statistical relationships in cases where no direct causal connection can be demonstrated by pathological or other evidence. Pertussis vaccine damage, which has yet to be reliably demonstrated pathologically, offers an obvious opportunity for the use of statistics to demonstrate cause and effect.

But when statistics are applied to the study of vaccines, political immunology demonstrates its infinite flexibility: statistical evidence demonstrating cause and effect is denied when this same evidence, applied to any other branch of medicine, would be accepted without question. For instance, the FDA document criticizing "DPT: Vaccine Roulette" (1982) maintained that "a statistically significant temporal association between two variables such as neurologic disease and immunization with pertussis vaccine does not necessarily prove that they are causally related. A causal relationship between DPT immunization and permanent brain damage would be supported by the finding that the illnesses were clinically distinctive, restricted to immunized children, closely related in time to immunization, associated with a biologically plausible hypothesis and without other causes."

This convenient reasoning was displayed with particular clarity in connection with the government's investigation of SIDS deaths in Tennessee. In 1978–79, eleven babies were found to have died within eight days of a DPT vaccination. Nine of the eleven had been vaccinated from the same lot of pertussis vaccine, Wyeth #64201, and five (four from the same lot) had died within twenty-four hours of vaccination.

A statistical analysis of the clustering of deaths revealed that the likelihood of observing four or more deaths occurring randomly on any of the first eight days after the use of lot #64201 was 3 in 100. This meant that such a clustering could occur purely by chance only 3 in 100 times.

In statistics a causal relationship is strongly suggested when only 5 out of 100 given events could have occurred by chance (meaning 95 out of 100 events did not occur by chance). In the Tennessee deaths, the possibility of random association with the vaccine was not 5 in 100 but 3 in 100. In fact, E. B. Mortimer, M.D., later reported that the probability of this being a chance association was even lower—between 2 and 5 in 1,000. And Daniel Shannon, M.D., thought it was even lower than that—between 4 and 5 in 10,000.

The statistical evidence in favor of a connection between the deaths and the DPT shot was strong. Would the medical authorities bite the bullet and admit that the vaccine was related to the deaths? Absolutely not.

An examination of the attempt to deal with this very unpleasant bit of statistical data tells much about the thought processes of political immunologists. At a March 19, 1979, meeting on the subject at the FDA Bureau of Biologics, one of the Tennessee public health officials called attention to "an apparent clustering of cases with the suspect lot shortly after vaccination."

The gathering of physicians and federal public health officials went over the ramifications of the situation during several hours of discussion. At one point Richard Naeye, M.D., asked, "I personally would know how to recommend if I knew . . . what would be apt to happen if the lot was withdrawn in terms of public reaction." After this question was asked, there was a discussion of the "swine flu" epidemic and Guillain-Barre syndrome, and CDC's Alan Hinman observed, "There remains a considerable body of feeling that there has been a major negative impact on immunizations in general."

Naeye then replied, "But the Guillain-Barré thing did not really touch the childhood population, did it? So, if we are going to balance a very small number of deaths, maybe one or two, against what may be a large number of deaths if the whole populace is suddenly sensitized to the fact that DPT might kill, then, you see, it gets to be a different issue. I think we are dealing with so little data here that it is going to be a very hard decision."

Hinman answered, "Obviously it is a very hard decision, or one presumes if it were an easy decision, it would have been made already."

CDC's Bernier added, "Are you suggesting that there might be, because of a reduced acceptance of DPT immunization, there might be a subsequent increase in deaths in that age group?"

Naeye replied, "Yes, due to pertussis, for example, right?"

After a short discussion of the British epidemic, Timothy Dondero, M.D., of the Tennessee State Department of Health, continued, "There are obviously political implications in this. What if this gets into the press?"

Toward the end of the meeting, FDA's John Robbins, in what appeared to be the consensus of participants, stated, "I think if we do make a decision that is hasty and not based upon sound data, then there will be enormous consequences to our whole program to consider."

The gathering of physicians did not recommend that the suspect vaccine lot be withdrawn from the market, perhaps heeding the suggestion of Jerome Klein, M.D., that "If a specific recommendation is made to remove this lot . . . the subsequent question that must be asked, we will be facing for a long time . . . and that is the present recommendations for immunization during the first year of life." So, instead, the group adopted a consensus statement drafted by Klein stating that "the most prudent course at this time would be to develop more information."

Meanwhile, the CDC announced, "The events in Tennessee raise questions for which we have no ready answers."

In fact, there *were* answers. At one point in the FDA meeting, the participants had discussed Shannon's work on the use of breathing monitors with "near-miss" SIDS cases (see Chapter 5) and Naeye observed: "When Dr. Shannon finally is able to get all his data out and publish it, it is going to haunt everybody, because the whole issue of immunizing children at high risk is going to be very, very pointed. . . . What is the manufacturer going to do? What is anybody going to do when Dr.

Shannon finally publishes his data, assuming it is correct? Everybody is going to be on a very hot seat, it seems to me. . . ."

On April 26, a meeting was held at the CDC headquarters in Atlanta to again discuss the Tennessee deaths. At the end of it, all the participants were provided with questionnaires and asked to answer in writing the question: "Is there adequate evidence of meaningful association between DPT vaccine lot 64201 and sudden infant death in Tennessee?"

After the answers had been received in June, CDC director Foege wrote a memo to the Surgeon General stating that the experts "did not feel that a causal relationship had been established between vaccination with DPT from Wyeth's lot 64201 and sudden infant death in infancy. However they did not feel that a causal relationship could be totally excluded." He urged that interviews be conducted with the parents of the infants who had died.

Foege concluded his report, however, by stating, "A suspicious clustering occurred, but there is no reason to believe that there was a direct causal relationship between vaccination with DPT vaccine Wyeth lot 64201 and the occurrence of sudden deaths in infancy." He did not indicate how the conclusion of the experts was to be reconciled with his own rather different interpretation of the events.

Three weeks later, Foege's interpretation of the events stated in this memo to the Surgeon General was used by Harry Meyer, Director of the FDA Bureau of Biologics, as evidence to oppose a request by Wyeth Laboratories to list among its pertussis vaccine contraindications circumstances thought to predispose to SIDS. Meyer told Wyeth in a July 11 letter, "While SIDS has been reported after administration of DPT vaccine, expert groups who recently reviewed the data did not find evidence of a cause-effect relationship."

Meyer found "particularly pertinent" Foege's statement that "there is no reason to believe that there was a direct causal relationship between vaccination with DPT Vaccine Lot 64201 and the occurrence of sudden death in infancy." Meyer advised Wyeth: "Based on the available data we do not see a medical basis for listing circumstances thought to predispose to SIDS as contraindications to the use of DPT vaccine. We do not agree, therefore, with your proposal on page 2 of the circular under 'Contraindications.' There is no evidence that such a change would prevent SIDS. . . ."

Wyeth yielded to Meyer's objection and dropped its proposal to include circumstances thought to predispose to SIDS as a contraindication to the pertussis vaccine.

Meanwhile, Wyeth withdrew its suspect lot 64201 from the market. This was done "out of an abundance of caution," reported *The New York Times*.

The investigation of Wyeth Lot 64201 was a striking example of political immunology's ability to draw conclusions from facts which do not seem to support that conclusion. Initially, the experts "did not feel that a causal relationship could be totally excluded." But after passage through several FDA and CDC memoranda, this doubt had been transformed into Meyer's statement that "experts . . . did not find evidence of a cause-effect relationship." In August 1982, Hinman was quoted by a news service as stating that the SIDS cases in Tennessee were all a "coincidence."

Almost incomprehensibly, a series of CDC meetings on SIDS deaths in Tennessee, which should have served to stimulate increased investigation into deaths occurring shortly after DPT shots, was actually used as justification for limiting contraindications to the pertussis vaccine and minimizing the connection between the vaccine and infant death. When the CDC's "Important Information" form for parents was revised the following year in 1980, it no longer told parents that after a DPT shot "death may occur . . ." but now read "Sudden unexplained infant deaths have occurred rarely after vaccination, but it is not known whether this has been caused by the vaccine."

The tombstone was placed on what happened in Tennessee three years later, in the September 1982 issue of the *Journal of Pediatrics*, when Bernier and his colleagues at the CDC wrote their epitaph on the infant deaths. To prepare readers, the editors announced, "The *Journal* has always attempted to publish promptly any article of unusual importance or current interest . . . articles that are particularly timely or that contain information of potential immediate importance to the health of children. . . . The following paper was selected for prompt publication."

Three years later? After another ten million children had received the vaccine? But what did the Bernier article state? While noting that there were only 3 chances in 100 that this clustering of SIDS deaths could occur randomly after a DPT shot, the authors concluded, "This evidence seems adequate to indicate an unusual temporal association between DPT vaccination with lot A [i.e., lot 64201] and SIDS." They then made this amazing statement: "Whether or not this temporal association reflects a causal relationship remains undetermined; we found no evidence to support such a causal relationship."

What evidence were they looking for, having already rejected evidence demonstrating statistical significance? They sagely remarked that "the question of whether or not lot A was causally associated with the deaths observed was examined in light of the more general question of whether or not any DPT vaccine can cause sudden infant deaths." Rather than trying to determine whether Lot 64201 caused these deaths, the researchers refused to draw any conclusions on this point without first resolving the general question of whether the vaccine can cause infant death in any case.

Bernier and his colleagues went on to rationalize, "Anecdotal evidence from foreign countries where different DPT vaccination schedules were used beginning at later infant ages . . . does not suggest an association between DPT and SIDS because the age-distribution curves of SIDS cases are similar, even though vaccination patterns are quite different." Were they talking about the Northern Ireland study again— the one that does not support the argument? And why is it scientifically acceptable to use "anecdotal evidence" to disprove a relationship between DPT and SIDS but not acceptable to use "anecdotal evidence" to prove that relationship?

The authors concluded, "More importantly, preliminary data from a National Institutes of Health-sponsored, multicenter, case control study on SIDS have failed to show any increased frequency of DPT vaccination among SIDS cases when compared to matched controls. The findings of our study, combined with the NIH results, provide no support for reducing efforts to immunize infants with DPT."

Why was this article analyzing the Tennessee SIDS deaths not published for three years? Could it have been to wait for the brand-new NIH study which was not designed to provide new information about the vaccine and SIDS, but to prove that the political immunologists had been right all along? But what about this new SIDS study?

The Cooperative Epidemiologic Study of SIDS Risk Factors conducted by the National Institute of Child Health and Human Development (NICHD) used a method called the "retrospective case-control technique." NIH collected a series of four hundred cases of SIDS from various regions in the United States over a fifteen-month period from October 1978 to December 1979. For each child who died a SIDS death, two living children or "matched controls" were selected. Each pair of controls was "matched" with each dead infant for birth date, birth weight, and race.

When the vaccination histories of the two groups were compared, it was found that 62 percent of the SIDS cases had never been vaccinated, while of the "controls" only 44 percent had not been vaccinated. This was supposed to "strongly support the view that DPT immunization is not a factor in the etiology of SIDS," and CDC Director Walter Dowdle stated this in testimony before a Congressional Committee on July 22, 1983.

But does it really? Obviously the 62 percent of SIDS cases who were never vaccinated could not have died from the vaccine. But what about the 38 percent of SIDS cases who were vaccinated? As Geraghty pointed out, "The study clearly answers the question as to whether DPT vaccine causes all SIDS events. The answer is obviously no. . . . The question as to whether certain SIDS events could be DPT causally related—a much more technically demanding proposal—is far more germane."

SIDS undoubtedly is due to a variety of causes, of which the DPT shot is only one. And yet the NIH SIDS study treated all the SIDS deaths as a uniform, homogeneous group.

Babies vary greatly from one another. In addition to different dates of birth, weights, and races, they have different birth histories, genetic predispositions, and other constitutional variables. Some may be more vulnerable to the pertussis vaccine, and others less so. And yet the NIH SIDS study treated them as a homogeneous group.

Who knows if the "cases" and the "controls" were truly matched for all of the significant variables? If the significant variable is an as yet undefined and undetected genetic predisposition of the sort being investigated by Steinman (see Chapter 7), the two groups could not have been truly matched in this way.

That *some* cases of SIDS may be due to the pertussis shot cannot be deduced from this study. That *some* children may be particularly vulnerable to the DPT shot also cannot be deduced from this study. But these are the very points which must be investigated in any study of the relationship between DPT and SIDS. Therefore, the authors' conclusion that the data "strongly support the view that DPT immunization is not a factor in the etiology of SIDS" is not borne out by the evidence.

The problem with any "case-control" comparison is that the two groups may not be identical or truly matched for the variables which are really significant. Evidently, the authors of the widely-acclaimed British NCES study on the pertussis vaccine understood this problem. They said in 1981: "The case-control method has the advantage of simplicity and speed. Its main disadvantage is that unknown factors related to the way in which controls are selected may influence their likelihood of being exposed to risk. For this reason, the results of case-control studies must be interpreted with caution. . . . In case-control studies the assumption that the case and control groups are random samples of the relevant population is rarely, if ever, satisfied."

Alvan Feinstein, professor of medicine at Yale and one of the foremost authorities on medical statistics, agrees. He wrote in 1967, "the persons under study may be subdivided according to age, race, sex, occupation, income level, and numerous other demographic variables— but not according to major factors responsible for hidden bias that can substantially distort the results."

Feinstein added, "The possibility that the data might be immensely distorted or wholly erroneous does not receive intensive discussion, perhaps because this technique has been the standard practice of leaders in the field."

When the "leaders in the field" are prominent government health officials in the CDC and FDA the case-control method becomes a useful tool in political immunology.

The UCLA-FDA Study: Minimizing Adverse Reactions

An outstanding recent example of an exercise in political immunology was the study, "Pertussis Vaccine Project: Rates, Nature and Etiology of Adverse Reactions Associated with DPT Vaccine," financed by the FDA and conducted at the University of California, Los Angeles, from January 1, 1978, to December 15, 1979, by Christopher L. Cody, M.D., Larry J. Baraff, M.D., James D. Cherry, M.D., S. Michael Marcy, M.D., and FDA project officer Charles R. Manclark, Ph.D. This study was published in *Pediatrics* in November 1981, but the unpublished contractors' "Final Report," submitted to the FDA on March 18, 1980, contains far more revealing data.

One purpose of the UCLA-FDA study was to provide—for the first time—a reliable estimate of the number of pertussis vaccine adverse reactions in America, so that medical researchers would have a scientific basis upon which to judge the safety of any new pertussis vaccine that might be developed in the future. Baraff, one of the study's principal authors, told television journalist Lea Thompson that the study was also commissioned because the FDA did not want American parents to refuse to give their children pertussis vaccine as parents in England were doing, saying, "The Food and Drug Administration was concerned that this sort of public panic might spread to the United States, [and] they wanted to document that the vaccine was in fact safe and not associated with severe consequences."

So the study was undertaken, at least in part, to prove that the FDA and the CDC had been right all along: adverse reactions are rare and nothing to worry about. This goal was not realized because the UCLA-FDA study found a higher incidence of reactions to the DPT shot than any previously reported in the literature. After it had been running for only nine months, the authors told participants in the 1978 FDA Pertussis Symposium, "The most striking finding in this preliminary analysis is the relatively high frequency of persistent crying, convulsion-like episodes, and collapse following DPT immunization."

The frequency of these more serious neurological reactions might have been one reason why the scope of the study was apparently curtailed. At the 1978 FDA Symposium the authors had announced that they planned to prospectively evaluate 50,000 DPT immunizations; ultimately they included less than one third of that number.

As published, the UCLA-FDA study revealed a significant number of DPT reactions. Minor and short-term reactions were high: local reactions occurred after 64 percent of the vaccinations, and minor systemic reactions occurred after 50 percent of the vaccinations. Neurological reactions were also high: nine children went into convulsions, nine suffered collapse, and about twenty had high-pitched (encephalitic) screaming, which is considered by many neurologists to suggest central nervous system irritation.

These were serious reactions, and they were occurring more frequently than anticipated. What is more, two infants died during the course of the study within four days of a DPT shot.

In the published report of the study, these reactions appeared less strikingly serious than they actually were, for the following reasons:

(1) the number of children enrolled in the study was not given. All data were given in terms of numbers of vaccinations, making this denominator value larger than it would have been if given in numbers of children; (2) conclusions drawn from the study group were applied to the United States infant population as a whole even though the group studied was prescreened to exclude high-risk children, an exclusion which does not occur in real life; (3) high-pitched screaming was not classified as a serious reaction, although many physicians consider this reaction to be a manifestation of cerebral irritation, and even the authors admitted that "the significance of this reaction is unknown"; (4) cases of serious reactions were not followed up for longer than a few weeks, even though the impact of the vaccine on the child's health might not be apparent until months or years later; and (5) the FDA placed an arbitrary time limit of forty-eight hours within which reactions had to occur in order to be included in the study. This eliminated from the statistical data the unknown number of neurological or other serious reactions which occurred more than forty-eight hours after the shot.

How Many Children Participated?

Perhaps the most unusual of these techniques was the first: the failure to report the number of children who participated in the study. In the published version, the authors state that the study included an analysis of "784 DT and 15,752 DPT shots." There was no mention of the number of children enrolled.

In a 1982 letter to Representative Daniel A. Mica, Assistant Secretary for Health Edward Brandt, Jr., M.D., stated, "There are a number of factors that make it impossible to produce a realistic number through simple division. Therefore rates are expressed as reactions per total number of injections."

The unpublished "Final Report" gave two figures for the number of children enrolled. The cover sheet states, "Sixteen thousand five hundred and thirty-six children aged 0–6 years received either DPT (15,572) or DT (784) vaccine." But inside, the report states that "approximately 7,000 children" were enrolled. This was not the only elementary mathematical error made by the study's authors (see Chapter 20).

In a 1982 interview with the *Journal of the American Medical Association*, author James Cherry, M.D., stated, "In almost 6,000 children there was no evidence of neurological damage." When asked in a letter in 1984 how many children were enrolled in the study, Baraff replied, "approximately 11,000." When asked the same question in that same year, Cherry finally explained:

"The number of children enrolled in the study was not mentioned in our *Pediatrics* paper because I don't believe we knew the precise number of children. The data was recorded by immunization, as this is the logical unit to study. Although I fail to see any great need to know the total number of children enrolled in the study, it seems to be so important to you. I will point out that we made a major mistake in coding our data for the computer and therefore we had no easy access to compare reactions in children who received more than one immunization. We have recently reprogrammed much of the data and will be looking at this in detail in the near future."

In fact, recording data by "immunization" is thoroughly illogical, and the reason is very simple: incidence expressed in terms of shots does not correlate with incidence in terms of children. To take a hypothetical example: if 5,000 DPT shots are given in a study in England and 5,000 shots are given in a study in America and both studies produce 100 convulsions, it could be claimed that both studies yielded the same reaction rate. But suppose the number of children enrolled in the two studies was different? Specifically, suppose that 1,000 children participated in the American study and 3,000 in the British study. The serious neurological reaction rate in the United States would be one in ten children, while in England it would be one in thirty children. This very real difference is obscured when reaction rates are given in terms of the number of shots administered instead of the number of children enrolled. This also makes it impossible to compare one study with another.

Charlotte Hannik, M.D., of The Netherlands wrote in 1969, ". . . I think it better not to correlate the total number of reactions with the total number of injections or the total number of doses released, but with the child itself."

It is misleading to give results in terms of shots administered. It is not disembodied shots that run high fevers, develop convulsions, become mentally retarded, or die. This happens to children, many of whom in America receive three to five DPT shots in the first five years of life. But how many DPT shots did each child enrolled in the UCLA-FDA study get?

It is not clear whether the authors randomly picked children from private practices and clinics, giving each child a single shot and never seeing the child again, or whether a portion of the children were vaccinated two, three, or four times. The published study in *Pediatrics* states, "approximately 75% of vaccinees returned for subsequent doses." If 75 percent returned for one shot only, the total number of children in the study would have to be no more than 9,000 (9,000 plus 75 percent of 9,000 equals 15,752). It seems probable, however, that in many cases infants returned for second, third, and fourth shots, since the study lasted nearly two years. Therefore, the 7,000 figure given in the unpublished "Final Report" to the FDA may be the most accurate.

The incidence of collapse and convulsions was given in the published study as follows: "Convulsions and hypotonic hyporesponsive episodes [collapse] each occurred in 1:1,750 immunizations." The rate for serious neurological reactions was made to appear innocuous—one chance in 1,750. In reality, if the number of children enrolled in the study was 7,000, it would be correct to state that serious neurological reactions were suffered by one in 389 children. This rate is much more representative of the facts and much less innocuous.

It is startling to realize that a study financed with public funds, which has been hailed by the federal government and the medical establishment as a definitive statement on pertussis vaccine reactions, does not even contain the most elementary scientific fact—the number of subjects participating. The final sentence of the published article reads, "This study supports the conclusion of others: that the benefits of pertussis immunization far outweigh the risks." For such a sweeping statement to be made, one which affects the life of every child in this country, it is especially important that those "risks" have been carefully calculated. This could only have been done if the number of children enrolled was known and taken into consideration.

The Study Population vs. the Real World

The second way in which the results of the UCLA-FDA study were minimized was through its prescreening of the participants. The study did not include "Children who had previously experienced severe adverse reactions following DTP immunizations, as defined by the . . . Red Book of the American Academy of Pediatrics. . . ." In addition, those children in the study who reacted to a DPT shot with convulsions, collapse, prolonged crying, or unusual crying (i.e. "high-pitched scream-ing") were not given more pertussis vaccine.

Therefore, the study was far from representative of what happens in the real world of pediatric private practices and public health clinics across America, where children who have had high-pitched or pro-longed crying, convulsions, collapse, etc., after a DPT shot are often—sometimes repeatedly—given more pertussis vaccine. While it would obviously have been unethical and dangerous to give more pertussis vaccine to children who had reacted to an earlier shot, the fact remains the population studied was not representative of the American infant population who receive DPT shots. The results of the study, therefore, would tend to underestimate the incidence of adverse reactions if applied to the whole population of the country.

What About High-pitched Screaming?

The third way study results were minimized is that the authors did not classify "unusual high-pitched crying" as a major reaction. What is more, there seems to have been confusion over just how many cases of high-pitched screaming there were in the study.

On one page, the published article states that after 11,051 shots, there were 22 cases of "unusual crying," which is the authors' definition of high-pitched screaming. The preceding page, however, states that after 15,752 shots had been given, 17 infants had a "truly unusual high-pitched cry." The same contradiction is contained in the unpublished "Final Report." Were there 17 or 22 cases or perhaps 33 cases (11,051 is two thirds of the total 15,752 shots) of high-pitched screaming? It is also interesting to note that the children in the study who had high-pitched screaming were not given further pertussis vaccine, but high-pitched screaming was not defined as a "major reaction" by the authors.

What Happened to the Eighteen Children?

The fourth way the UCLA-FDA results were minimized is that the eighteen children who were described as having "more serious" col-lapse and convulsion reactions were not followed up to determine whether or not they eventually showed major or minimal brain dam-age, such as a seizure disorder or learning disabilities. The published report stated: "No evidence of encephalopathy or permanent brain damage was seen in any vaccine recipients. In view of lack of neurologic sequelae and death associated with DTP immunization in the study, it seems prudent to continue the routine utilization of pertussis immunization in infancy and childhood."

Although the authors indicated that these eighteen children were seen by a neurologist within a few weeks of their reaction and that every one of them had a normal EEG at that point, there was no systematic attempt to evaluate their growth and development after that.

Interiewed on "DPT: Vaccine Roulette," the FDA's John Robbins stated, "The funds for contractual arrangements . . . there are just no funds within the FDA for that now." Lea Thompson asked him, "They were only followed for forty-eight hours. There is some reason to believe that some children develop complications after that. It seems that you have them in your grasp. Wouldn't you like to know what happened to them?" Robbins responded, "I think so . . . sure . . . it's just not the only thing that's been cut back, unfortunately."

Two years later, in March 1984, Robbins was quoted in the *West County Times* (San Francisco Bay Area) as justifying the lack of follow-up of the eighteen children who reacted neurologically because "most were Hispanic families from the UCLA [sic], which made the chances of follow-up almost nil."

Avoiding official knowledge about the fate of these eighteen children has taken up a disproportionate amount of bureaucratic time. At a November 10, 1983, FDA meeting attended by twenty-six physicians and scientists from the FDA, NIH, CDC, National Academy of Sciences, and six universities, there was discussion of an "unsolicited" study proposal from an unnamed researcher to follow up the eighteen children.

An internal FDA memorandum summarizing the meeting reveals that the proposed study suggested comparing the eighteen children "to matched controls" and giving study subjects a "neurologic examination, psychometric evaluation, and HLA typing for 70 antigens." (HLA, or human lymphocyte antigen, typing is a technique for determining an individual's genetic makeup and resembles the work being done by Steinman on identifying high-risk children, as discussed in Chapters 7 and 13.)

According to the memorandum, the study proposal was not received well by those attending the FDA meeting: "The general conclusion of the participants was that it is highly improbable that useful information could be obtained from the proposed study. Data for some of the parameters, such as neurologic examination and psychometric evaluation, would be uninterpretable because of the lack of comparable baseline data for the study subjects, thereby making it impossible to control the study for these variables."

This same reason for not following up the children was given by UCLA-FDA investigator Cherry in a letter to the authors. He wrote: "Followup in this group really is meaningless because there is no adequate control group for comparison. Since neurologic disease is relatively uncommon in young children, it is necessary to have a control group, or otherwise you will assume a cause-and-effect relationship when one really doesn't exist."

What Cherry and some others attending the FDA meeting seem to be suggesting is that their interpretation of medical science prevents them from evaluating the present health of these eighteen children without locating a "control" group of eighteen other children of the same race, sex, weight, and birth date who received a DPT shot for comparison.

Does this mean that a physician cannot evaluate the health of a single child in his practice unless he compares that child with a "control"?

Nevertheless, the FDA memorandum reveals that "one or two attendees at the meeting . . . believed that even with the deficiencies in the proposed study, the relatively quick access to subjects warranted support of the HLA part of the study because, even though there was a low probability that it might yield useful information, there was the feeling of interested parties that 'something' should be done. This view was not shared by the majority of the attendees. . . . It was the consensus of all consultants present, in addition to participants from NIAID, NINCDS, and CDC that the proposed study did not have scientific merit."

Even so, at least one participant urged, "although the proposed study did not deserve support from the standpoint of the science involved, an argument could be made that followup would be reasonable as a matter of medical care."

The "majority" view evidently prevailed because the follow-up has not yet been done. The FDA and the American public still do not know what happened to the "UCLA-FDA Eighteen" and whether any of the children have continuing health problems. Why is the FDA so reluctant to conduct the follow-up? Is it because officials suspect some of the children have seizure disorders, learning disabilities, or developmental delays?

The FDA's failure to discover what happened to the eighteen children and its decision not to proceed with HLA typing is particularly surprising in view of a public statement made only six months earlier by William Jordan, M.D., of the National Institute for Allergy and Infectious Diseases. A major voice in government-funded medical research, Jordan was present at the November 1983 FDA meeting and stated at the April 1983 Open Meeting on Pertussis and Pertussis Vaccines: "I would like to speak to the problem of identifying high risk, which is, if we had an HLA marker or some other genetic tool, it would certainly be a useful one. There is none in sight at the moment."

At the May 3, 1984, Senate hearings called by Senator Hawkins on the National Childhood Vaccine Injury Compensation Act, the Senator asked government officials if there were plans to follow up the eighteen UCLA-FDA study children. CDC's Alan Hinman stated that the FDA was considering an in-house project rather than one that would be performed by an outside contractor.

However, a call to the FDA Public Information Office in June elicited the response that, according to Dr. Paul Parkman, Scientific Director of the FDA National Center for Drugs and Biologics, the decision had not yet been made to conduct this investigation.

It seems incredible that the FDA should be uninterested in the fate of these eighteen children. The agency has claimed that there was no long-term neurological damage from the vaccine in the UCLA-FDA Study, but how do they know if no long-term follow-up of serious reactions in the study has ever been done? In actuality, such an investigation should also include the seventeen (or was it twenty-two?) children whose neurological reaction took the form of high-pitched screaming.

Since the UCLA-FDA Study ran for almost two years, it should at least have been possible to maintain contact for an extended period with those children whose serious reactions occurred early in the study. And even today, as the November 1983 memo indicates, the FDA can gain "relatively quick access" to these children, which should facilitate any follow-up effort.

How Many DPT Reactions Were Excluded?

The final technique that minimized undesired results in the UCLA-FDA study was deciding at the outset to include only reactions occurring within forty-eight hours of the DPT shot even though the medical literature is full of reports of vaccine reactions occurring days or even weeks later. The British National Childhood Encephalopathy Study (NCES), published in 1981, found a significant association between the DPT shot and neurological illness occurring within seven days of the shot. Retrospectively, this factor alone calls for a reanalysis of the raw data in the UCLA-FDA study.

When asked why the study adhered to the cutoff period of forty-eight hours, Cherry wrote: "The 48 hour cutoff point was, I believe, a contract requirement, although I am not certain of that." He also criticized the NCES seven-day cutoff period as excessive, since the bulk of the reactions occurred in the first three days.

Baraff, when asked the same question, wrote: "The rationale for the 48 hour cutoff was arbitrary. It was our belief that by choosing a shorter time period there would be less controversy regarding the validity of a temporal association between DTP reactions and immunization. I believe in retrospect that this decision was appropriate. The majority of reactions in fact occurred within the first 24 hours. Illness which began more than 48 hours post immunization in all cases which we investigated did not appear to be related to the vaccine. Whatever time is chosen is strictly arbitrary. There is no scientific proof that any of these reactions is causally related to the vaccine."

This makes good sense politically. The shorter the time period, the fewer the reactions and the better the statistics look. But it makes little sense scientifically. The FDA's John Robbins stated at the 1982 FDA Symposium, "Many of these activities, such as the histamine-sensitizing activity, persist for many days after injection of the LPF, indicating a phase of altered host reactivity characteristic of many other bacterial toxins." And there are numerous references in the literature to vaccine effects manifesting later than forty-eight hours after the shot.

The distortion which such an "arbitrary" cutoff can produce is made sadly evident by the fact that the deaths of two babies, which occurred within ninety-six hours of a DPT shot, were not mentioned in the published study. These two deaths were diagnosed as SIDS and, quite correctly, the UCLA-FDA study was able to state: "no deaths occurred within 48 hours of immunization."

Closer examination of these two "SIDS" deaths raises serious questions, not only about their diagnosis as SIDS, but also about the lack of any mention of the cases in the published report. The unpublished "Final Report" submitted to the FDA described them as follows:

"The first child was a two-month-old male who had no problems for 48 hours following his first DPT immunization. At 72 hours post-immunization he developed coryza [runny nose]. At 84 hours he was found dead in his crib. No pathologic cause for death was found on post-mortem examination by the L.A. County Deputy Coroner.

"The second infant was a two-month-old female who received a DTP immunization in the nursery at two days of age [sic] and another DTP immunization at two months of age. Following the second DTP immunization the mother stated the child slept more than normal, ate less than usual and was somewhat lethargic. The child developed loose bowel movements approximately 24 hours post-immunization. These symptoms began to resolve approximately 48 hours post-immunization, but continued until four days post-immunization when the child was found cold, blue, and lifeless in bed by the father. The post-mortem examination by the L.A. County Deputy Coroner revealed no pathologic cause for death."

These two deaths were explained, or rationalized, by the authors of the UCLA-FDA study in the unpublished "Final Report" as follows: "SIDS is estimated to occur in approximately one in 500 infants by age six months. It is most frequent in the four-month interval between two and six months of age. Therefore, in any 96-hour period, approximately one in 15,000 infants in the age group would be expected to die of SIDS. Therefore, two such deaths in this series are not unexpected."

Even if the above calculation of spontaneous or random SIDS deaths is correct, this statement appears to be based upon a denominator of 15,000 infants, not 15,000 vaccinations. If 1 in 15,000 infants in the age group can be expected to die of SIDS every ninety-six hours, the estimated 7,000 infants in the UCLA-FDA study actually had an SIDS incidence more than four times higher than expected. Is this just another elementary mathematical error by the authors of the study?

The incidence of neurological damage from the pertussis vaccine found in the UCLA-FDA study was quite considerable, as is further discussed in Chapter 20. This fact, however, seems never to have registered on the minds of practicing pediatricians who read the report in *Pediatrics*. Perhaps this is because the resulting data seems to have been presented in such a way as to make the vaccine appear as harmless as possible.

The authors of the UCLA-FDA study concluded: "This study supports the conclusion of others: that the benefits of pertussis immunization far outweigh the risks."

No Room for Dissent

An even more alarming aspect of political immunology is the medical establishment's suppression of unfavorable adverse reaction data, and its unwillingness to give a forum to physicians who point out flaws in vaccination programs. Medical publications in Britain and America share responsibility for this attempt to silence those who have the courage to dissent from the majority view.

The medical establishment is powerful. When a doctor discovers evidence about risks associated with a popular medical procedure and stands up for his convictions despite disapproval from his colleagues, history has shown that he is in danger of being ostracized by his colleagues. If he does not stop his rebellious behavior, attempts are made to discredit him. It is a long-standing tradition that a doctor does not contradict his colleagues. And this is part of the reason why the pertussis vaccine has not been improved, why reactions have not been recognized, and why children continue to be hurt.

Yet these "medical heretics" are sometimes prophets. Some doctors who have had the courage to stay the course and not back down from what they know to be true have eventually proven to be correct, even if not in their own lifetimes.

In the 1860s the great Hungarian physician Ignaz Semmelweiss pointed out that hospital doctors were killing women by performing autopsies and not washing their hands properly before they delivered babies. Although he proved he was right by requiring medical personnel to wash their hands in chloride of lime before examining women in labor or performing deliveries, thus cutting the deathrate from "childbed fever" (septicemia) from 120 to 12 deaths per 1000 births, he was laughed at and brutally criticized by his colleagues. Doctors of the day did not like being told they were responsible for the deaths of their patients. Semmelweiss was so harassed and ostracized by the medical establishment that he fled from his hospital in Vienna and eventually died in an institution.

Gordon Stewart, who has studied the pertussis vaccine and whooping cough for more than a decade, began publishing controversial articles about the vaccine in British medical journals during the 1970s. Although he was and still is severely criticized by other doctors, he was able to publish his adverse reaction and epidemiological data in British medical journals until the past few years. Commenting on his inability to get data published today, Dr. Stewart wrote in a letter to the authors:

"As far as the Establishment goes, there seems to be no difference in the attitudes taken in Britain and America. I still do not know why, but as soon as questions begin to be asked about this particular vaccine, the ranks close with amazing unanimity. . . . The editors tend to print pro-vaccine articles which can be challenged only in letters—they will not print anti-vaccine articles."

Manipulating the Facts and the Media

When all other attempts to suppress the reality of vaccine reactions fail, the last resort for political immunologists is to assure the public that things would be much worse in the absence of a mandatory mass vaccination program.

In 1979, a hypothetical cost/benefit analysis was published in the *New England Journal of Medicine* by Jeffrey Koplan and others under the auspices of the CDC and the Harvard School of Public Health. It attempted to compute the value of a vaccination program by estimating the numbers of lives that would be lost, and the amount of permanent disability from whooping cough, if there were no pertussis vaccine program in America. By overestimating the benefits and underestimating the costs, the authors were able to conclude "our analysis supports continuation of vaccination."

Koplan and his colleagues estimated that without a vaccination program there would be 71 times as many cases of whooping cough as there are today, and 25 times as many deaths. But they totally ignored the experience of West Germany, where the number of deaths from whooping cough declined from 36 in 1970, when 58 percent of children were vaccinated, to 7 in 1979, when less than 10 percent were vaccinated. They ignored the experience of Sweden where some 19,000 cases of whooping cough occurred in 1977–79 and no deaths were recorded. They also ignored the experience of Britain, where health authorities have claimed that a whooping cough epidemic has raged since 1977 because so many parents have rejected the pertussis vaccine. In 1982, approximately 65,000 reported cases of whooping cough resulted in 14 deaths, and it is not clear that all 14 of these deaths were laboratory-confirmed cases of whooping cough.

Stewart criticized the Koplan analysis for being "based, unfortunately, upon obsolete data and projections which are disproved by events in Britain, West Germany and Sweden. I have offered current, verifiable data for testing in the same model but this offer has been refused by the [*New England Journal of Medicine*] and ignored by CDC."

A perhaps unwitting accomplice in the practice of political immunology has been the American mass media, especially the press. Mass vaccination programs are heavily promoted and supervised by the federal and state governments and, while the press has no trouble scrutinizing other governmental activities, it has generally taken a hands-off approach to the pertussis vaccine controversy.

Several months after "DPT: Vaccine Roulette" was shown in the spring of 1982, the Maryland Health Department suddenly issued press releases announcing a whooping cough "epidemic" in Maryland with the implication that the upsurge in cases was due to parents not having their children vaccinated. The major newspapers in Maryland and Washington, D.C., repeated the health department's account of the epidemic.

How many cases does it take to make an epidemic? Every year between one and three thousand cases of pertussis are reported, but the CDC estimates the total number of cases to be ten to twenty times that number. There is obviously very serious underreporting. Did the total of seventy-nine reported (but not bacteriologically confirmed) cases of whooping cough in Maryland in 1982 constitute an "epidemic"?

Timothy Johnson thought so. On his *Healthbeat* program he intoned, "officials are concerned about the State of Maryland where an epidemic . . . is currently being fought. Cases there are running ten times the normal rate for that state. More than 60 cases have been recorded so far this year."

On the program with Johnson was Robert Ancona, M.D., chairman of the Maryland Medical Society Committee on Immunization and Infectious Diseases. He agreed: "This epidemic has been several fold times the usual reported incidence of pertussis and is clearly an epidemic. We feel that some of these cases, at least, were due to a lack of immunization on the part of the patients."

And the CDC *Morbidity and Mortality Weekly Report* of July 1983 carried an article on the Maryland whooping cough cases which appeared to imply that "DPT: Vaccine Roulette" was connected to the "epidemic." It stated, "Following a television presentation on pertussis vaccine side effects, DTP vaccine sales by one pharmaceutical company to the private medical sector in Maryland decreased 45 percent in April, 1982, compared to average monthly sales for the preceding months. . . ."

The small detail left out of the press releases and statements of health officials is that it was epidemiologically impossible for the Maryland epidemic to have been caused by a fall-off in the vaccination rate due to the television documentary. There is a three-year lag between the time a population stops vaccinating and the occurrence of a substantial rise of whooping cough cases. In the intervening three years, herd immunity prevents bona fide epidemics. At the 1982 FDA Symposium on New Pertussis Vaccines, A. H. Griffith explained why this is true, using the British experience as an example:

". . . as you vaccinate the children under the age of one year, and whooping [cough] is spread mainly at the ages of three or four years, you need cohorts of three or four years of vaccinated children to develop before you have an effect on the incidence of whooping cough. And this is what has happened in the U.K.; as the vaccination rate increased, so did the incidence of whooping cough come down. . . . Then after the adverse publicity, the vaccination rate dropped dramatically. You have to wait three years and then you start having an epidemic. And this is what has happened. We have whooping cough three years after vaccination [rates dropped]."

So the 1982 whooping cough "epidemic" in Maryland that occurred barely three months after the broadcast of "DPT: Vaccine Roulette" could not have been caused by parents refusing to vaccinate their children because they watched the television documentary (see Chapter 11). In fact, a good part of the Maryland "epidemic" was due to increased reporting because of publicity surrounding the pertussis vaccine in 1982; furthermore, many of the children who came down with pertussis had been vaccinated. Lea Thompson commented in a TV interview:

"The reporting of pertussis is up because doctors know about it and are thinking about it. Parents know about it and are thinking about it. It could be, and probably is true, that there has always been that much whooping cough out there, and we just didn't know about it before."

Later in 1982, the Wisconsin Health Department also announced a whooping cough epidemic in that state—this time the "epidemic" consisted of 43 cases (see Chapter 11). It too was shown to be occurring primarily in vaccinated children. The reporting of these so-called whooping cough epidemics in Maryland and Wisconsin appeared to be designed to discredit Lea Thompson and WRC-TV for having dared to point out problems in a mass vaccination program promoted and operated by the American medical establishment.

But while daily newspapers and magazines have generally tended to take the denials and reassurances of government health officials and doctors at face value, television has played a major role in increasing public awareness of vaccination problems.

Lea Thompson scored the first breakthrough, alerting parents to some of the tragic cases of vaccine-damaged children in this country. She showed how difficult it can be for parents who must devote their lives to caring for retarded, epileptic, and physically handicapped children injured by the pertussis vaccine. She introduced several of the physicians who have been warning about pertussis vaccine risks, such as Gordon Stewart of Scotland and Robert Mendelsohn of Chicago. She pointed out that the virulence and incidence of whooping cough had started to decline before the introduction of the pertussis vaccine and that West Germany and Sweden had stopped recommending the vaccine years ago.

As soon as the documentary appeared, NBC was bombarded with telephone calls from doctors complaining about the show. But Lea Thompson stood by her story. She said, "There was a lot of pressure put on [this station] by doctors who called us irresponsible and yellow journalists. . . . [The station was] getting a lot of hot letters from fairly important people. . . . I have been criticized for every line in that documentary, and if I had to do it again, I wouldn't change any of it. . . . I have three children. Almost everyone who worked for more than a year researching this documentary had children. We did it for our kids and for everybody's kids. I would still do it all over again."

And parents who saw "DPT: Vaccine Roulette" were grateful. Some were referred by the station to Dissatisfied Parents Together in Washington, D.C., the parent group that formed after the documentary was broadcast. One mother of a child who had suffered uncontrollable screaming for hours after two DPT shots, wrote, "After viewing the DPT program . . . my husband and I learned for the first time that there can be serious neurological reactions to the pertussis vaccine in some children that can result in neurological defects and permanent brain damage. We were also unaware that contraindications exist . . . we realized that our son's background included three of these contraindications. We discussed the matter with our pediatrician, and it has been determined that our child will not receive further pertussis inoculations. . . . Who knows if perhaps a terrible tragedy was averted by the education that we received through that program?"

A 1982 *Phil Donahue Show* also alerted many parents to the risks of vaccination. Parents of some children with seizure disorders and other neurological problems realized for the first time what had happened to their children.

One mother described her feelings after she watched the show. "I was really angry when I saw the *Phil Donahue Show*. So much time had gone by from the time my son and I were going through the pain of his reaction to the DPT shot. I was very much alone at the time. I didn't know what was happening, and the doctors didn't know what was happening. After I saw the *Phil Donahue Show*, I said to myself: 'Hey, they should have known what was happening.'"

A 1983 *MacNeil-Lehrer Report* highlighted the pertussis vaccine controversy, and one of the most interesting exchanges in the show was when MacNeil tried, unsuccessfully, to pin down CDC director Walter Dowdle on the number of children damaged by the vaccine each year.

MACNEIL: I'm just trying to put a figure on how many small children would be at risk of serious brain damage in a year, typically, statistically, in this country.

DR. DOWDLE: That I wouldn't have the figures for, except to say how many vaccine doses are actually available to be given.

MACNEIL: I see. . . .

The CDC does not know how many children are killed or brain damaged by the pertussis vaccine in the U.S. each year; but it does know how many DPT shots are "available to be given." It is the practice of political immunology at its very best.

15

Profile:
Four in One Family

And now abideth faith, hope, love, these three;
but the greatest of these is love.
I Corinthians 13:13

Harriet and her husband Don had always wanted a big family. James, Paul, and Amy were beautiful, healthy babies. And so was Michael when he was born in 1970.

Michael was in perfect health except for a number of allergies, including an inability to tolerate milk. He projectile-vomited milk and had to be placed on soybean formula. He was also allergic to rice cereal, which made him vomit and break out in a rash. When Harriet breast-fed Mike, she could not take aspirin or he would break out in eczema from head to toe.

Mike reacted to his first three DPT shots at three, four, and five months of age with a fever of about 102 degrees and what Harriet described as "deep sleep that lasted for about sixteen hours." In the weeks following his third shot, Mike's eyes started to cross, and he stopped using the right side of his body.

"We took him to an eye doctor, and they put a patch over his right eye. I asked the doctor why Mike was holding his right arm at a funny angle against his side and dragging that right leg when he tried to crawl. The doctor assured me that Mike would outgrow it. When he kept it up, we just put it down to his eye problems."

As Mike grew, he continued to be very clumsy and only use his left

260

hand. While he was playing, he would sometimes stop and stare blankly for several seconds as if he had lost touch with reailty. "At the time, we didn't realize he was having petit mal seizures. We didn't know anything about seizures then. When all of a sudden he would stop jabbering and stare off into space, we thought he was daydreaming."

Seven years after Mike was born, Harriet gave birth to fraternal twins, Cathy and Theresa: "We learned that if Theresa rolled over this week, Cathy would roll over next week. From birth, Theresa was ahead of her sister in everything."

Theresa, however, was very allergic to milk and had to be put on soybean formula to prevent her projectile vomiting. Like Mike, she was also allergic to rice cereal. Cathy was not allergic to milk or anything else. But to avoid confusion, Harriet placed both babies on soybean formula.

The twins received their three DPT shots when they were four, six, and seven months old. After each one, they ran fevers of from 102 to 103 degrees, and after crying hard for several hours, lapsed into a deep sleep that lasted for more than fifteen hours.

"I brought them home, gave them aspirin to keep the fever down, and they slept all that afternoon and until the next morning without waking up. They slept like they had been knocked out. I always blamed it on the aspirin," said Harriet.

In the weeks following her third shot, Theresa's eyes started to cross, and Cathy overtook and surpassed her in mental and physical development. "All of a sudden Cathy pulled ahead. Cathy sat at seven months, and Theresa couldn't sit alone until she was thirteen months old. Cathy stood alone at ten months, and Theresa couldn't stand until she was four years old. Cathy walked at fifteen months, and Theresa couldn't walk until she was six years old."

When Theresa was eleven months old, doctors diagnosed her as a spastic diplegic with epilepsy. She was found to have an abnormal EEG and was put on Dilantin. At the same time, doctors took another look at Mike, now eight years old, and told Harriet that he was blind in his right eye, had an abnormal EEG, and had cerebral palsy. He was also put on Dilantin to control his petit mal seizures.

Harriet and her husband were devastated by the news that two of their six children were neurologically damaged. Doctors ran extensive tests on both Mike and Theresa, but could find no genetic reason or any cause for their condition.

"We just kept hunting and hunting for a reason for all of this. We went through the 'who is to blame?' period. There are no neurological problems anywhere in our family, and the doctors kept assuring us that there was no genetic reason for what happened. So we decided to go ahead and try again to have another child," said Harriet.

Harriet gave birth to another set of twin girls, only this time they were identical. "We were so excited and happy because they were just perfect babies. They had no problems except they were both allergic to milk and rice cereal. We put them on soybean formula, and they were fine until they got their third DPT shot," Harriet said.

Mary and Rebecca received their first two shots at three and four months of age. Two days after their second DPT shot, Harriet noticed their eyes crossing for brief periods of time. She immediately made an appointment with an eye doctor. But by the time the eye doctor saw the twins a week later, their eyes seemed to be fine.

When Mary and Rebecca were given their third DPT shot at five months, they began screaming hysterically before they even left the doctor's office.

"They screamed almost immediately after they got the shot. Before we left the doctor's office, the nurses asked me if they were going to be okay, and I said that I thought they were just mad. We went to my mother's and I gave them Tylenol because they were still screaming. Then they fell into a deep sleep until the next morning," said Harriet.

The next day both girls awoke and began screaming again. That night they ran temperatures of 104 degrees. For three days and three nights they screamed on and off. "They would scream until they collapsed in exhaustion and went to sleep. Then when they woke up, they would scream some more. I kept giving them Tylenol for their fever."

The fourth day after their shot, they stopped screaming, but they were restless and fussy for three more days. Seven days after their shot, Harriet noticed that Rebecca was acting strangely.

"She began startling like a newborn baby, and her eyes wandered and moved in strange ways. I picked her up and looked over my shoulder at her reflection in the bathroom mirror, and I saw her gasp like she was hiccuping, cross her eyes, roll them back up into her head, and then bang her head down on my shoulder."

The next day Rebecca repeated her strange eye and head movements three or four times, and so Harriet took her to a neurologist. It had been nine days since her third DPT shot. Harriet remembers the horror of watching Rebecca go into a series of myoclonic seizures. "While we were waiting in the neurologist's office, Rebecca rolled her eyes to the left, across the top of the room, and down to the right side of her face. She stiffened her right arm, right leg, left leg, and left arm. Then she started smacking her lips and making a high 'oo-oo-oo' sound as she rolled her eyes and rhythmically stiffened one limb after another. It was awful."

Rebecca was admitted to a hospital, and while she was there, she continued to have seizures. "Before the nurses padded her crib, she bruised her forehead from slamming her head into the bars of the crib while she was seizing," Harriet said. "She was there for thirteen days and by the time she left, she was in a coma. She just lay there with staring eyes and her body was as stiff as a board. She looked like she was dead. She couldn't eat or even suck on a bottle anymore. When the doctors discharged her from the hospital, they told me to take her home and love her."

The doctors announced that Rebecca had infantile spasms with hypsarrhythmia and myoclonic seizures. They prescribed powerful steroids, ACTH, to try to stop the convulsions.

When Harriet arrived home with Rebecca, she immediately noticed that her twin sister Mary was acting strangely. Her eyes were wandering all over her head, and from time to time she would startle and stiffen her body.

"I asked my husband and mother if they had noticed Mary doing this while I was with Rebecca in the hospital, and they said yes, but they thought it was just because she was upset that I was gone. I called the neurologist, and he immediately put her on ACTH. Soon Mary lapsed into a coma and was as unresponsive as Rebecca was most of the time."

Rebecca and Mary went into and out of comas for the next three months. Harriet did not know if they were going to live or die.

"I sat by their beds for three months waiting for them to recognize me. Some of the doctors told me that if they pulled through, they would probably be vegetables. There was a point when we thought Mary was blind and deaf she was so unresponsive. The steroids they both were taking caused them to grow black hair all over their bodies. They had pubic hair so thick I was embarrassed to change them in public. Their eyebrows grew together, and long black hair grew down their noses and all over their arms and legs."

After the twins were taken off the steroids, the doctors decided that the reason they were having infantile spasms was because they could not tolerate the amino acid valine. "The doctors did not immediately connect their condition to the pertussis vaccine. They told me they thought Rebecca and Mary had a metabolism disorder that prevented them from digesting certain amino acids. They put them on the 'maple-syrup disease diet' instead of formula. They were so miserable they cried day and night."

On this diet, Rebecca and Mary remained at the weight of nineteen pounds for a year. Their heads stopped growing. Their gums began bleeding and filled with pus. Harriet took them to a general practitioner who diagnosed malnutrition and placed them on a regular diet. "They began getting better within a day or two of being placed on a regular diet. They started growing and developing," Harriet said.

At the age of three, Mary and Rebecca cannot sit, stand, or walk. Their attention span is almost nonexistent. They are classified as mentally and physically retarded. They will probably need full-time care for the rest of their lives.

Harriet and her husband have been locked in a battle with their state public school system to win the right for Theresa, now in first grade, and Mike, now in seventh grade, to receive special education services. Theresa has just learned to walk, but in addition to her physical handicaps, she is learning-delayed. She also has an extremely short attention span. Easter Seals worked with Theresa for a year and a half before she attended kindergarten to train her to sit still for two or three minutes at a time.

Mike has been evaluated as intellectually gifted, but he has specific learning disabilities, possibly including dyslexia. Like Theresa, Rebecca, and Mary, Mike is left-handed (everyone else in the family, including Harriet and her husband, is right-handed) and has visual-perception problems. It takes him twice as long to write down what he sees on a blackboard or in a book as it does a normal seventh-grade student.

"If I could only turn the clock back," said Harriet. "If I had only been informed to look for signs other than just a fever or a sore leg after the DPT shots. If I had only been told that a history of neurologic problems in one child put his brothers and sisters at risk with the pertussis vaccine. If I had only known the definition of a seizure, so I could have done something sooner. Nobody told me. That is what makes me angry. It didn't have to happen four times."

❅ ❅ ❅ ❅ ❅

The three-bedroom trailer sits on a gently rolling hill just outside a small town in Arkansas and seems to sway slightly as a strong winter wind whips up from the surrounding fields. Inside, eighteen-year-old Amy is holding Rebecca, and sixteen-year-old Paul is feeding Mary a bottle.

The three-year-old twins have their golden hair tied in pigtails, and they are dressed almost identically in brightly colored overalls. Their blue pinstriped blouses with wide white collars heighten the pale beauty of their angelic faces. Like marionettes, they hold their thin arms and wrists at odd angles, and their fingers momentarily freeze in crooked positions. They are drooling, squirming, and occasionally shouting while they take turns smiling at their brother and sister who are caring for them.

Six-year-old Theresa, all giggles and tousled blond hair, shuffles over to the door where her twin, Cathy, is standing. Wearing a pink polka-dot blouse and matching pink pants, she flashes a toothless grin at her mother as she slowly makes her way across the living room. Her legs are bent at the knees, and she walks on the inside of her collapsed ankles.

Like any other teenager, Michael is dressed in blue jeans and tennis shoes. The brace on his teeth, which is held onto his head by a black strap, does not seem to bother him as he drinks a glass of soda. He talks slowly, enunciating every syllable in every word. Despite his unusually deliberate speech pattern, the vocabulary he uses shows his intelligence.

Harriet is fixing lunch. Looking at her, there is no question about where her daughters got their big blue eyes and blond hair. Tall and strong-boned, she laughs easily but sometimes nervously. Her shyness gives her a girlish quality that immediately puts strangers at ease. Her children call her "Momma," and she always seems to have time to answer every "Momma" that they call out to her.

"It has been hard coping with what happened to the children. But what we went through in the last town we lived in was such a terrible, terrible nightmare that I look back on it now, and I can't even believe it actually happened. It almost destroyed us and our marriage," Harriet says. She has finished making sandwiches and finds a chair in the crowded living room.

"It all started when we tried to get the public school to help Theresa by giving her special education, so she could learn. She is handicapped, and she needs the kind of special education that is spelled out in Public Law 94-142, which was passed in 1975 and requires equal education for handicapped children. But the school told us they didn't have the money or the facilities to give her special education even though they had been receiving federal funds for years to educate handicapped kids. Then they refused to categorize her as handicapped so they would not have to provide it. When I told them it was a law, that they had to do it, they got mad at us. That is when it all began."

Harriet and her family had lived in the town for ten years, and Don worked for the owner of a local catfish farm that provided catfish to everyone in town. As part of his salary, Don was allowed to take home all the catfish his family could eat, and his boss also paid part of his utility bills. But when Harriet and Don tried to get special education for their handicapped daughter, everything changed.

"At first, Don's boss told him that unless he stopped pressing for special education for Theresa, he would dock his pay twenty dollars a week. When we still didn't stop, he refused to let Don bring any catfish home. Then he stopped paying a portion of our utility bills. And when that didn't work, he said, 'I told you to drop it and you didn't drop it and so you are fired.'"

The family had always faithfully attended the town's Methodist Church, and Harriet recalls what happened after they asked the school to provide special education services for Theresa: "There was a women's group in our church and many teachers and members of the school board belonged to it. They told the group that Don and I had asked for a wheelchair lift for the bus and thirty-five thousand dollars worth of therapy equipment for Theresa, which was not true. They accused us of saying we wanted the whole school remodeled for Theresa, which was also not true. At the time, all Theresa was using was a big rubber ball and two broomstick poles for her physical therapy which would have totaled no more than thirty dollars."

Paul is tall and dark-haired like his father. There is a gentleness about him and a maturity that makes him seem older than his sixteen years. He remembers what happened to him at school: "The kids stopped talking to me. I was told by the school superintendent to get Theresa on and off the school bus every day because she was in a wheelchair and needed help. One day, when I got up to leave class to help Theresa, the teacher said, 'If you leave this class again, don't you ever come back.' "

"We shed many a tear," Harriet said sadly. "Every day one of the children would come home crying because a teacher or one of the kids said something to them at school. They were blackballed. All we wanted was meaningful education for Theresa."

When Harriet and Don refused to give up their fight for their daughter, the school's special education supervisor summoned a psychologist to evaluate Theresa.

"The psychologist said Theresa was not in need of special education, and we were shocked," Harriet said. "We asked for a hearing to review the decision. At that hearing, the psychologist admitted she gave Theresa a "below-average" score on a test in which Theresa could not successfully perform any of the problems. It didn't matter that she admitted she misrepresented Theresa's abilities. We lost the hearing."

Harriet says that word went out throughout the small town that the family was to be ignored. "When we would go to church and sit down in a pew, people would get up and leave the two pews in front of us and the two pews in back of us empty. People can be cruel in small towns. They are run by a certain group, and if you cross them, you had better beware."

Finally, it got too much for the family. Without any way to educate Theresa or to earn money and without any friends left, they decided to pack up and leave the town they had lived in for ten years.

"We went to church until the very last Sunday before we left and reminded them by sitting in that pew that we were still there. They were not going to tell us that we couldn't go there," Harriet explains. "We did have one neighbor who came and sat in the pew in front of us that last Sunday and talked to us. It was the first time anybody in the church had talked to us for months. When I left, I wrote a note to the church and said I was sorry so many of them would be glad we were leaving and that I hoped someday they would understand why we did what we did for our daughter."

Harriet and Don moved thirty miles away, back to the Arkansas town where Harriet had grown up and her family had been prominent for generations. Harriet's mother was convinced things would be different for them now they were back home.

"Things were different as far as the church and friends were concerned, but it took a year before the public school system agreed to test Theresa for special education and physical therapy. The word was that we were troublemakers and that there was nothing wrong with our kids, that we just wanted them 'labeled.' Even though Theresa was the only child in the class who could not write her name, hold a pencil correctly, use scissors, or tie her shoes, the Arkansas Special Education Agency told us all over again that we had to prove that Theresa had an educational deficit. They refused to accept any medical records or results of earlier tests that Theresa had taken and showed the extent of her handicaps."

With the help of Easter Seals, Crippled Children's Service, and a lawyer from the Handicapped Advocacy Service, Harriet finally pressured the school into putting Theresa into a resource room to help her fine-motor and perception problems. After a physical therapist convinced the school that Theresa could not learn to write or gain fine-motor control unless she was given physical therapy, the school agreed to transport her for therapy once a month.

Mary suddenly squirms and cries out, trying to wriggle out of Paul's lap. She pushes away the bottle and kicks her legs, which are encased in plastic braces. Hearing her sister, Rebecca begins to shout and the room is filled with sharp cries.

"We're going to take everybody out, Momma," Paul says matter-of-factly. Carefully he puts Mary down on her stomach on the floor, and she begins to wail even more loudly. She screams and tries to pull herself along the floor, using her arms because she cannot move her legs.

"Can I go, Momma?" asks Theresa excitedly. "Can I go walking, too?" She tries to move quickly to the door, but her twisted legs will not cooperate, and her gait becomes even more awkward.

Amy has almost finished washing the lunch dishes in the kitchen, and she calls out to Paul, "I'll go with you."

As poised and mature as Paul, Amy does not complain about the daily responsibility of caring for her handicapped sisters, because as she says, "I have really never known much different. Cathy was the only one younger than I who wasn't affected."

"Get Theresa's wheelchair," Harriet reminds Paul.

"My wheelchair," Theresa repeats happily, trying to contain her excitement.

Paul picks up Mary, and Amy picks up Rebecca; Theresa hobbles out with Cathy and Mike behind her. Their laughter and chatter fade into the distance, and the room becomes unusually quiet.

"Mike tests as borderline gifted, but his learning disabilities keep him in the third level of seventh grade," continues Harriet. "He understands everything, but he can't transfer what he sees and knows to paper fast enough to finish his tests in time. We think he may be dyslexic because he scrambles his words.

"The school will not allow him to use a tape recorder to take down his notes or use a typewriter to take tests. He works four to six hours every night just to get his homework done. And because he is in the third level, he is not qualified to go out for off-season football. He desperately needs sports for his physical development, to keep the weakness on his right side from getting worse."

After Easter Seals told Harriet that Mike should not have time limits placed on him during tests and should learn to use a typewriter, Harriet appealed to the school. "They told me no student can take typing until he is in high school. They don't want me to teach him at home. I can't believe it because schools all over the United States are giving learning disabled kids access to typewriters even in elementary school."

Mike's teachers are giving him A's and B's on his report card. One day Mike brought home a health spelling test that was graded "96." When Harriet checked the test, she found many misspelled words. "There were twelve misspelled words and yet they gave him a 96. You see, they don't want to admit he has enough of a problem to give him individualized help. They told me the school will not evaluate children for special education unless they are failing. He is failing in certain areas, but they won't officially admit it. Governor Clinton has just announced his new educational program for Arkansas, and he says that parents and teachers will be held responsible if children are not educated properly. How can I be held responsible when I cannot get the school to admit Mike has a learning disability and help him to deal with it?"

Harriet believes her problems with obtaining special education for her handicapped children stem from the reluctance of public school systems to use federal, state, and local funds earmarked for special education for that purpose. Under P.L. 94-142, Arkansas received more than ten million dollars of federal funds in 1983–84 to educate the state's 46,231 handicapped children.

"Maybe the money schools get to educate a handicapped child doesn't pay for the actual costs. I do know they are receiving funds. I have heard that sometimes the number of handicapped kids in a school is inflated—they call them 'phantom kids'—so that the federal appropriation will be larger, but the money is used for things like athletics or administrators instead of educating the real handicapped kids in the school like my children."

Money is always a worry for Harriet and Don because their income cannot increase as the years go by, or they will lose the benefits they now receive to pay their medical bills. Mike, Theresa, Mary, and Rebecca receive SSI income and Medicaid to pay for doctor and drug bills and financial support from Crippled Children's Service to pay for medical equipment. Don cannot make even twenty-five dollars more a week in his job, or they will lose their eligibility.

"If we lost our eligibility, we couldn't begin to pay the medical bills we have every month. Physical therapy is forty dollars an hour, and the twins go two hours a week. We spend a fortune in gas traveling back and forth to Little Rock several times a week to see eye doctors, orthopedists, neurologists, and orthodontists. And this is multiplied times four, because they all have to go. Rebecca and Mary need leg braces, which cost five hundred dollars apiece, and have to be replaced as they grow. When a boy kicked in Theresa's wheelchair on the school bus, the metal bar he bent cost fifty dollars to replace. Each of them has had eye surgery to straighten their crossed eyes. Theresa has had two eye operations, and each one cost one thousand dollars. She has also had heel-cord surgery."

There are sounds of the children coming home, and soon Paul walks through the front door carrying Rebecca in his arms. Amy follows with Mary in her arms; then come Cathy and Mike. Theresa is the last, and she stumbles into the living room smiling as usual, her toothless grin a reminder that she knocked her front teeth out during a bad fall several months ago. Mike removes the brace that he wears day and night to correct his crooked teeth, which were damaged by the anticonvulsant he took for five years, and searches the refrigerator for a snack.

As soon as Rebecca and Mary are put down on the floor, they both begin to shriek inconsolably. Harriet picks up Rebecca, who arches her back and continues to sob. "What's wrong, Becky? Do you want Momma? Come here." She offers Rebecca a bottle.

Like their parents, sisters, and brothers, Rebecca and Mary are tall for their age. Harriet awkwardly tries to balance three-year-old Rebecca on her lap as she gives her the bottle.

"What is really incredible," she says, "is that at the beginning of this school year, the school sent home a note with Paul that told us that he had to get a measles, mumps and rubella shot or he would be thrown out of school. The only way he could be exempted is if he had already had measles, mumps, and rubella and this was documented in a doctor's medical records. Paul has had all three, and I rushed over to my doctor and asked him to write Paul a letter to exempt him."

But the Arkansas Department of Health insisted that Harriet drive to Little Rock, which is a hundred miles away, and personally deliver the doctor's letter so it could be reviewed before Paul would be exempted. "I was introduced to Dr. J. P. Lofgren, the state epidemiologist, and he told me, 'I really wish you would go ahead and give Paul the MMR shot because we can't guarantee he is immune even though he has had the diseases.' I asked him if he could guarantee Paul would be immune if he got the MMR shot. He said, 'No, I can't promise that but I recommend he get the shot because he will be the first person to be sent home from school if there is a measles or mumps outbreak in the school.' I asked him how much of an outbreak there could be if only one percent of the children were not immunized, and he said, 'Well, sometimes the shots don't work.'"

After Harriet explained about her four vaccine-damaged children, Paul was granted a medical exemption from the MMR shot. "I'll tell you one thing," says Harriet calmly. "My kids aren't getting any more shots. They will have to kill me first."

Cathy is trying to console Mary, who is still shrieking and attempting to pull herself over to Harriet. "What's the matter, Mary? Do you want me to hold you?"

With the wisdom of a six year old, Cathy announces wistfully, "They can't sit up alone. You have to watch them."

Harriet smiles and runs her fingers affectionately through Cathy's hair. "Yes. You are a pretty good watcher aren't you. You are a good helper."

Amy takes Rebecca from her mother's arms. Harriet lifts Mary into her lap and holds her close. "I don't know what will happen to my children. Mary and Rebecca may eventually have to be placed in an institution. We are in court right now trying to reach a settlement with the manufacturer of the DPT vaccine that hurt them. We have many doctors testifying that their condition is due to the pertussis vaccine. But we could lose our case and end up with nothing, with no way to provide for them when we get too old to care for them. It scares me. It makes me so sad," finishes Harriet softly.

Mary stops crying and melts into her mother's arms. She bends her head back, her mouth wide open, and gazes into her mother's face. It is silent for a moment in the Arkansas trailer that is home to a remarkable family with a capacity for love and endurance that is a tribute to them all.

16

Who Is Responsible?

> If there ever could be a proper time for mere catch arguments,
> that time is surely not now. In times like the present, men
> should utter nothing for which they would not willingly be
> responsible through time and in eternity.
>
> *Abraham Lincoln*

In the multifaceted story of the pertussis vaccine, it is difficult to answer the inevitable question, "Who is responsible for what has happened?" The answer is as complex as the pertussis bacterium itself.

Some place the blame on the federal government, because it has the authority to regulate vaccine quality, monitor adverse reactions, develop a safer vaccine, and decide research priorities.

Others believe that vaccine manufacturers are primarily responsible, because they actually produce the vaccine and should have been more diligent in monitoring adverse reactions and improving their product.

Still others, including many parents, blame the doctors who administer the vaccine improperly, often repeatedly giving it to children who have suffered a previous severe reaction.

But many hold practicing doctors blameless because they were only following the confusing and ever-changing guidelines issued by eminent physicians sitting on the American Academy of Pediatrics' Committee on Infectious Diseases and the Public Health Service's Advisory Committee on Immunization Practices.

In reality, they all share the blame, along with legislators who made the decision to require almost every child in America to receive a vaccine of unknown toxicity before entering school. Parents are perhaps the most innocent and have the most to learn from this story. But parents must re-evaluate the role they played in allowing doctors to inject children with a vaccine about which so very little is known, and permitting elected representatives to pass laws requiring it.

The Role of the U.S. Government

The Food and Drug Administration's John Robbins, M.D., once remarked, "The concept of safety for vaccines is much different than the concept of safety as applied to many other things. Vaccines are given to healthy people; our goal should always be 100 percent safety."

Charles Manclark, Ph.D., who is the FDA official responsible for pertussis vaccine research as well as for testing all pertussis vaccine lots released by drug manufacturers for administration to the public, maintains that the government takes steps to attain this goal of safety, and stated in an interview that "the pertussis vaccine is the most thoroughly monitored substance in the whole of drug manufacturing. Our Division of Product Quality Assurance checks and monitors every pertussis vaccine lot of every manufacturer."

The role played by the federal government—the regulator—and the handful of manufacturers who produce the pertussis vaccine—the regulated—lies at the very heart of this story and has shaped the history of vaccination in this country.

The Division of Biologics Standards

The federal government's responsibility for vaccine regulation began in 1902 when Congress established the Public Health and Marine Hospital Service. One of the duties of this newly formed agency was to regulate the sale and transport for human use of serums, toxins, antitoxins, and related products.

By the 1950s, the agency had changed names several times, and in 1955 it was reorganized and named the Public Health Service's Division of Biologics Standards (DBS) after it was learned that some of the Cutter Laboratories' lots of Salk vaccine had caused paralytic polio in nearly 200 children. During the next seventeen years the DBS was the major driving force in the standardization, upgrading, and testing of the pertussis vaccine.

For most of those seventeen years, the DBS conducted its work in the obscurity loved by federal bureaucrats. But in 1971, one of its better known and more distinguished scientists, J. Anthony Morris, Ph.D., assisted by lawyer James Turner, a former associate of Ralph Nader, charged the DBS with many violations of its vaccine-regulating role. Senator Abraham Ribicoff of Connecticut helped keep the issue on the front page of America's newspapers for several years. It was a period remembered even today by surviving DBS employees as a time of unending turmoil, heartbreak, and misunderstanding.

Between 1960 and 1966, Morris, who is a specialist in influenza virus vaccines, had been responsible for testing this vaccine on the population of the Caroline Islands. He said in a 1983 interview, "we found that the incidence of protection afforded by vaccination against the strain that was active was about 20 percent . . . the 20 percent range is so low that you could say with validity the vaccine afforded little or no protection against influenza."

Morris vividly recalled what happened when he reported to DBS director Roderick Murray that after six years of study, he found the influenza vaccine to be ineffective: "He stripped me of my technicians. He stripped me of my lab facilities, so it was impossible for me to proceed further. It ended up that I had only one person working for me, instead of the ten people I had had for the past six years."

Morris explained why he thought Murray reacted so negatively to his suggestion that the influenza vaccine was not effective. "Influenza vaccine is the only vaccine administered annually. This is a tremendous market. At that time, about twenty million doses of influenza vaccine were being produced and sold yearly. If you took that vaccine market away, it would have left a tremendous hole, and I believe that the administrators within NIH were not willing to see that market disappear. Certainly, the pharmaceutical companies were not willing to see that market disappear. Where do you think vaccine experts go when they leave the government? They either go to a related medical field, or they go to work for a pharmaceutical manufacturer."

Every lot of vaccine produced is supposed to be tested for safety and potency by the manufacturer and then submitted to the government for retesting. Once the government determines that the lot has passed these tests, permission is given to the manufacturer to release the lot to be administered to the public.

In 1971, Morris charged that the DBS was releasing lots of flu vaccine which were failing DBS potency tests. His claim was upheld by the General Accounting Office (GAO), which reported that some of the vaccine lots had a potency of less than 1 percent of the established standard. A DBS official made a memorable statement at a 1971 congressional hearing: "The manufacturers would sell water if they could get away with it."

Morris and others demonstrated that Murray had ordered DBS personnel to accept the manufacturers' test results without requiring that vaccine lots pass the DBS standards. In the mid-1970s, Morris refused to endorse the DBS's "swine flu" mass vaccination campaign and warned the public that not only would there be no "swine flu" epidemic but that the vaccine had the potential to cause serious side effects. He was subsequently fired by the new DBS director, Harry Meyer, M.D.

Morris was eventually proved to be right: the "swine flu" epidemic never materialized, and the vaccine caused cases of Guillain-Barre syndrome—a type of paralysis. Political pressure eventually forced the government to set up a compensation system for "swine flu" vaccine victims.

The DBS defended itself against Morris's charges by arguing that the science of immunology was imprecise and that it was unjust to hold the agency to a higher standard than the state of the art permitted. This view was echoed in the 1979 report of the Panel on Review of Bacterial Vaccines and Toxoids: "It is important for the public and its agencies to appreciate the tentative and evolving nature of the science of immunization, particularly to combat the notion that decisions made in the public interest at one point in time are necessarily valid and binding at another."

Bureaucratic Empires Built by Distinguished Scientists

What did this mean for the pertussis vaccine? Since it was introduced into the United States without large-scale clinical trials, clearly the DBS had a responsibility to scrutinize and follow up reports of adverse reactions, to press forward with improved safety and potency tests, and to develop a better vaccine. But the record does not indicate that it vigorously pursued these goals. While the DBS cannot be accused of sins of commission, it may well be faulted for sins of omission.

When an agency comes under fire, attention is first directed to its leader. Since 1955, the DBS had been run by one of its own well-regarded scientists, Dr. Roderick Murray. No one ever criticized Murray's integrity or competence, but many accused him of being overly conservative. A former associate, Dr. Vernon Knight, chairman of the Microbiology Department at the Baylor University College of Medicine in Houston, said, "He has a record of absolute honesty and total devotion to protecting the public. If there is any criticism, it is that he has been overdeliberate. But, frankly, that is the way to stay alive in this business."

Murray himself was in a peculiar bureaucratic bind. The mission of the DBS was to develop new vaccines and also to regulate the production of existing vaccines. The U.S. Congress, which had given the DBS these two responsibilities, may not have realized that the business of developing new and safer vaccines might come into conflict with the business of regulating existing ones. But the truth is that they often did come into conflict. And at every turn Murray opted for regulating existing vaccines rather than aggressively trying to develop new and safer ones.

As a result, the research end of the DBS was underfunded, understaffed, and underproductive. Another former DBS associate, Dr. C. W. Hiatt, said in 1972: "The intellectual attitude of the DBS management was not hostile as long as your research didn't rock the boat. We only got ourselves tangled up when we got involved in any way with control responsibilities. The occasions when actual findings were ignored were very, very few. But there were incipient instances of that, when the organization would prefer you didn't get into a given area."

Dr. Bobby Young, whose comments on the DPT vaccine have become a part of the public record and who was also an alumnus of the DBS, said in 1972 that the agency's attitude toward research was one of "suppression, harassment, and censorship of individual investigators such as Morris. . . ." In the 1972 hearings before Senator Ribicoff's Subcommittee on Executive Reorganization and Government Research, Dr. Leonard Hayflick, of the Stanford University School of Medicine, observed:

"My final point concerns a host of criticisms that have been leveled at DBS by many eminent scientists, for the most part bearing on its image as an agency that rarely acts but only reacts. Instead of assuming a leadership role in the area of biological products control, in the view of many, DBS has assumed a role subservient to its constituency. . . . The DBS has acted in many major areas by simply not acting at all, thus fomenting controversy and exacerbating differences that could have been aired and easily resolved. The tragedy is that the avoidance of major decisions by the DBS is unjustifiable for a regulatory agency, for it inevitably works to the disadvantage of the public it is charged to protect."

As a result of these hearings, the DBS was transferred in 1972 from the Public Health Service (PHS) to the Food and Drug Administration (FDA), where it became the Bureau of Biologics (BOB) headed by Meyer. Although HEW Secretary Elliot Richardson denied that the move was motivated by any dissatisfaction with the scandal surrounding the DBS and its problems with vaccine regulation, this was seen as a face-saving gesture.

A DBS employee who played a major role in the unfolding drama of the pertussis vaccine was Dr. Margaret Pittman, a distinguished bacteriologist and specialist in pertussis vaccine research who was director of the DBS Laboratory of Bacterial Products from 1957 until her retirement in 1971.

It was Pittman who had helped Pearl Kendrick develop the intracerebral challenge test for pertussis vaccine potency in 1948 and who helped improve it in 1953. In a 1984 interview she stated that this test was her major scientific accomplishment, since it "for the first time related potency to clinical efficacy of the vaccine." Pittman's name is also associated with the mouse weight-gain test for toxicity.

However, as discussed in Chapters 3 and 19, these tests developed more than thirty years ago have remained essentially unchanged and are today thought to be very poor measures of the vaccine's toxicity and potency. The unanswered question is why there has been so little apparent movement in refining these tests or in pertussis research generally.

Do the Tests Measure Anything?

With the challenge tests, scientists and physicians thought they had finally laid to rest the problem of pertussis vaccine adverse reactions that had been so dramatically demonstrated in the 1948 article by Byers and Moll. The medical world was convinced such articles would no longer be written because there would no longer be any adverse reactions. Dr. William McLean, director of microbiological research for Parke-Davis, stated in 1968 that he himself, Dr. Pittman, and others at the NIH and the CDC at the time felt that these tests, "which are part of standards for all pertussis [vaccine] made in this country had eliminated the encephalopathic type of reaction."

In fact, the medical world was mistaken. As the record shows, the mouse weight-gain test for toxicity, despite reformulations and revisions, did not eliminate a substantial incidence of adverse reactions to the vaccine.

In 1963, C. N. Christensen, medical director of the Eli Lilly Company, wrote to the *American Journal of Diseases of Children* that he had sent questionnaires to 104 heads of hospitals and departments of pediatrics asking about their experience with the pertussis vaccine since 1955, when the new standards for vaccine production first came into effect. He found that "twenty-two children with some type of encephalopathy following pertussis vaccine administration were observed in thirteen institutions from 1955 to 1961." Of these, fourteen had neurological sequelae, including "moderate to severe mental retardation, . . . recurrent convulsions, . . . and cerebral palsy." He concluded that "some hazard" still attended the use of the vaccine.

An unpublished version of this letter delivered at a DBS meeting stated even more strongly, "It is obvious that severe neurologic reactions have occurred in children after immunization with pertussis vaccines which have passed the toxicity and potency tests currently in use." Also, "Two informants volunteered that in their institutions, the incidence of neurological reactions in the past five years appeared to be about the same as it was ten or fifteen years ago."

As part of a Pharmaceutical Manufacturers Association meeting in March 1964, a group of vaccine producers came together to discuss problems with the tests. A summary of the meeting was prepared and one participant reportedly said, "Dr. Pittman's mouse test hasn't gotten rid of encephalopathy." Another observed that "Pittman claims she has reduced encephalopathy, but there has been a dosage control coincident with the institution of the toxicity test." And finally, "Why hasn't Pittman accepted the obvious problems with this toxicity test?"

The group was asked, "Does anyone here have a whole cell vaccine that is not reactive in children?" The answer, to a man, was "no."

The memorandum (written twenty years ago) concluded, "It has long been felt by those companies preparing pertussis vaccines that the mouse toxicity test bears no relationship to the clinical reactivity of a particular lot of vaccine."

Pittman discussed this very matter in a 1965 article: "In the preparation of pertussis vaccine there is a delicate balance between detoxification and preservation of potency. Control of toxicity would be facilitated if there were satisfactory answers to the following questions: (i) Is mouse-measured toxicity correlated with untoward reactivity in children? (ii) What are the best methods to produce a vaccine of minimal reactivity for children? (iii) What laboratory assays best reflect toxicity? . . . Information on the relation of animal assays to reactions in children is inadequate."

But while scientists were pondering these significant unanswered problems and questioning the value of the one test that was supposed to protect babies from death and injury, these same babies were steadily being vaccinated.

Pittman went on to state, "It is anticipated that a cooperative field study will be initiated after a base line of reference has been established. It is hoped that the clinical study will determine whether or not there is a correlation between the laboratory assay and untoward reactions in children." But while plans were being laid (or not being laid) for the cooperative field study, a nationwide experiment with the vaccine was being performed every day, as states started to pass laws calling for compulsory mass vaccination as a requirement for school entry. Evidently it was not considered unwise to inoculate millions of children with a vaccine that could not accurately be measured for toxicity by any existing test.

The potency and toxicity tests, which were the key to improving the vaccine, were Pittman's major professional accomplishment, and she was perhaps the foremost authority on this issue. As director of the Laboratory of Bacterial Products reporting directly to Roderick Murray, whom she described in an interview as "a very devoted scientist, brilliant man, and a good administrator," she had the position and power to press for improvements in these tests and in the vaccine itself.

Apparently, Pittman took a strong, even a proprietary interest in pertussis vaccine issues during her tenure of power. Lawyers for Eric Tinnerholm, a child damaged by the DPT-Polio Quadrigen vaccine manufactured by Parke-Davis, complained at the subsequent trial that it was difficult to obtain evidence that Quadrigen was more toxic than the DPT vaccine "because Dr. Pittman, who alone possesses the necessary information, has regarded this lawsuit and her role in it as an attack or criticism on her and her department."

And yet there was very little progress. Griffith of Burroughs-Wellcome remarked at the 1982 FDA Symposium: "This uncertainty of the question of whether the mouse potency test provides a reliable [measure] of the protective efficacy of pertussis vaccine in children is and will remain a considerable handicap to the development of new pertussis vaccines."

It could be argued that the state of the art in vaccine research simply did not permit any upgrading of the potency and toxicity rests. But the state of the art in any scientific discipline advances rapidly or slowly depending upon the emphasis it is given.

And the pertussis vaccine apparently was not given a high enough priority during these years to permit major scientific advances to be made. Why? The answer was given by Manclark in a 1983 interview: "Since the pertussis vaccines on the market have been certified as safe and effective, it is difficult to obtain funds for work on improving these vaccines. Governmental budgetary resources, which are always tight, will obviously be directed into areas of seemingly greater need. The manufacturers are in the same position. Their vaccines have been certified safe and effective. Why should they expend funds on improving them?"

Especially in connection with these tests, the cart got placed before the horse. Once the vaccine had been mandated for mass compulsory use, the tests could not be discarded, even though everyone knew that they were deficient. They had become indispensable to the process of certifying lots of pertussis vaccine safe for public use.

This was brought out in an exchange at a 1980 vaccine conference in Israel. One participant declared with exasperation, "It seems to me the essential reason which prevents the development of an effective and safe pertussis vaccine is this barbarian and irrelevant mouse protection test. . . . What we should do is to get away from this 'marriage' with the intracerebral challenge and search for relevant assays. . . ."

To this the FDA's John Robbins responded, "I agree with every single thing you say, including the grammatical punctuation, but it is not so easy to make a 'divorce' from the mouse protection test if you have to sign your name to a protocol to be released for pertussis vaccine."

The vaccine had to pass safety and efficacy tests, even if these tests proved little or nothing.

What is more, the existence of these tests even inhibited potential research on improving the vaccine. Scientists in private laboratories, who decide what problem they want to research and then spend a significant amount of their time writing and applying for government grants to finance this research, assumed that scientific questions about whooping cough and the pertussis vaccine had long been settled and were no longer an issue.

After the initial research in the 1950s and up until the past few years, there has been little interest in funding whooping cough or pertussis vaccine research. Daniel Levitt, M.D., Ph.D., of the Guthrie Reseach Institute, in a 1983 interview stated: "I could study basically the same situation and the same interests in a research project, and if I directed it at Chlamydia, it would very likely be funded. Most researchers feel that the effects of pertussis, the influence of pertussis on the immune system, have been pretty well evaluated in the 1940s, 1950s, and 1960s. Chlamydia is a hot microorganism right now. . . ."

Adverse Reactions Ignored

The very fact that the vaccine was pronounced safe and protective effectively inhibited aggressive research into improving it. The only factor which could have galvanized the DBS into an active program to refine the tests as a first step to improving the vaccine would have been a frank recognition of adverse reactions. But the record does not suggest there was recognition of vaccine reactions. It suggests just the opposite.

Pittman wrote in 1965: "Fortunately, encephalopathy after vaccination is relatively rare." And when the GAO looked into vaccines in 1971 as a result of the Ribicoff hearings and consulted DBS officials, it concluded: "There is no generally accepted or definitive evidence that pertussis vaccine does, in fact, cause serious adverse reactions . . . [there are] no problems associated with the safety, purity, potency, and efficacy of pertussis vaccine that would require any HEW action."

By this time, of course, the vaccine had been in general use for more than two decades and reports of serious adverse reactions had appeared from time to time in the scientific literature. Physicians were supposedly expected to notify the manufacturers of reactions and, as can be seen from the 1979 *Report* of the Panel on Review of Bacterial Vaccines and Toxoids, reaction reports had been trickling in since the early 1960s.

It was a well-known fact, even in the 1960s, that the reporting of adverse reactions was minimal to the point of being nonexistent. The 1979 Bacterial Vaccines Panel pointed out that doctors were not routinely reporting reactions to manufacturers and that many doctors not only were unaware that reporting was important, they did not know the clinical features of a reaction.

Another reason was that doctors and manufacturers were afraid of lawsuits. The Panel's *Report* stated, "both physicians and manufacturers may be held liable for damages in suits brought by patients who may suffer adverse reactions from established vaccines. All of these factors undoubtedly discourage reporting."

The 1979 Bacterial Vaccines Panel found that, in the category of "major reactions," a grand total of three deaths and one case of permanent neurological damage had been reported to manufacturers. Even the picture of "minor" reactions was clearly deficient. To take one example among many in the Panel's *Report*, Merrell-National Laboratories was able to provide only "six reports of adverse reactions, all of minor consequence . . . during a five year period when many hundreds of thousands of doses of this vaccine were distributed."

This sort of incidence of major and minor reactions is so grotesquely out of line with what has been reported in the literature and what can be learned from interviews with parents that it would be almost comical if not for the numbers of wasted lives it represents. But for decades, no one was concerned enough to rectify the situation and in 1976, Red Book Committee chairman Vincent Fulginiti could remark, "Amazingly, we do not know the incidence [of adverse reactions] in the United States, despite the recommendation that every child receive the vaccine."

In 1979, the Panel reached strong conclusions and recommended that the reporting system be substantially upgraded: "Without maximum reporting or some other form of surveillance, definition of the rates and significance of untoward reactions to current and future vaccines cannot be ascertained. . . . The Panel is convinced that currently employed surveillance systems to identify adverse reactions to pertussis vaccine are inadequate and recommends that definitive steps be taken by the appropriate subdivisions of the Public Health Service [DBS and CDC] to improve them."

It is inconceivable that DBS personnel in the 1960s and early 1970s were unaware of these serious weaknesses in the data-gathering program for adverse reactions. Manufacturing facilities were inspected annually and DBS personnel had the right to look at adverse reaction files. Furthermore, manufacturers were providing some reports.

But there is no evidence that priority was ever given to investigating these reaction reports or ensuring that they were comprehensive and accurate. The bureaucratic sluggishness of a federal regulatory agency known familiarly as "the boat that never rocked" seems to have blocked a systematic search for the unwanted side effects of the pertussis vaccine.

Until the transfer of the DBS from the Public Health Service to the FDA in 1972, there was not even a separate file for reports of adverse reactions coming in from manufacturers. They were all classified with "general correspondence."

Without recognition of adverse reactions by scientists and doctors in positions of authority in the federal government, there has been little recognition of them by leaders of the AMA and the AAP. By extension, there has been little awareness by the ordinary practicing physician of vaccine adverse reactions and little incentive to report them. Without a systematic effort to collect and describe vaccine damage cases, there was no pressure for change. No pressure for change meant no incentive to upgrade the vaccine.

Because of this, the journal *Science* could state in 1972: "Without doubt the DBS has capably fulfilled its minimum function, that of ensuring the immediate safety of vaccines. What is at question is whether the DBS has adequately carried out such broader responsibilities as improving the quality of vaccines and assessing the longer term risks and benefits associated with vaccine use. . . . Specific research areas in which the DBS coverage is most commonly faulted are the improvement of existing vaccines, particularly . . . pertussis."

Although cutting down on brain damage and death caused by the pertussis vaccine should have been a primary goal of DBS during the early decades of mass public use of the vaccine, this goal was undercut by political, legal, economic, and public relations considerations. There was always the possibility that if word got out to the public that the pertussis vaccine was causing serious reactions, the public would reject the mass vaccination program. Since 1974, federal agencies, physicians' organizations, and manufacturers have been especially obsessed by the fear that American parents would follow the lead of British parents and abandon the pertussis vaccine. Perhaps this is why the government seems to have actively discouraged discussion of vaccine reactions.

In 1970, George Dick observed, "It is surprising that information about serious reactions to pertussis vaccine is neither generally available nor openly discussed. Yet the reactions to other vaccines, such as smallpox and measles, are freely acknowledged." A year later, Peter Isaacson and Allen Stone said, "There has been a tendency on the part of certain higher government circles to play down any open discussion of problems associated with vaccines. This is on the quite reasonable basis that the public would become alarmed, begin to doubt the proven efficacy of most vaccines, and make final disease eradication more difficult. Perhaps this has been overdone. Scientists now find themselves in a position of balancing the benefits of a vaccine against the risk, yet are in no position to judge what the long-term risks are."

Abram Benenson, M.D., chairman of the Department of Community Medicine at the University of Kentucky, stated at the same time that merely by discussing the risks and benefits of vaccines, "We are conditioning the public to reject measures that sometimes, in some situations, are very important."

The 1972 *Science* article noted that "the picture is also blurred by a reluctance among vaccine workers to discuss problems openly when they arise. This is because of the understandable fear that public confidence in vaccines—and vaccine authorities—will be eroded."

Dr. Pittman herself stated in a 1984 interview, "I don't think it is wise to upset the public about these things."

Are Vaccines Drugs?

The minimizing of vaccine reactions was made easier by the lack of a legal requirement that vaccines undergo clinical trials in order to be cleared by the government for release. If large-scale clinical trials had been conducted with the vaccine in America before it was released, data on reactions would have been collected, as they were by the UCLA-FDA study in 1979. But as has been discussed in Chapters 3 and 5, such trials were never conducted.

The reason for this peculiar state of affairs is rooted in the history of food and drug law. In 1902, Congress gave authority to the PHS to regulate vaccines, but authority to regulate drugs was given to the FDA. Up until 1962, vaccine manufacturers had to demonstrate the "safety," "purity," and "potency" of their vaccines, while drug manufacturers had only to demonstrate "safety."

In 1962, however, the Kefauver amendments to the Food, Drug and Cosmetic Act required manufacturers of drugs to prove their "efficacy" by clinical trials as a precondition of licensing, and the question immediately arose: Must vaccine manufacturers also prove efficacy of vaccines by clinical trials? In other words, would the intracerebral challenge test in mice continue to be accepted as proof that the vaccine was effective in protecting children against whooping cough, or would manufacturers have to run clinical trials on the vaccine in the same way that manufacturers of drugs had to run clinical trials?

Strangely, almost a quarter of a century later, this question has still not been answered because of the government's Hamlet-like indecision. Although HEW legal counsel advised Roderick Murray in 1969 that the Kefauver amendments gave DBS the authority to require manufacturers to conduct clinical studies to demonstrate vaccine effectiveness, Murray rejected the position of the HEW general counsel and refused to implement it. Perhaps he feared this change would lead to abolition of the DBS and incorporation of its functions into the FDA.

So, a purely bureaucratic, civil service concern—the desire to maintain the separate administrative autonomy of a minor governmental agency—is apparently one of the reasons why vaccines administered to every child in the country do not have to be demonstrated effective by clinical trials. Ironically, when the DBS was finally swallowed up by the FDA in 1972, the FDA bought the DBS position that manufacturers should not be required to prove vaccine efficacy in clinical trials. Today, the FDA still does not require that vaccines be proved clinically effective.

In September 1980, FDA Commissioner Jere Goyan explicitly stated this in response to a petition filed by a consumer organization calling for clinical testing of vaccines: "While the agency has affirmed many times that biological products are drugs within the meaning of the [Food, Drug and Cosmetic] Act, they are not subject to the new drug provisions . . . the specific statutory criteria governing new drugs, 'adequate and well-controlled clinical studies,' have not been applied to biological drugs."

To be or not to be a drug, that is the question. Awesome confusion still prevails. In 1982, in an attempt to blunt the effect of "DPT: Vaccine Roulette," J. Michael Lane, M.D., of the FDA's National Center for Drugs and Biologics (the most recent name for the DBS), wrote to all state and territorial health officers: "Before vaccines are licensed, they must undergo clinical testing to demonstrate safety and efficacy." The right hand doesn't seem to know what the left hand is doing.

It is just one more twist in the tortuous history of the government's regulation of vaccines. If large-scale clinical trials had been required, the vaccine's reactivity would have been revealed as it was in the UCLA-FDA study. Americans would not have had to wait forty years after the vaccine was introduced to understand the risks involved.

Today the FDA requests that manufacturers perform clinical tests of any vaccines licensed since 1962 on a "voluntary" basis, and the companies working on new vaccines are planning to conduct clinical trials. But there is still no legal requirement. The ghost of the DBS still haunts the halls of the Department of Health and Human Services.

While many factors contributed to this abdication of regulatory responsibility by the government, the most significant was its historic lack of interest in vaccine reactions, which left these reports mouldering away in files instead of being collected and analyzed for ways to improve the vaccine and cut down on reactions. This made it easier for officials to toss off "benefit/risk calculations" whenever the vaccine was criticized without any idea of the true magnitude of the risks.

Perhaps officials thought the problem would just go away. Perhaps they thought a safer vaccine could eventually be developed and gradually phased in, permitting criticism of the previous product to be dismissed as ancient history. But an improved vaccine has not yet been made available to U.S. children, and adverse reactions still occur.

Monitoring Adverse Reactions and "Hot Lots"

Today the Centers for Disease Control (CDC) and the FDA are supposed to work together to protect the public health and safety by monitoring vaccine reactions. The FDA tests vaccines for potency and toxicity, while the CDC surveys the incidence of whooping cough in the country (which indirectly measures vaccine efficacy) and collects reports on vaccine reactions (which indirectly measures vaccine safety).

The CDC's involvement with vaccine reaction monitoring dates from 1978, when the Public Health Service set up the Monitoring System for Illness Following Immunization (MSIFI), which has been discussed in Chapter 9. Unfortunately, MSIFI was not designed to provide comprehensive statistics on reactions so that an accurate benefit/risk analysis could be made. Its primary mission is to flag suspicious clusters of reactions to warn the government and manufacturers that a particular lot of vaccine is "hot" and should be withdrawn from the market.

Roger Bernier, of the CDC, told a 1982 FDA Symposium, "The current surveillance systems for vaccine reactions depend on vaccinees or their guardians remembering to report reactions as instructed to their local public provider and depend on these, in turn, reporting through their state health departments to CDC. This system is designed primarily to serve as an early warning system for detecting unusual reactions or an increase in expected reactions, and is not designed to provide reliable incidence rates of reactions following immunization."

But even this partial and imperfect mission of MSIFI is not always carried out properly, as can be seen from the story of Lederle DPT Vaccine Lot 585–181.

The MSIFI guidelines define a potential "hot lot" as one which generates at least ten reports of illness, or two reports of seizures, or two reports of deaths. Such reports are supposed to trigger a thorough investigation of the vaccine lot and withdrawal of one that appears to be especially toxic. Lederle Lot 585–181, distributed in 1980, met these "hot lot" criteria but was not withdrawn from circulation. It remained on the market until all vials had been sold.

According to internal FDA and CDC memos, on March 20, 1980, CDC's Bernier called FDA's John Robbins to report that the CDC was getting an unusual number of severe reaction reports associated with DPT vaccine from Lederle Lot 585–181. This lot, which had been manufactured by Connaught Laboratories, had passed the FDA safety and potency tests, and subsequently had been purchased from Connaught by Lederle for distribution in August 1979, under the Lederle label.

On March 28, an internal Lederle memo reported a telephone conversation with Marjorie Pollack, of the CDC, in which she spelled out precisely what kind of adverse reactions, including deaths, had been associated with this lot: "28 serious adverse reactions reports from six states."

The memo continued: "Of the 28, four were reported as Sudden Infant Death Syndrome (SIDS): 1) Six weeks old, SIDS five days post-vaccination—November/December, 1979; 2) Eight weeks old, diffuse diarrhea one day after vaccination, SIDS 15 days after—? [sic]

date; 3) Six weeks old, symptoms of URI [upper respiratory infection], SIDS five days post vaccination—January, 1980; 4) Eight weeks old, SIDS less than 24 hours post vaccination—September, 1979.

"Twelve had systemic reactions involving, variably, fever, skin rash, respiratory distress, CNS [central nervous system] depression, somnolence, seizures, vomiting, irritability. One seven-month-old child had seizure on two separate immunizations with the same control number. An eight-month-old child had seizure and respiratory arrest, recovered spontaneously. A third child is thought to have had a neurological reaction, and irritability has persisted since vaccination in early March. A fourth child, three months old, had fever and seizures nine hours after vaccination last September, and has had recurrent seizures since. Two children with respiratory distress and shock-like reactions were treated successfully with epinephrine. The remaining twelve of the 28 reports concerned severe local tissue reaction."

The memo described the conversation further: "The State of Colorado PHS reports an incidence of reaction to batch No. 585–181 of 45/100,000 doses. Public sector incidence figures for Colorado and the U.S. as a whole for all of 1979 were 6/100,000 doses. This suggests that 585–181 is unusually highly reactive."

Lederle Lot 585–181 was clearly associated with enough serious reactions to alert the MSIFI and stimulate an in-depth investigation. This was supposed to happen but it did not. A Lederle memo of March 20 revealed that John Robbins at the FDA "stated that, in his opinion, this was nothing to worry about" and that "the CDC was overreacting to this situation."

On April 9, Carolyn Hardegree of the Public Health Service wrote her own memo for the record, stating that "a total of nine seizures have been associated with this lot. . . . Dr. Pollack has calculated that the reported reaction rate for this lot in Colorado is 45/1000,000 doses. . . . With all other DPT given to children under 1 year the rate is 6/100,000." She concluded, "There is no statistical data to show that this lot is associated with more seizures than another lot of Lederle DPT."

Another memo "for the record" from Carolyn Hardegree, dated April 15, 1980, states that the reported adverse reactions were now being calculated at 16/100,000 doses and that, according to Dr. Pollack, 585–181 "does not appear more reactive" than other lots.

To date, at least six children are known to have died or been left with permanent brain damage after reacting to vaccine from Lederle

Lot 585–181. All six received the vaccine after the April 15 meeting at which the subject was closed. One child has already cost her family and the state in which she lives more than $80,000. It would have cost the manufacturer approximately the same amount of money to withdraw the lot from the market.

Compared to the government investigation of Wyeth Lot 64201 associated with the SIDS cases in Tennessee discussed in Chapter 14, very little was done to investigate Lederle Lot 585–181. The question naturally arises: Was the suspect Lederle "hot lot" treated so delicately because FDA officials did not want to provide a public already sensitized to the connection between SIDS and the DPT vaccine with yet another opportunity to suspect that the vaccine was injuring and killing children?

Evidently other suspected "hot lots" are not routinely being investigated, as can be seen from a 1982 article by CDC's Harrison Stetler stating: "Over the past three years, several potential hot lots have been detected, and a few have been investigated by the CDC."

Is Stetler referring to the "investigation" of Lederle Lot 585–181? More importantly, why haven't all suspected "hot lots" been investigated?

The SIDS connection, which was so evident in the Wyeth lot implicated in the Tennessee deaths, also played a role in Lederle Lot 585–181. According to the March 28 Lederle memo, Pollack had noted that four deaths occurring shortly after a DPT vaccination were reported as SIDS. Was any effort made to investigate each death fully for substantiation that these deaths were not SIDS but were DPT-related? Were health departments and coroners informed of this possibility?

Another problem highlighted by the Lederle Lot 585–181 incident was the FDA's inabilty to readily trace all vaccine doses from a given lot. A Lederle official pointed out in the March 20 memo that John Robbins "had requested complete distribution data for this lot. He also made a request for distribution data of all future lots of DPT and indicated that Connaught Laboratories had agreed to such a request. This means, then, that the Bureau of Biologics would have in hand the distribution of every lot actually in use and, if a problem arose, they would simply check their records to see in what parts of the country the lot in question was located. This is a new twist to adverse reaction reporting and management will have to approve such a plan. I advised Dr. Robbins of this fact."

It appears that as late as 1980, vaccine manufacturers were not required to inform the government exactly how vaccine from different lots was being distributed in the country. Added to this confusion is the fact that manufacturers make the vaccine in "batches," from which "lots" are drawn to be poured into vials and released to physicians. But the batch and lot numbers are different. Consequently, if severe reactions are associated with a particular lot, other lots drawn from what may have been a defective batch cannot easily be found and checked for unusual reactivity.

The problem of quickly tracing "hot lots" of vaccine is made worse by the fact that most doctors do not keep records of the manufacturer's name and the lot and batch numbers of vaccines they purchase and administer. Bernier of the CDC stated at a 1982 FDA Symposium, "Another difficulty in postmarketing evaluation is the documentation of pertussis vaccination history by exact type of vaccine received. Currently, most vaccine records are maintained by antigen only. And ensuring that providers include the manufacturer and lot number of vaccines on all records does not appear feasible."

On May 29, 1984, however, the State of Maryland adopted a law requiring physicians to maintain records of lot and batch numbers of all vaccines administered to children and to record any vaccine reaction in the child's permanent medical record. This bill, which was supported by Dissatisfied Parents Together, was opposed by the Maryland Medical and Chirurgical Faculty and the Maryland Chapter of the American Academy of Pediatrics.

Does U.S. Pertussis Vaccine Contain More Bacteria?

One of the contributions made by Pittman was to determine the number of pertussis bacteria in the total human immunizing dose. In 1954 this was set at 96,000 million bacteria and assigned the value of twelve "protective units" or "opacity units." And the way in which this bacterial content of a suspension of B. pertussis was determined was by measuring its grayish color, or "opacity."

European manufacturers and the WHO, however, subsequently developed a different opacity standard which is apparently lighter than the American one. In 1973 the United States agreed to adopt the WHO standard, but this has yet to be implemented.

The result is that the U.S. adsorbed (i.e., with an adjuvant) vaccine may contain 1.6 times as many bacteria as those made to the WHO standard. Some scientists have theorized that because the American vaccine appears to contain more bacteria, it may also be more reactive.

Confusion has long reigned on this point. At a meeting of vaccine producers held in 1964 under the auspices of the Pharmaceutical Manufacturers Association, one participant allegedly stated (according to an unpublished memorandum), "If reactions are high, then the opacity unitage may be high." Another asked, "Can there be a variation in the opacity unit test? We found a lot of vaccine with an opacity unitage of 30, and it was intolerable in humans; 20, however, was okay."

Cameron observed in 1978 that the existence of two opacity standards in the world raises several questions: "Does this mean that vaccines adjusted to the WHO standard are twice as potent and half as toxic, organism for organism, as those made to the U.S. standard? If the U.S. vaccine were made to the WHO standard, Cameron continued, "Another advantage [would] be the additional safety factor introduced by halving the number of bacteria per dose."

The question of the number of bacteria in a dose of vaccine is not inconsequential. At a 1980 vaccine conference in Israel, a Netherlands scientist announced that the Dutch had recently reduced the bacterial content of their vaccine from twelve to ten opacity units (even though the Dutch vaccine was already being made to the lighter WHO standard), "Until now this seems to work reasonably well. The Dutch have, I think, a couple of hundred thousand of vaccinations without encephalitis."

Why hasn't the United States investigated lowering the number of the bacteria in the vaccine to make it less reactive?

One fact is clear: the pertussis vaccine used in the United States is different from that used by the rest of the world. Whether the U.S. vaccine is more potent and more toxic should have been resolved long ago by the governmental agencies responsible for protecting the health of children.

The Vaccine Manufacturers

The 1979 Bacterial Vaccines Panel made a distinction between the liability of an individual vaccine manufacturer and that of the federal government. It concluded, "The former should comply with the regulations of production and marketing procedures. If these obligations are fulfilled and the vaccine is administered correctly, responsibility for immunization accidents should rest with the official agencies recommending them."

Does this mean that manufacturers are less responsible for vaccine damage than the government health agencies regulating the production of vaccines and recommending mass immunization, namely, the CDC and the FDA?

The Panel seemed to think so. It noted that, although animal models are needed for accurate and reliable safety and efficacy tests, "manufacturers are not primarily responsible to implement the quest for animal models, and the development of such models will require public research support."

The Panel pointed out that concerning standards for measuring safety, efficacy, purity, immunogenicity, and immune response, "the motivation and impetus to accomplish this is unlikely to come spontaneously from pharmaceutical manufacturers unless review of vaccine licensure is conducted periodically."

From the beginning the manufacturers were very aware of the reactivity of the pertussis vaccine, as can be seen from their comments at the 1964 PMA meeting discussed earlier which was devoted entirely to this issue. Typical comments by participants were: "We may be giving too large a dose. Possibly we can reduce the dose and reduce reactions." "There certainly is a difference in lots of vaccine." "If Pittman believed her potency test, then this problem would not have happened." "There is no doubt we need a laboratory test which will bear a direct relationship to the subsequent clinical findings, particularly fever and encephalopathy." "All one needs to do is look at the complaint file, and we see a fluctuation in the incidence of reactions, and yet nothing changes as pertains to the media, strain of organism, or protein nitrogen."

But vaccine production is one of the most highly regulated businesses in this country, and manufacturers are forced to adhere to federal government standards. Therefore, if a vaccine is to be upgraded, the push usually has to come from the government.

This does not mean that vaccine manufacturers are more ethical or less selfish than other producers of goods and services in the marketplace. A look at just one case of vaccine damage that went through the courts in the 1960s reveals what can go wrong with vaccine manufacturing.

The Quadrigen Fiasco

In 1957, Parke-Davis decided to combine the new Salk polio vaccine with its existing DPT vaccine, Triogen. The new product, called Quadrigen, was licensed by the government in July 1959. When it was withdrawn from the market nine years later, more than eight million doses had been injected into nearly three million babies.

The Quadrigen story reveals how the government's testing procedures for new vaccines may fail to protect the public's safety. But it is more than that. It is also a clearcut example of a vaccine manufacturer ignoring unfavorable preliminary test data and elementary safety precautions in its haste to market a new product.

The Quadrigen case raises the legitimate question of how often the government's testing procedures have failed without this coming to the public's attention. It also raises legitimate questions about the ethics of vaccine manufacturers.

One of the first babies to receive Quadrigen in 1959 was Eric Tinnerholm, who was left paralyzed on his right side with a permanent seizure condition and an estimated I.Q. of 5. A suit was brought by his parents against Parke-Davis, and a judgment of $650,000 was confirmed by the U.S. Court of Appeals.

At the trial it was brought out that the polio component of Quadrigen deteriorated from contact with the preservative, Merthiolate, used in all DPT vaccines at that time. Parke-Davis, therefore, had decided to use a different preservative—benzethonium chloride (known as Phemerol in the trade). The trial court found that, under certain circumstances, Phemerol had the ability to degrade the pertussis component of the vaccine, making it more toxic at a rate of about 6 percent per month.

The lawyers for the Tinnerholms charged that this was probably due to destruction of the B. pertussis cell wall by Phemerol, causing "autolysis," i.e., release of intracellular toxins into the solution, and a simultaneous decline in potency through loss of the cell wall antigens. If this did, in fact, happen, how did Quadrigen ever pass the DBS safety and potency tests?

Margaret Pittman testified that degradation took place when the vaccine was accidentally warmed and then cooled during its many stages of transportation from trucks to warehouses to pharmacies before reaching doctors' offices. She asserted that the vaccine tested by DBS had been maintained at a constant temperature and had not undergone alteration.

What is certain is that Parke-Davis did not test the effect of its new preservative on Quadrigen under typical conditions encountered in the marketplace, which included the temperature changes the vaccine underwent during transportation. This would have taken weeks or months to do, and as the lawyer for the Tinnerholms stated, "Faced with a product that had the potential to destroy the brains of small children to whom it was intended to be administered, reasonable care required of Parke-Davis extreme vigilance in its manufacture. Did Parke-Davis exercise such vigilance? We think the evidence demonstrated a lack of vigilance amounting to almost indifference and a rush to get the product to market that overwhelmed all other considerations."

What did Parke-Davis actually do in the way of testing Quadrigen before releasing it to American doctors? After performing one cursory study of the vaccine's efficacy on a group of babies in inner-city Detroit, it applied to the FDA for a license. Two other studies were underway, one particularly designed to test for adverse reactions, but Parke-Davis did not wait for the results.

In early 1960, the Massachusetts Department of Public Health found that Quadrigen was not passing the state's potency tests. The company's response was to abruptly increase the number of pertussis bacteria per unit of the vaccine! This was an almost incomprehensible step, since it meant changing the composition of the vaccine after the license had already been issued.

It was also a very risky step, and Parke-Davis knew it. The head of the company's Biological Division wrote to the DBS in 1960, "As I mentioned, we have decided to increase the bacterial count on each lot from 15 to 20 opacity units, with the thought that this should enhance stability as well as potency. We realize, of course, that this is a two-edged sword, and we may be encouraging toxicity problems by this action."

The addition of more pertussis bacteria increased the potency and toxicity above the DBS limits, so Parke-Davis then cut the bacteria back to the previous level. Again the vaccine had trouble passing the potency test. This seesawing back and forth ultimately meant that only one vaccine lot was accepted out of six submitted to the DBS between August 1961 and November 1962. Quadrigen was apparently a product that could not be made both safe and effective.

Eventually Parke-Davis realized that Quadrigen was unstable in its initial formulation, and it marketed a different one: a dual-chambered syringe with the DPT on one side and the polio vaccine on the other.

The U.S. Court of Appeals held that Quadrigen was an "unreasonably dangerous" product, and that Parke-Davis was responsible for the consequences. It refused to enter into the question of the manufacturer's alleged negligence in using Phemerol as a preservative without testing it. However, the conclusion that Parke-Davis behaved in a medically irresponsible way appears to be warranted.

This same hit-or-miss approach to vaccine manufacturing and distribution is seen in the way Parke-Davis distorted the data on Quadrigen's safety. The package insert for the vaccine stated:

"When given in accordance with suggested methods, local and systemic reactions following the administration of Quadrigen are usually mild. The incidence is usually no greater than is normally experienced with trivalent vaccine. . . . The final product represents triumph over technical difficulties of formulation and incompatibilities. Foremost among the problems solved is the concentration of the full potency of each antigenic compound in an individual dose volume of 0.5 cc. This was achieved without increasing the incidence of side effects."

Upon what data did Parke-Davis base this glowing tribute to Quadrigen's safety? Witnesses testified that the clinical trial Parke-Davis conducted in inner-city Detroit, prior to obtaining a license from the DBS, had not been designed to study reactions but only to determine if the vaccine was protective against whooping cough. Furthermore, the reporting system for reactions was largely passive. Parents were simply urged to report adverse reactions, which notoriously leads to underreporting. And though parents were questioned at succeeding clinic visits, no temperatures were taken. Even so, the parents of 30 out of the 298 babies—one tenth of all children in the study—reported reactions.

But the most astonishing fact to emerge at the Tinnerholm trial was that the pertussis component of the Quadrigen used in the Detroit clinical study was different from the pertussis component in the Quadrigen eventually marketed to doctors. It was taken from a batch of vaccine that had been stored for a year without any preservative at all and was added at the last minute to the mixture containing Phemerol. The authors of the published account of this clinical study made no bones about this fact and observed that the pertussis suspension "had diminished in potency" during its year of storage. So the adverse reactions reported by parents of 10 percent of the children participating in the clinical trial were from a pertussis component of *reduced* potency.

Parke-Davis then performed a second study on the same inner-city population of Detroit. This time Quadrigen was compared with the Parke-Davis DPT vaccine, Triogen. Instead of relying largely on passive reporting, as in 1958, public health nurses went into the homes of babies and took their temperatures. It turned out that the babies receiving Quadrigen had a higher incidence of temperatures over 102 F. than those receiving Triogen.

Parke-Davis did not publish this information. It was never mentioned in the published account of the clinical studies. At the Tinnerholm trial, Parke-Davis claimed that its statisticians had decided that the difference between Triogen and Quadrigen was within the normal range of statistical error.

The actual extent of the difference between the reactivity of Triogen and Quadrigen was brought out in a 1959 article by pertussis vaccine pioneer Louis Sauer. This was a study of Quadrigen conducted on "large groups of young institutionalized infants (mostly under six months of age) . . ." and as Sauer concluded, ". . . without any adverse reactions. There was no rise in rectal temperature in approximately 60%; 101 F. in 12%; 102 F. in 10%; 103 F. in 8%; 104 F. in 5%; and 105 F. in 2%. All temperatures were back to normal within 36 to 48 hours, regardless which dose was administered."

Thus, Sauer seemed to suggest that a temperature of 105 F. for forty-eight hours did not qualify as an "adverse reaction." By his conclusion, the 7 percent of the babies with temperatures of over 104 F., and 2 percent over 105 F., were not experiencing adverse reactions.

A witness at the Tinnerholm trial did not regard these temperature elevations as normal or the difference between Triogen and Quadrigen as well within the normal statistical spread. Joseph H. Lapin, M.D., an expert on whooping cough and pertussis vaccines, testified that he had never seen temperatures that high in twenty years of using Triogen.

Eric Tinnerholm had a temperature of 108 F. after his shot of Quadrigen.

Parke-Davis had no basis in its own clinical trials for absolving its product of adverse reactions on the package insert. In addition, it was getting a steady stream of messages from its "detail men" (company salesmen) that the new four-in-one vaccine was highly reactive.

One of these messages was reproduced in the trial transcript: "Joe Bauer has reported to me that three (3) of his best pediatricians have stopped using our product because of systemic and local reactions. One of these physicians is V. Larkin of Forest Hills, a man who holds Parke-Davis in high esteem. Ben Rogers reported the loss of two of his best users. Dr. John DeHoff of Flushing, who has used our product since its introduction and used on an average 20 vials per month has reported to Rogers *severe temperatures in almost every patient,* and he will not use Quadrigen in the future. Four of the above physicians are important influential pediatricians in both areas and could affect the future of Quadrigen locally."

Quadrigen's package insert did not refer to data that would have weakened the commercial position of Parke-Davis in the vaccine market. In particular, there was no mention of one baby who died during the 1959 testing of the vaccines, even though the diagnosis of vaccine-related death was made by a professor of pediatrics.

This apparent disregard of scientific evidence suggests that Parke-Davis treated the pertussis vaccine as just another product, like a new toothpaste or deodorant to be brought on the market as quickly as possible. No hint was given that such a product might be lethally dangerous to babies.

The last lot of Quadrigen was sold in 1968.

Testing "Hot Lots" of Vaccine on Children

At the 1964 PMA meeting of vaccine producers, one participant asked: "Is it feasible to suggest that before commercial lots are released, that the manufacturer send enough material to a clinic and have the reactogenicity evaluated before release of the entire lot?"

This actually happened in Michigan in 1975. A defective lot of DPT vaccine was deliberately tested in children.

Michigan and Massachusetts are the only two states that manufacture their own DPT vaccine. In 1975, Michigan was reportedly producing 800,000 doses annually and was one of the nation's major distributors. Before any of it could be sent to other states, however, it had to meet potency and toxicity standards set by the FDA for commercial manufacturers.

In July 1975, DPT vaccine Lot 1182 was sent to the FDA for routine testing prior to release. The FDA found that Lot 1182 was three times more potent than the regulations allowed and refused to allow Michigan to distribute it outside the state.

Rather than immediately destroy the defective lot, which represented about 400,000 doses, Michigan health officials decided to see just how reactive it was by testing it on several hundred children in Ingham County. An internal memo from the Michigan State Health Department reveals that state health officials knew that "Lot 1182 is potentially more reactive than the material [Lot 1180] tested in July" but decided to "release the vaccine without license, enclosing a note with the suggestion that Lot 1182 may be somewhat more potent than prior lots and suggesting that if there are problems, that a .25 ml dose for booster (only) immunizations may be in order."

This was done, but as Michigan health officials later decided, "This has caused some confusion among physicians and apprehension to use the vaccine. It was decided to withdraw the statements from further shipments of Lot 1182 because this lot has shown no greater reactivity than other lots of DPT."

To date, court records show that at least three children injected with vaccine from Lot 1182 suffered reactions which left them with seizures, paralysis, and brain damage. Their parents sued the Michigan Department of Public Health, describing the department's use of the vaccine as "potentially lethal misconduct" showing "callous disregard for human life."

Dr. Maurice Reizen, the state's Public Health Director, insisted that the vaccine was safe and was quoted in the *Detroit News* as saying, "I seriously question the FDA's rationale (for rejecting Lot 1182) and the accuracy of their testing. We're prepared to defend the allegations. . . ." The State of Michigan asked that the parents' suits be dismissed, protesting that the doctrine of sovereign immunity protects the state government from claims arising from services that only the government can provide. Attorneys for the children argue that citizens in the state could just as easily obtain the vaccine from commercial manufacturers, and that if the state is not willing to accept responsibility for damage, it should stop manufacturing the vaccine. This case is still in the Michigan courts.

The story of Lot 1182 is one more depressing example of the indifference with which the lives of children have been treated by those in positions of responsibility within the vaccine establishment. A defective lot of vaccine was tested on children. The destruction of Lot 1182 would have meant a loss of money as well as an admission of error on the part of the Michigan Department of Public Health. For these officials, apparently it was an unacceptable price to pay for the certainty that no harm would come to the unsuspecting children receiving the vaccine.

But the story does not end there. In February 1984, the NIH awarded the Michigan Public Health Department a three-year $486,674 contract to produce an improved pertussis vaccine for human testing (see Chapter 19).

Are There Any Incentives To Upgrade?

Vaccine manufacturers are subject to the same temptations as other producers to cut corners and sacrifice quality for the sake of profit. But unlike other manufacturers, vaccine producers derive little economic benefit from improving their product.

The makers of cars, television sets, or computers want to produce a better product because this will yield a larger share of the market. In the past, the makers of vaccines have not had this incentive, particularly since there has been a historic unwillingness on the part of the manufacturers and the government to admit the vaccine is highly reactive. Without a reason to improve the vaccine, there has been no incentive to improve it.

Doctors and patients alike have viewed vaccines as "generic," meaning that all DPT vaccine is alike no matter who manufactures it. Therefore, competition among producers has usually has been based on price. This keeps profit margins down for all of them.

In this way, vaccines differ from drugs. A manufacturer can patent a drug which is then advertised to the public and the profession as being safer or better. Holding exclusive rights to this drug during its patent life, the producer can recoup the investment made in its improvement. Doctors and patients will develop loyalty to a particular firm and its products. But vaccines are very rarely patented and cannot usually be offered to the public as safer or more potent than competing products because physicians and the public are aware that vaccines are all manufactured to the same federal standards.

And why should a manufacturer want to improve its vaccine? Each major change in a vaccine's composition can require a new series of federally-mandated tests for safety and potency. Once a vaccine has passed federal safety and potency tests and been licensed for distribution in interstate commerce, the manufacturer must only maintain the status quo. The fact that the pertussis vaccine is legally mandated in forty-one states assures producers of a ready-made and stable market. The FDA Bacterial Vaccines Panel in 1979 observed that "emphasis upon proof of efficacy and upon critical standards of the scientific quality of vaccine data may inhibit the motivation to modify and improve current vaccines and to introduce new ones."

Biological products, such as vaccines, play a very small role in the U.S. drug industry. In 1977, all vaccines and toxoids for human use accounted for just 3 percent of the pharmaceutical industry's gross output. Most producers make far greater profits on any one of the drugs they market than on vaccines.

While vaccine manufacturers generally have not tried to voluntarily improve their vaccines, a major exception was Eli Lilly, which did attempt to improve its DPT vaccine in the early 1960s and called its new product Trisolgen. It was marketed as a "split cell" or "extract" vaccine and was an example of a vaccine manufacturer trying to gain a bigger share of the market through technological innovation.

Eli Lilly stated that the extraction process permitted the "cellular debris" to be discarded from the pertussis vaccine, and Trisolgen was promoted as less reactive than its competitors. This claim was generally accepted by physicians, and Trisolgen was thought to have captured nearly half the market despite a slightly higher sales price (the sales figures and market shares of individual manufacturers are closely held trade secrets).

Despite its excellent market position, in the late 1960s Lilly stopped producing Trisolgen and sold the rights to Wyeth Laboratories. In a 1984 interview, the former medical director of Eli Lilly, C. N. Christensen, M.D., stated that this move was part of a corporate decision to withdraw from the manufacture of biologicals entirely (except for rabies vaccine and one or two others for which Lilly was the sole supplier). Dr. Christensen stated: "The vaccine market was very fragmented and unstable. There were a lot of suppliers and not much money to be made from DPT."

Even though it may have held about 50 percent of the market with a product that was reputed to be safer than the other DPT vaccines available, Lilly was willing to sacrifice Trisolgen. "There was a lot of soul-searching" about that decision, said Dr. Christensen.

The Trisolgen story suggests that even a successful vaccine is a relatively unimportant element in the sales and marketing strategy of a major drug manufacturer. But while Trisolgen was on the market, and thought to be less reactive than other vaccines, it represented a threat to the producers of these other vaccines. How did Lilly's competitors react? Did they attempt to copy the Lilly process or develop a "split cell" or "extract" vaccine of their own? Internal documents from one major manufacturer show that this challenge was simply ignored.

This manufacturer ran a trial comparing its own vaccine with Trisolgen, testing the two vaccines on 335 children. In all categories— pain, swelling, redness, nodule formation, irritability, vomiting, anorexia, and temperature elevation—Trisolgen was less reactive.

A detail man selling this manufacturer's vaccine to physicians wrote in 1971 that the doctors in his area preferred Trisolgen. He was worried about what to do with the vials of vaccine that nobody wanted to buy. He said, "Two of my good clinics have given me the same story . . . the children get elevated temperatures, red arms, and in general are just sick after immunization. . . . As a result they are switching to Lilly's Trisolgen. I am sitting here with about 250 vials. . . . How can I answer this complaint and retain my sales?"

The product service manager wrote back that "both our Medical Advisory and Quality Control staffs state that there is no reason to suspect that our [DPT] is any more reactive than Lilly's." In 1975, a proposal to upgrade the pertussis component of the company's DPT vaccine was shelved because "the product line could not support it."

Each manufacturer is protected by its license, which only compares its vaccine with the federal standard. Vaccines are not compared with one another, and there is no economic or regulatory inducement for a manufacturer to improve its product just because the competing vaccine might be better.

The lower economic benefits of manufacturing vaccines coupled with even further loss of income from lawsuits has caused many drug companies to abandon the field. In 1948, there were about a dozen DPT vaccine manufacturers in the United States; today only two produce

DPT for national distribution (the states of Massachusetts and Michigan, as we have mentioned, also produce DPT for the citizens of their states).

Why concern about profitability has prevented manufacturers from producing a less toxic pertussis vaccine is discussed in Chapter 19.

Manufacturing and Distribution Problems

The Quadrigen case raised the question of what happens to the vaccine once it has been shipped. Quadrigen deteriorated because of temperature variations during the long journey from the manufacturer's storage plant to the physician's hypodermic needle. Just how often is this "cold chain" broken?

Federal regulations provide that DPT vaccine must be maintained at a low temperature but not allowed to freeze. If the vaccine freezes, it becomes discolored.

It only takes one weak link in the "cold chain"—from manufacturer to wholesaler to retailer to doctor to patient—to affect the quality of the DPT vaccine. A member of the DPT litigation group of the American Trial Lawyers Association stated in an interview, "I have seen more than four hundred letters in one manufacturer's file complaining of discolored DPT vaccine, and in only one case did the manufacturer admit this possibility and offer to replace the lot of vaccine."

In a letter to the *New England Journal of Medicine*, Howard H. Frankel, M.D., warned doctors about the effects of temperature changes on killed vaccines, such as the DPT vaccine:

"According to personal communication, major pharmaceutical companies ship killed vaccines, such as DPT . . . at 2 to 8 C. [35–46 F.] to regional, company-owned distribution centers, where they are stored under the same conditions. However, the vaccines are subsequently shipped from the distribution centers to wholesalers by common carrier, i.e., under noninsulated, nonrefrigerated conditions for up to 72 hours, at temperatures between 10 and 52 C. [50–126 F.] The wholesale-drug suppliers store the vaccines at 2 to 8 C. until they are again shipped without refrigeration to pharmacies and physicians. Upon arrival at the final medical facility, the medications are once more refrigerated at 2 to 8 C. Official regulations clearly state that killed biologic vaccines must be stored at 2 to 8 C. throughout their 'dating' periods. One wonders, therefore, whether these delicate vaccines are weakened, inactivated or perhaps even altered so that they have harmful effects, as a result of alternating extremes of heat and cold."

DPT vaccine, which is supposed to remain at a constant temperature of between 35 F. and 46 F., is subjected twice to temperatures fluctuating between 50 F. and 126 F. for up to three days at a time because it is shipped under the same conditions as a postcard! How many vials of vaccine have gone bad after cooking in 115-degree heat in the back of a truck in the middle of July?

This is just one more example of the carelessness and lack of concern with which vaccines are treated. In other areas of life, carelessness merely leads to inefficiency. In the case of the pertussis vaccine, it can lead to death.

Douglas's mother still wonders if a "break" in the cold chain was what killed her baby, who began reacting within five hours of his first DPT shot and died twenty-three hours later (described in Chapter 5): "My father-in-law looked into my son's death because we definitely felt it was due to the shot. He called either the state or county health department and one of the employees said that their refrigerator had gone off. They even told one of our attorneys this. They said their refrigerator had gone off for the weekend and they had come back to work and they noticed it was off. They said they sent back some of the DPT vaccine in the refrigerator but not all of it. They didn't feel it was all bad."

The Medical Establishment

Along with the federal government and vaccine manufacturers, the medical establishment must bear a share of the blame for what has happened. Physicians occupy a privileged and respected position in our society and must assume extra responsibility for what they do and say. The record shows that prominent members of the medical establishment have often evaded this responsibility on the pertussis vaccine issue.

From the beginning, the medical establishment ignored the Hippocratic maxim that has guided physicians for more than two thousand years: "First, do no harm." It accepted the vaccine uncritically and dispensed it on a broad scale well beyond the time when whooping cough was epidemic and life-threatening. The momentum that built up from the programs of Sauer in Evanston and Sako in New Orleans was allowed to continue without comment or reevaluation. Because whooping cough had been a terrifying disease in the 1920s, physicians ignored vaccine risks in the 1950s.

The failure to acknowledge vaccine risks began with the AAP's recommendation during the 1950s that the first DPT shot be given at one month of age. The only clinical evidence supporting this decision was Sako's 1945 trial on 4,000 infants aged two to twelve weeks (see Chapter 3). Sixteen of those babies were reported as having "severe reactions." What happened to them later? The record does not say. But if that .04 percent of "severe" systemic reactions were applied to today's American infant population of three and one third million undergoing vaccination each year, it would suggest that more than 13,000 vaccinated babies suffer "severe" reactions annually.

The AAP 1950s recommendation to vaccinate at the age of one month may have been primarily based on the convenience of the pediatrician, not on the considered well-being of the child (see Chapter 3). A similar frame of mind persisted into the late 1970s, as is seen in the 1979 Report of the Bacterial Vaccines Panel which states: "Ideally immunization should begin at 2–3 months of age, or at the time of a six-week checkup if that is more practical." Of course, six weeks is more practical for the pediatrican, but is it best for the baby?

This early start with vaccination enabled Parke-Davis in 1960 to suggest a schedule which would have allowed a baby to receive five shots by his first birthday. Common sense should have suggested that this was overkill. The British policy of encouraging physicians to start vaccinating between three and six months of age, with a total of only three shots, shows much more wisdom.

Confusing Contraindications

Another dangerous policy pursued by the AAP was to minimize the issue of adverse reactions and contraindications. And when it did give guidance on these very important matters, its advice in the *Red Book* was so contradictory and unclear that the ordinary physician was often left bewildered.

Red Books throughout the 1960s told doctors to give partial doses of pertussis vaccine when a baby reacted with fever, somnolence, or other unusual symptoms to a previous shot. This advice was not backed by research demonstrating that partial doses of the pertussis vaccine are less harmful than full doses once a severe reaction has occurred.

The only clear contraindication listed in the 1960s was "convulsion or severe reaction," and then "no further injections of pertussis vaccine should be given." There was no definition of a "severe reaction" and no guidance as to the time period within which the reaction must appear to be counted as a severe reaction.

In its sixteenth edition (1970), the *Red Book* took a step backward from an already dismal position. Now "the occurrence of a severe reaction" was only "cause for caution in subsequent injections." If there is a "prolonged convulsive episode," the next injection "should be deferred"; then fractional doses should be used as test doses "and immunization completed slowly." The thrust was to give the vaccine at all costs.

The seventeenth edition, published in 1974, repeated the above recommendation but did state that pertussis vaccination should be stopped if any central nervous system disorder develops.

The eighteenth edition in 1977 again changed course: high fever (105 degrees F.), convulsions, and other severe reactions were now definite contraindications. But by 1982, doctors were told that children suffering from a high temperature, somnolence, screaming, and persistent crying—which were absolute contraindications in 1977—now "probably should not receive additional doses of pertussis vaccine, although these phenomena are of unknown significance."

In both 1977 and 1982, the physicians on the Red Book Committee reassured doctors throughout America that "frequently only a temporal association is noted between reaction and vaccine administration, with no proof that pertussis vaccine caused the reaction."

The history of the *Red Book* on the pertussis vaccine issue is one of confusion, which has resulted in bewildered doctors hurting children. In 1970, for instance, the *Red Book* editors urged doctors not to vaccinate a child with an active infection "until the infection is properly controlled." Did this mean that a sick baby taking antibiotics to "control" an infection was considered a fit subject for vaccination?

In 1982, the editors concluded, "Convulsions that . . . are well controlled do not contraindicate pertussis vaccine." Did this mean that a baby taking Phenobarbital to control convulsions was also a fit subject for vaccination? Is a baby undergoing treatment for an infection or under continual medication for seizures the equivalent of a healthy baby as far as vaccination is concerned?

In 1970, the *Red Book* advised doctors to "proceed with caution, using fractional doses when inoculating children with a history of neurological disease" and added that aspirin or Phenobarbital may be given "for three days following the immunization procedure to minimize febrile reactions." Here again is the question of the wisdom of half doses for high-risk children. Is this suggestion scientifically valid? Hannik in The Netherlands noted in 1978 that infants who reacted violently to a full dose "show a recurrence after further injections with half a dose or even with one tenth of a dose." In 1967, Ström reported a similar case in which a temperature of 103 degrees F. recurred after one tenth of a dose.

Dr. Janice Cockrell's 1982 comment remains true today: "The immunologic response to half-dose DPT regimens has never been scrutinized, and the necessity of three DPT immunizations during the first year of life is being questioned." One important question that has never been answered is whether the infant receiving half doses should have the prescribed number of shots or double the number. Reports from parents of vaccine-damaged children suggest that doctors ought to consider the following advice: If a serious reaction has occurred and the baby can't be given a whole dose, don't give any at all.

These are all vitally important issues, but they remain unresolved forty years after the start of the DPT vaccination program. The conflict among the experts over the significance of half doses is one more sign of the prevailing confusion about the pertussis vaccine.

The Failure To Exclude High-risk Children

With all the unknowns, the AAP seemed compelled to urge pertussis vaccination of virtually every child under nearly all circumstances, instead of advising physicians: "When in doubt, don't vaccinate." What harm would have been done if a small portion of high-risk children had been spared the pertussis vaccine?

It is apparent that the members of the Red Book Committee knew perfectly well that vaccinating children with neurological or convulsive disorders was risky. Philip Brunell, current chairman of the Red Book Committee, who attended the 1982 FDA Symposium on New Pertussis Vaccines, raised the subject there by asking A. H. Griffith of Burroughs-

Wellcome in England the following question: "I would like to sort of see if I could get you to stick your neck out and tell us what you would advise practitioners who have to immunize children with neurological disorders or convulsive disorders. The Red Book Committee has been wrestling with this problem for years and years and we still don't have a satisfactory answer."

Griffith replied: "Well, as a vaccine manufacturer I would take the safest course. Obviously, I am going to advise not to vaccinate where the child is liable to get a convulsion. . . . The easiest way out is to avoid those cases where there is going to be a convulsion. And that is why the exclusion is there. And this is fair. If you can get a 90 percent coverage of vaccination in the country there is no need to vaccinate those children. They are protected by the herd."

The United States today has achieved almost 96 percent DPT vaccination coverage. According to Griffith, that is 6 percent higher than is really needed to prevent whooping cough from gaining a foothold in a vaccinated population, which is what is meant by "herd immunity." Six percent of American children would come to 210,000 children each year, which leaves room for excluding high-risk children from the vaccination program with no effect on the protection of the rest of society.

Griffith's comment is typical of the more cautious attitude of European physicians to the pertussis vaccine and whooping cough. They seem to be more willing than American physicians to take contraindications seriously and, in case of doubt, they prefer not to vaccinate rather than risk the death or injury of a child. Writing in a 1981 issue of the *British Medical Journal*, David Hull, M.D., of the University Hospital in Nottingham, observed that British physicians feel "considerable uncertainty on how the contraindications should be interpreted." The result? "This is probably one factor responsible for the fall in the rate of whooping cough immunization in the United Kingdom."

Why are American physicians different? Is is because they were never taught differently in medical school? Is it because the men and women on the AAP Red Book Committee, ACIP, CDC, and FDA who tell doctors how the pertussis vaccine should be given are mainly academic epidemiologists and infectious disease researchers, whose primary goal is eradicating disease from society—not practicing pediatricians, whose primary goal is the total health and well-being of the individual children they treat in their offices every day? Is it because the pertussis vaccine is mandated by law? Or is it a subconscious fear of discrediting the vaccine and threatening its public acceptance by admitting that not every child should get it? Perhaps it is all of these.

After the airing of "DPT: Vaccine Roulette," one veteran pediatrician from Maryland's Eastern Shore wrote to Lea Thompson that he "always holds his breath for the first twenty-four hours after giving the shot." His fifty years of experience taught him that reactions do occur and can be dangerous. But many physicians seem unwilling to believe that harm could come from the pertussis vaccine. Even when the child is in uncontrollable convulsions within hours of a DPT shot, they refuse to see the connection.

Mothers, who observe their children far more carefully than any doctor, became increasingly suspicious of the DPT shot when they found their babies sick or dying shortly after being vaccinated. But doctors rejected their logical conclusions. One mother said: "I have always felt it was the shot because her convulsion came just one hour after it. But no doctor would admit it. I would go to a hospital and she would be having something wrong and I would tell them her story and they would look at me like I was crazy. They kept telling me she would have gotten seizures anyway, that it was just coincidental that the seizures happened so close to the shot."

The mother of this little girl, who now has an uncontrollable seizure disorder and is developmentally delayed, reports that the doctors did not give her daughter more pertussis vaccine but at the same time adamantly denied that the shot caused her condition. A doctor who consulted the 1970 *Red Book* for guidance would have been told to continue vaccinating.

After bewildering American physicians all these years, the leadership within the AAP now seems to be blaming them for ignoring contraindications and adverse reactions. Louis Cooper, M.D., the New York State Chapter Chairman of the AAP, who appeared on the *MacNeil-Lehrer Report*, engaged in the following exchange:

MACNEIL: Is the system geared to efficiently exclude the minority who shouldn't get it? Do doctors know the risk and are they careful at excluding those who shouldn't get it?

COOPER: It's hard for me to imagine that every American doctor knows the detail of the risks that he should, but I think in general . . .

MACNEIL: Whose fault is that if he doesn't?

COOPER: I think ultimately the doctor's. Certainly the medical literature and all of the educational programs of our universities and teaching hospitals, the Academy of Pediatrics, the Academy of Family Practice, the Centers for Disease Control make these data widely available. So if a physician doesn't know the risk, I can blame no one but that individual physician.

Former AAP Red Book Committee Chairman Vincent Fulginiti, M.D., made a similar statement in commenting on the WRC-TV documentary: "It was stated that many doctors are not aware of the risks and reactions from the shot. No evidence for this generalization was given except to follow with a few interviews with parents implying that 'doctors' and 'interns' are unaware of DPT reactions. To generalize to 'many' doctors is fraudulent at worst and deceptive at best. I personally know more than thirty pediatricians in our city and all are aware of the side reactions to pertussis vaccine, as are most of the groups of physicians to whom I have lectured throughout the U.S. in the last twenty years."

Such statements appear to be the first signs of nervousness by vaccine policymakers, who may now be setting out to blame the nation's physicians for following their lead over the last four decades.

Ignoring Adverse Reactions

The medical establishment's first failure was to flout the Hippocratic maxim that the physician must avoid doing harm. Its second failure was to ignore the evidence of vaccine damage when it started coming in.

For two thousand years, physicians have known that careful observation and description of a disease are the first steps toward its treatment or prevention. But this was not done with pertussis vaccine reactions. American medical literature can be searched in vain for detailed case histories of vaccine-damaged children, descriptions that were once the hallmark of any medical investigation. Since the invaluable Byers and Moll study in 1948, perhaps one substantive article describing the pertussis vaccine reaction in full clinical detail has appeared in American medical literature.

How could the medical establishment evaluate vaccine reactions if no one was willing to observe and describe them? Clinical descriptions are the raw material of medical science. But this raw material was apparently not to the taste of the AAP's Red Book Committee. Instead, when mothers and fathers of vaccine-damaged children came forward with their stories, they were dismissed as "anecdotal."

These physicians do not seem to realize that important medical information is found not only in the pages of *Pediatrics* or the *New England Journal of Medicine*. They do not seem to understand that paying careful attention to what mothers have to say about their children is not a waste of time. They appear to have trouble grasping the concept that by accumulating "anecdotal" evidence, they might come up with findings that would clarify their questions about the pertussis vaccine.

It seems odd that not one of America's thirty thousand pediatricians has recently come forward with an article or publication disclosing personal experiences with the vaccine. One reason is the fear of potential lawsuits. Another is that few are willing to expose themselves to personal criticism, extending to vituperation and even ostracism from the medical establishment. An even more powerful reason is the virtual impossibility of getting opposing views published in American medical journals headed by leaders of the medical establishment, or even getting the research performed in the first place.

Funding for Medical Research

This raises the question of how medical research in the United States is organized and, in particular, how it is funded. According to the Association of American Medical Colleges, in fiscal year 1981–82, 1.24 percent or $18 million of all medical school research was funded internally by the medical schools themselves. Another 1.38 percent or $20 million was funded by state and local governments. Just over one sixth or $249 million was financed by drug companies. And the largest amount—80 percent or more than $1 billion—was funded by the American taxpayer in the form of federal grants.

To get a share of the internal funds from a medical school is very difficult. Therefore, a physician interested in infectious disease research might first turn to one of the companies that manufactures vaccines. But these companies are naturally not anxious to fund research on adverse reactions to the vaccines they sell—which is one reason why this subject has been so neglected over the past decades.

If the physician cannot obtain funding from a drug company, he can apply to the NIH. It is the rare medical researcher who has not applied at some time in his life for a federal grant or does not hope to apply for one in the future. But the applicant for such a grant must take care not to antagonize those who control the purse strings. This means not pursuing lines of research which run counter to government policy or dominant medical opinion.

Federal grant money can serve to reinforce conformity of views on medical issues while invisibly censoring those with contrary opinions. Members of the vaccine policymaking bodies, such as the AAP and ACIP, are awarded federal grants no less than those of other official and semiofficial medical organizations.

For example, of the twelve members of the 1982 Red Book Committee, at least six were recipients of federal research grants totaling nearly $1 million. Some of the 1982–83 grants were directed at the development of new vaccines and others have run for a decade or longer.

Intimate ties between nongovernmental organizations such as the AAP's Red Book Committee and the federal government are a pervasive fact in medicine today. At least eight of twenty-three members of the editorial board of *Pediatrics*, the official journal of the AAP, received federal research grants in fiscal year 1982.

The federal government's counterpart to the Red Book Committee is the CDC's Advisory Committee on Immunization Practices, known as the ACIP. More than any other organization in the vaccination establishment, the ACIP exemplifies the way physicians and scientists are brought together and persuaded to give support to each other and to a common vaccination policy. The overlap between the ACIP and AAP is obvious. Three of the members of the ACIP are from the Red Book Committee. Another, who is designated as a "liaison," is on the Red Book Committee and was on the editorial staff of the 1982 *Red Book*.

The ACIP is also filled with government employees in high positions within the NIH, FDA, and CDC. The executive director of the ACIP is an employee of the CDC and another ex officio member not only dispenses federal research grants in NIH but is also an ex officio member of the Red Book Committee. Yet another ex officio member of ACIP is involved in the regulation of vaccines within the FDA.

Four of the ACIP members were recipients of NIH research grant money in 1982 totaling just under $600,000. The obvious point here, as in the case of the AAP Red Book Committee, is that there is an appearance of a conflict of interest.

On the one hand, there is a legitimate desire to include a representative group of what are thought to be the best minds in disease and vaccine research. On the other hand, it is quite obvious that the majority of the ACIP members, like the members of the AAP, are tied to the existing vaccination policy and committed to it by their whole careers.

The AAP and the ACIP do not differ from one another about vaccine policy, nor do they depart from the overwhelming consensus of the medical establishment for continuing business as usual. Members of the vaccine establishment have a common interest in presenting a united front, speaking with a common voice, and avoiding independent thought about vaccination questions.

Any researcher with ambition will think long and hard before taking the lead in an assault on federal health policy. A physician caught up in the research game must exercise a degree of self-censorship. Otherwise, the doors of the medical establishment close, the research funds dry up, and a promising career may be at an end.

Publish or Perish

Suppose, finally, a vaccine researcher decides to forego funding from either a drug company or the federal government and to go it on his own by collecting vaccine damage cases, describing them in detail, and publishing an article. His chances of having it accepted by a reputable journal are almost nonexistent for two reasons.

First, the idea that a vaccine is causing significant damage is not scientifically respectable. The prejudice against it has been so strong in the medical community that an article pointing out the dangers of a particular vaccine would probably be turned down by the editorial board, of which one-third or one-half of the members might themselves be recipients of federal research grants. But the editorial board would not have to dismiss the article because of a belief that the vaccine is harmless. It would only need to point out that the research is below accepted scientific standards.

Such an article would necessarily contain careful clinical descriptions of vaccine-damaged infants. But prevailing opinion in medicine today has turned away from the close and careful disease descriptions which were once the highest ideal of medical research. Truth is now believed to be obtained by comparing groups and not by describing individual cases. Here sick people have value only as part of a "sample" of sufficient size to possess statistical significance. The individual child has meaning only when matched to a "control." The only research recognized as valuable, as "scientific," is that which compares "test groups" with "control groups."

This kind of thinking led Gerald Fenichel, M.D., to write in 1983: "There are many lessons to be learned from the ongoing pertussis immunization controversy. . . . The most important lesson is that case reports are often misleading." And it was this same kind of thinking which led senior officials of the FDA and the CDC to reject a proposal to follow up the eighteen infants in the UCLA study who reacted (see Chapter 14) unless a "control group" could be assembled.

But comparing large groups in this currently fashionable way costs money, hundreds of thousands, even millions, of dollars. The individual researchers, the solitary geniuses—today's Jenners and Pasteurs—are effectively blocked from pursuing unpopular lines of research and making unique contributions to medicine. Their research will never get funded. And without funding, their ideas will never be published.

In this way, the production of new medical knowledge is controlled by a system of interlocking directorates of the kind which were banned from the production of goods and services by the antitrust laws. Members of one committee sit on other committees. Editors of medical journals move on to become professors in medical schools, and vice versa. High officials in the federal health bureaucracy take equally high positions in the drug industry.

Gordon Stewart, discussing this state of affairs in an interview, noted that the interlocking directorate is, in fact, worldwide. "It is a very closed circle. The international health authorities are controlling it as well. It means that something like one hundred people are pretty well controlling what goes on in the entire world of vaccines. They are all in cahoots with each other and with the pharmaceutical companies."

Members of the medical establishment cannot attack a federal vaccine policy without suffering professionally. In spite of the billion dollars per year spent on federal medical research grants, no sum has been great enough to reveal how much damage is being done by the pertussis vaccine.

The unhealthy connection between medical thought and federal funding should be broken. The problem is not easy to resolve since the brightest and most aggressive physicians gravitate toward positions of authority and also take the lead in research. But the American public and its elected officials should realize that the existing pattern of inter-connecting relationships among vaccine policymakers may be doing as much harm as good to the progress of medicine. There should be a greater awareness of the blinding effect of money on the way physicians and scientists think about medical issues.

A Conflict of Interest

There is an emerging realization that scientists and doctors can be as short-sighted in pursuing the public interest as the businessmen of an earlier time who so ferociously fought antitrust laws. In March 1984, a conflict of interest story reported in the *Washington Post* stirred the medical world. Miles Weinberger, M.D., Professor of Pediatrics at the University of Iowa, appeared as an expert witness in 1983 before an FDA panel evaluating asthma preparations, and sharply criticized a certain asthma medicine on the ground that some people absorbed it badly and became ill. He then took his per diem and travel expenses and went back to Iowa City.

Months later, the news came out that the drug Dr. Weinberger criticized was made by a competitor of Key Pharmaceuticals, Inc., the company which was paying him $31,000 per year in consulting fees and research grants plus $95,000 in stock options. The *Washington Post* reported that this had never been revealed by Dr. Weinberger to the FDA panel or to the *New England Journal of Medicine*, which had accepted an article by him on the asthma drug.

Dr. Weinberger responded that his contact with Key Pharmaceuticals was sufficiently revealed by footnotes in supporting materials submitted to the FDA panel. He added: "I can see where the appearance of conflict of interest is there. All I have to fall back on is my own integrity." But the secretary of the FDA panel said later, "Maybe the rules should be changed."

In June 1984, the FDA did change its rules requiring those testifying before its advisory panels to disclose—in advance and in writing—any financial or professional interest that might affect the issue under discussion.

The medical establishment today is rife with conflicts of interest.

Dr. Weinberger defended himself by stating, "paid consultation to industry by experts in academic settings is an extremely common activity, is considered permissible and ethical, and is fully encouraged by America's colleges and universities."

This practice clearly appears to be extensive throughout the medical establishment. But the direct financial links are not the only element in this apparent conflict. Equally significant is the fact that vaccine policymakers appear as expert witnesses for vaccine manufacturers in lawsuits brought against them on behalf of vaccine-damaged children. Manufacturers make frequent use of the services of prominent present or former Red Book Committee members and one lawyer who represents parents of vaccine-damaged children commented, "Whether they are in conflict of interest is something we trial lawyers talk about all the time."

The reason for the appearance of a conflict of interest is inherent in the situation. For example, Red Book Committee members decide what are and what are not contraindications and adverse reactions to vaccines. They may also be in a position to receive research grants from manufacturers or large fees for testifying on their behalf. Under such circumstances, it is possible that the temptation may exist to do the manufacturers a favor in return and narrowly restrict the definition of adverse reactions and contraindications in their capacity as vaccine policymakers. (A narrow interpretation of the contraindications and reactions would also help any physician who finds himself involved in a lawsuit for damaging a child with the vaccine.)

Who, in all this, is minding the public interest? These vaccine policymakers who do double duty as expert witnesses for manufacturers may well say, "All we have to fall back on is our own integrity." But will anyone believe them?

A Reluctance To Record and Report Reactions

The Red Book Committee has recently become more sensitive to parents' need for information about vaccine risks—but much of the reason is apparently to protect doctors from having to face malpractice suits. In a *Red Book* "update" issued in November 1982, the Committee declared, "Recent court experience in suits alleging injury from oral polio vaccine have emphasized the attention given by judges and juries to the actual procedure and language used at the time of immunization by physicians and their surrogates. In some jurisdictions it has been decided in specific cases that a warning about vaccine risks is important in deciding liability. The Committee does believe that information should be provided to patients (parents) at each vaccine encounter."

Some private pediatricians are now requiring parents to sign consent forms before a child is vaccinated. But what are parents getting in return for promising not to sue the physician should vaccine damage occur? The least they could expect would be a commitment by physicians to be more responsible about reporting adverse reactions and keeping vaccine records.

But the FDA has rejected any obligation to require physicians to report reactions. Walter Dowdle wrote in 1983, "FDA/HHS believes that requiring mandatory reporting of adverse reactions by physicians would be a significant additional burden, would be difficult to enforce, and thus would be regarded as controversial." In fact, he also noted, the FDA does not even possess this authority.

Evidently only new laws like the one adopted in Maryland in 1984 will force doctors to give parents information on vaccines and report and record reactions. At legislature hearings on the proposed law, the Maryland Medical and Chirurgical Faculty (MEDCHI) voiced its opposition to being forced to write down reactions. MEDCHI's representative, Robert Ancona, M.D., stated in an interview:

"We are strongly opposed to the legislature telling physicians what to put in the patient's medical record. The medical record is a private document between physicians and patients and we don't want the legislature to be practicing medicine and getting involved in areas where it is not competent. Next thing the legislature will be mandating is that we write down penicillin reactions and a lot of other things. We just don't want the legislature telling doctors what to do."

It did not seem to occur to Ancona that physicians in the past have been sufficiently satisfied with the medical judgment of legislators to entrust them with the passage of laws mandating compulsory vaccination programs. Evidently, it is perfectly acceptable to force parents to give their children a potentially toxic vaccine, thus risking death or brain damage, but it is not acceptable to force doctors to record and report adverse reactions, so that the precise dimensions of this risk can be evaluated.

Future Vaccines: More Scandals?

Other vaccines are being developed in the research pipeline, and there will undoubtedly be a move by physicians in the AAP, ACIP, and state health departments to require at least some of them for entry to school. Every year, NIH hands out grants for research on vaccines for chicken pox, hepatitis, influenza, gonorrhea, herpes, pneumonia, rheumatic fever, croup, cancer, and even dental cavities.

One vaccine that has been developed and is now being tested is for Haemophilus influenzae Type B., which causes a virulent form of bacterial meningitis in young children. Lance Gordon, of Connaught Laboratories, was quoted in a 1982 *Chemical Week* article as stating, "If the tests go as planned, this could eventually become a general-use vaccine. It could be incorporated as part of the standard DPT vaccine now given to all children."

In the spring of 1984, Merck Sharp & Dohme announced the creation of a chicken pox vaccine that it hoped to make available to the American public in several years. However, concern about the possibility that the vaccine might have side effects including Reye's syndrome, an occasional complication of chicken pox disease (and influenza), has been expressed by several observers.

NIH is working with the Uniformed Services University of the Health Sciences to investigate the deadly *E. coli* bacteria, and, using genetic engineering, to develop a vaccine for dysentery and other childhood diarrheal diseases. But anti-genetic engineering activists have protested that the project could lead to the development of a biologic weapon. There is also concern over the possibility that genetic engineering might inadvertently create a new organism that would prove more dangerous than the bacteria already present on earth.

On the list of vaccines the National Academy of Science wants to develop are ones for bacterial pneumonia, bacterial intestinal tract diseases, rabies, malaria, tuberculosis, chlamydial infections, dengue fever, and Japanese encephalitis. It has been suggested that MMR boosters be required for students entering college. Finally, the FDA has been working on a pertussis vaccine to give to pregnant women.

But what guarantees are there that the herpes or meningitis vaccine of tomorrow will not prove to be like the "swine flu" or the Quadrigen vaccine of yesterday or the crude pertussis vaccine of today? To ensure that the same disastrous story is not repeated with each new vaccine, the dimensions of the medical establishment's responsibility for the pertussis vaccine must be recognized.

Because of their power to influence the health of whole generations of Americans, individuals holding positions of authority in the government, vaccine manufacturing companies, and the medical community have an extra duty to perform. That duty should extend beyond carefully observing the rules of bureaucratic game-playing or the economic bottom line. Unfortunately, this extra vigilance, this extra willingness to forego immediate profit or professional advancement for a long-term benefit to society, has not always marked the decisions of these vaccine producers, researchers, and policymakers. As a result, children have suffered.

17

Profile:
A Fight for Freedom of Choice

> . . . the precedent set here that permits the taking of the children *at all* is the vice that opens a Pandora's box which may haunt this court for years to come. In my view, one of the foreseeable spectres is the unfettered interference by the State Welfare Department in areas where it has no legal standing whatsoever. In its apparent zeal to protect the immuned from the unimmuned I believe the majority has given meaning to the word *neglect* which no amount of rationalization can justify. This is the door that has been left open. History reveals that once a door is open to an administrative agency that door is not easily closed. Whose children under what pretext will be taken next? Will they be kept forever? For the reasons stated, I respectfully dissent.
>
> *Justice James D. Johnson*
> *Arkansas Supreme Court*

She stood there, staring coolly into the face of a burly policeman, who had at least twelve inches and a hundred pounds on her. Another policeman, smaller and thinner than his partner, watched the confrontation uneasily. Jo Ann Cook, a mother from Pine Bluff, Arkansas, did not move. Her feet were firmly planted on American soil, blocking the entrance to Broadmoor Elementary School.

Six-year-old Justin Douglas Cook was beyond that door, in one of the tightly shuttered classrooms. He knew his mother was fighting for his right to stay in school. Despite letters from doctors expressing concern that Douglas was at risk of reacting to further vaccinations, the

Arkansas Department of Health insisted that he must either be vaccinated or expelled from school.

Jo Ann remembers what happened next. "I told the policemen I wasn't leaving. I told them 'Douglas is here under his constitutional right to an education. I have to protect my baby. You are going to protect him for me, aren't you?' But they just looked at me without changing expression and one of them answered, 'No, we have come to get you.'"

Jo Ann recalls that School Superintendent Jack Robey, who had summoned the two policemen, was nodding his head in agreement and reporters and television crews were gathered around her waiting for something to happen.

"The big policeman moved toward me and said, 'I am going to arrest you if you don't leave.' I took two steps back and he grabbed my arm. Then I yelled, 'Get your hands off me!' and tried to pull my arm away. But he grabbed my arm again and said, 'I told you I was going to have to arrest you.'"

"Then," said Jo Ann, "he took the handcuffs and hit me in the face with them and cut my cheek and eyelid. I guess it kind of knocked me out because the next thing I knew I was on the ground. He had the handcuffs on my wrist, and my wrists were so small that they went all the way through, so he was leaning on the bar where the handcuffs lock. He was pushing up on one side of the cuffs and down on the other. He really tried to break my arm."

Her arm was not broken, but the ligaments in her wrist were so badly torn that her arm was still in a brace months later, and corrective surgery will probably be required. And then Jo Ann Cook, mother of three, was taken to the county jail where she was charged with disorderly conduct and resisting arrest.

The day after Jo Ann was arrested, her lawyer filed a suit against the Arkansas Department of Health in a U.S. District Court asking for an injunction barring public school officials from expelling Douglas until a hearing could be held. Judge William R. Overton refused to issue the injunction, and two months later, Jo Ann and her husband James were served with a petition by the Juvenile Court of Jefferson County charging them with having "willfully failed or refused to provide proper and necessary education and medical care essential for the health and well being of the child. The child being the age required by law for attendance in school has not attended school. That such failure to attend school is a detriment to the care and nurture of the juvenile."

The petition went on to order that Justin Douglas Cook be removed from his parents "to insure that the child's educational and medical needs are met."

How is it possible that a child could be barred from attending school for not being vaccinated after doctors have indicated that further vaccination could threaten his health? How is it possible that his parents could have been charged with child neglect and threatened with having the child taken from them to be placed in a foster home and forcibly vaccinated? Doctors in a state health department cannot legally take children from parents and force them to be injected with a biological they cannot guarantee will not kill or injure them. Or can they?

Back in the late 1950s, a father of eight children dared challenge the Arkansas mandatory vaccination law. Archie Cude, a Polk County farmer, waged an eight-year battle with the State of Arkansas to prevent three of his children from being vaccinated against smallpox. A Christian, he objected on religious grounds and maintained that the Bible indicated that vaccination was a violation of divine law.

The State of Arkansas did not see it that way. After refusing to allow three of his children to attend school because they had not been vaccinated, the Arkansas Welfare Department tried to take the children away from Archie and his wife and have them vaccinated. Archie Cude then got a lawyer and fought all the way to the Arkansas Supreme Court. But when his case reached the court in 1964, the majority opinion went against him. It was ruled that parents do not have the legal right to refuse to have their children vaccinated because of religious beliefs.

Governor Orval E. Faubus took custody of the children. They spent three days in the governor's mansion and the Governor even took them to the Ice Capades. But the Cude children were eventually taken, kicking and screaming, to a doctor's office by the Polk County sheriff where they were forcibly vaccinated.

"I am not Archie Cude," said Jo Ann. "I am fighting the state's vaccination laws on medical grounds because Douglas is at high risk of reacting to the vaccines and I have letters from doctors who agree with me. I am fighting to save my child's life and his right to an education. I am not going to let anyone take him from me."

Jo Ann has good reason to be afraid for Douglas. She herself was born and raised in Pine Bluff, Arkansas. Her struggle with the medical establishment began after her first son, James D'Wayne, was given DPT and oral polio vaccine at nine months of age. As a baby he tended to spit up and have colic so badly he couldn't even drink soybean formula, and within hours of his DPT shot he started high-pitched screaming and ran a fever of 103 degrees.

"He screamed a high sounding scream like he was in so much pain he couldn't stand it," Jo Ann said. "He would maybe have an hour rest and then start in again. The day after his shots, he was diagnosed as having bronchial pneumonia. And after the shot, most nights he wouldn't sleep for more than a few hours at a time. He would just scream. He kept screaming on and off at night until he was almost three years old."

Because D'Wayne was constantly sick, he did not receive another DPT shot and oral polio vaccine until he was nearly four years old. Within two hours, he had a fever of more than 105 degrees and the left side of his body had begun to swell and turn bright red.

"I called the public health clinic and they told me that I was just a young mother and there was no problem and to put ice packs on him and it would go away. But we knew there was something wrong, and we rushed him to Dr. Julius Foster at University Baptist Hospital in Little Rock, a doctor my family knew. He treated him for three weeks, which was how long it took for the redness and swelling to go down and the knot to leave his arm. Dr. Foster told us never to give him vaccines of any kind and never to give our other children the vaccines because the allergic reaction could be hereditary."

Their second son, Joseph Dewight, was a very healthy baby. He did not have colic and was thriving. The Cooks had moved to Oklahoma by now. When Dewight was nine months old, he cut his leg, and a pediatrician insisted that he be given a DPT shot. Jo Ann and her husband did not want to take the chance of his having a bad reaction.

"We told him that Dr. Foster had warned us about giving our children vaccines. But he assured us that reactions were not hereditary and that he could stop any reaction that Dewight might have. Besides, he told us Dewight could die from lockjaw if he didn't get the shot. So he gave him a quarter dose of DPT vaccine, and we sat there for an hour."

But they left an hour too early. Within two hours, their once-healthy baby was running a 104-degree fever, coughing, and having trouble breathing. His leg had also developed a hard lump at the site of the injection. They rushed him to a hospital emergency room, and the doctors sent him home with Benadryl and cough medicine.

"He was wheezing and couldn't catch his breath. You could hear him clear across the house. By the next day, his throat had become so swollen it was almost closed and his fever was near 105. He couldn't lay down flat because he couldn't breathe. The pediatrician who gave him the shot put him on the antibiotic Keflex. But four weeks later he was still so sick that we came back into Arkansas to see Dr. Foster, who diagnosed asthma."

Dewight continued to have severe asthma attacks. The lump in his leg where he had received the DPT shot did not go away. Although he had been a good sleeper in his first nine months of life, after the shot, he would not sleep for more than an hour at a time.

"He would wake up and scream like he was terrified. Nothing would comfort him. He kept this up night after night until he was almost six years old. When he could talk, sometimes he would scream and tell us that his leg hurt, the leg which still had the knot in it from the shot. He is eight years old now, and he still has a knot in his leg where that shot went in."

At three years of age, Dewight was given oral polio vaccine and went into a severe asthma attack. He is still being treated for asthma and is allergic to a variety of medications.

When Justin Douglas came along, he was also a healthy baby with no colic or other health problems. When he was six months old, and a pediatrician insisted that Douglas be given a DPT shot, the Cooks said no. But again the pediatrician assured them that vaccine reactions were not hereditary.

Douglas was given a one-half dose of DPT vaccine and oral polio. Within two hours, he started running a fever of almost 105 degrees. He broke out in a rash that covered his body with red blisters. The pediatrician gave Douglas a shot and prescribed Benadryl. For four days, Douglas threw up and had diarrhea.

"He had diarrhea so bad that we couldn't put a diaper on him," said Jo Ann. "He just lay on a pad on the floor for four days. I kept calling the doctor, but he said it was just a virus and not the shot. Doug couldn't keep anything down, especially milk."

Before the shots, Douglas had drunk milk and had a good appetite. Afterward, he was unable to drink milk because he would break out in a rash on his armpits and neck. He also began having constant throat and ear infections. Finally Jo Ann took him back to Dr. Foster in Arkansas for treatment. Today Douglas is allergic to a variety of medications, insect bites, and foods, including milk.

In 1982, the Cooks moved back to Pine Bluff, Arkansas, after James got a job there. The Arkansas Department of Health agreed to exempt the older two Cook boys from vaccinations, but they would not accept the letter written by an Oklahoma doctor exempting Douglas.

"In fact," said Jo Ann, "the Oklahoma doctor, who wrote a letter exempting Douglas, was contacted by a doctor in the Arkansas Department of Health and told he should have his medical license removed for not giving Doug all his shots. The doctor in Oklahoma is so scared now that he won't talk to anyone about our case."

Gordon P. Oates, M.D., medical director of the Immunization Program for the Arkansas Department of Health, told Jo Ann that Douglas would have to receive all the required vaccines unless she could find an Arkansas doctor to write him an exemption. Jo Ann tried.

"By this time, Dr. Foster had died and so I had been seeing another doctor, James A. Lindsey, M.D., who did not want Douglas to have any more vaccines because he could not guarantee he wouldn't have a reaction that could injure him. But the pressure from the Department of Health was starting to build and the best that Dr. Lindsey would do was to write a note saying Doug had a history of allergies, and he wouldn't immunize Doug in his office."

The Arkansas Department of Health would not accept Dr. Lindsey's note as an exemption. Jo Ann received a letter stating that Douglas had to be vaccinated within thirty days or he would be suspended from kindergarten. The Cooks hired a lawyer, who managed to get the Department of Health to give Douglas an exemption from having more DPT shots but not from the measles, rubella, and polio shots. Douglas was ordered to leave kindergarten in March 1982.

That summer Douglas was stung by a bee and was given Benadryl to help control his allergic reaction to the sting. But he also reacted to the Benadryl. "The doctor treating him told us that he didn't know what he could give to Doug to counteract an allergic reaction he may have to a foreign substance. He said Doug was a highly allergic child," said Jo Ann.

By the fall of 1983, Douglas was scheduled to enter first grade and James Farrell, the new director of Immunization of the Arkansas Department of Health, contacted the Cooks. James Farrell, who is not an M.D., was actually on the payroll of the CDC acting as an advisor to the Health Department.

"Jim Farrell writes us a letter telling us that Doug cannot go to school. So I called him and asked him why he wrote the letter to us. He said, 'All the other letters kept him out of school, what is wrong with one more?' So I got mad. I asked him if he was an M.D. and he said he wasn't. I told him, 'Arkansas state law states you have to be an M.D. to tell someone they can't have an exemption. You can't tell my son he can't go to school.' "

For more than a year Jo Ann had been pleading with the Arkansas Department of Health to grant her youngest son a medical exemption so he could attend school. She had complied with the Arkansas mandatory immunization law which indicates if "any person to whom this Act applies shall be deemed to have physical disability which may contraindicate vaccination" that "a certificate to that effect" issued by "any physician licensed to practice by the three (3) medical boards" may be "accepted in lieu of a certificate of vaccination."

Jo Ann Cook decided that she had had enough. On Thursday, September 29, 1983, she took Justin Douglas to school. She sat him down in a first-grade classroom, gave him a piece of paper and a pencil, and for seven days either she or her mother sat outside the classroom to make sure nobody took Douglas away. He went to school like all the other children until the police arrived to take his mother to jail on October 3.

By this time, the duty of accepting or rejecting medical exemptions had been taken over by J. P. Lofgren, M.D., a 1976 graduate of Harvard Medical School, former employee of the CDC in Missouri, and now "state epidemiologist" for Arkansas. When the state put Dr. Lofgren in charge, he proceeded to review the medical and religious exemptions on file at the Arkansas Department of Health and notify many parents that their children's medical or religious exemptions were being withdrawn or were not being accepted.

He refused to give a medical exemption to the son of Jim and Theresa Taylor, even though five-year-old Zachary has a liver disorder, constant respiratory infections, and a possible immune deficiency. Zachary's mother is so severely hypoglycemic that she has convulsions. In addition, she is allergic to milk and many medications.

Zachary was removed from kindergarten. The Taylors then submitted a religious exemption and were given a five-month temporary exemption. Zachary was put back in kindergarten to complete the last three months of the school year, but his parents will be faced with the problem of submitting another request for a religious exemption before he will be allowed to enter the first grade.

Dr. Lofgren defended his actions. He said, "It is my job to enforce the immunization laws in this state and not give out medical exemptions which are not backed up by medical evidence. We adhere to the list of contraindications defined by the ACIP of the Centers for Disease Control. If we give out medical exemptions to every parent who asks for one, we put our state at risk of seeing a reoccurrence of childhood diseases."

Referring to Jo Ann Cook's struggle to obtain a medical exemption for her son, he said, "In the case of Jo Ann Cook's child, you have to keep in mind that health conditions that occur after the shot are not necessarily related to the shot. For example, the asthma that occurred after her second son's shot was probably just a coincidence. Asthma occurs in children quite independently from a vaccination."

Later that October, the Cooks took Douglas to Illinois, where he was examined by Dr. Robert Mendelsohn. Dr. Mendelsohn wrote a letter detailing the results of his examination: "Based on authoritative references in the medical literature specifically citing allergies as a contraindication to immunization, and based on my assessment of this child, all further immunizations of any nature are contraindicated. Any further administration of any immunization carries grave risk."

But Dr. Lofgren rejected Dr. Mendelsohn's medical opinion and said, "This letter contains no new information. Nor does it give a valid reason for Douglas to be exempted from polio, measles or rubella vaccine. The rash lasting three weeks which Douglas had after the one-half dose DTP was probably not due to the DTP vaccine. If it was related, it would most likely be the pertussis component. Although I will not at this time withdraw the exemption for diphtheria and tetanus vaccine, I encourage you to also have him immunized with these vaccines for his health."

On December 19, 1983, Jo Ann Cook was convicted in Pine Bluff Municipal Court for resisting arrest and disorderly conduct and fined $350. She appealed, asking for a jury trial.

On January 12, 1984, U.S. District Court Judge William Overton ruled that the State of Arkansas had not acted "capriciously" in expelling the child from school because Douglas was not vaccinated.

During the course of the hearing, both Dr. Lofgren and the State's expert witness, Russell Steele, M.D., admitted that they could not guarantee that Douglas would not react severely if he were vaccinated. Dr. Steele told the Court that "we counsel all recipients of any medication that there are adverse reactions."

During the course of the hearing, Dr. Lofgren admitted that he was not board certified in pediatrics or preventive medicine. On the witness stand, Robert Mendelsohn, M.D., stated, "This is the first time I have ever seen the responsibility for determining who is going to get immunization delegated to a doctor who is not board certified in either pediatrics or preventive medicine. I would suggest that your state health department has to answer some questions because every other state department to my knowledge . . . insists on certain minimum qualifications for doctors before they can reach these decisions."

Judge Overton, however, said he was "satisfied" that Dr. J. P. Lofgren had "expertise . . . and can form a sound judgment on whether Douglas Cook needs to be immunized." The Cooks appealed to the Eighth Circuit Court.

On January 17, Jo Ann and James Cook were convicted of "child neglect" by Judge Jimmy Joyce in the Jefferson County Juvenile Court and ordered to surrender their son to the state Social Services Division on January 27 so that he could be placed in a foster home and vaccinated. After Judge Joyce convicted the Cooks of child neglect, he tried to convince Jo Ann to have her son vaccinated.

"He told me the doctors were going to take Doug to a very secluded place and that they would have a lot of medication ready in case something happened and they were going to give Doug just a little bit of vaccine under the skin. I told him to tell Lofgren that if he wants to put just a little vaccine in Doug, he is already admitting there is a big risk. There is no way in hell I am going to let him do that. There is no medication to stop a vaccine reaction and he knows it. All you can do is deal with the damage afterwards. And we are still dealing with the effects of the DPT shot on all three of our sons years after they got it."

The Cooks appealed their conviction but Judge Joyce and other officials continued to make statements that led Jo Ann and James to believe Douglas might be taken from them and vaccinated, even though the case was being appealed to a higher court. Afraid for their son's safety, Jo Ann and James decided Douglas should be taken out of

Arkansas. They enrolled him in a school in Louisiana, where he could live with relatives.

"We had no problem getting him into the public school system in Louisiana. They accepted one letter written by one doctor indicating Doug should not receive any more vaccinations. Finally, he was able to get the education he deserves without being harassed," Jo Ann said.

Separated from their son by more than two hundred miles, Jo Ann and James commuted on weekends to visit Doug. Jo Ann said, "It hasn't been easy. But the price of freedom is high, and no one ever said that we weren't going to have to fight for it."

On April 25, 1984, Circuit Court Judge Randall Williams ruled that Jo Ann and James Cook were not guilty of neglecting Douglas's medical or educational needs because the Cooks had enrolled him in school in Louisiana. But he also ruled that the state health department regulations requiring that Douglas be immunized were not unreasonable. He maintained that Douglas would have to be vaccinated before being allowed to attend school in Arkansas.

❋ ❋ ❋ ❋ ❋

It is cold and rainy at Little Rock Airport. The grayness of the day seeps into the airport cafeteria overlooking the airfield as Jo Ann and James Cook talk with Steve and Donna Kudabeck. Steve has been convicted of truancy after three of their six children were banned from attending public school in Hot Springs, Arkansas, because they were not vaccinated.

Donna is holding her nine-month-old son as she speaks, and explains why she and Steve have not vaccinated their six beautiful, healthy children. "We have a family health history that seems to strongly contraindicate the administering of vaccines. However, our decision not to vaccinate is based on our deep, personal, scriptural beliefs. Although not a tenet of our church, these beliefs are ones we have held with conviction for more than fifteen years."

Steve continues, "We are not members of one of the few churches from which exemptions are accepted, and we do not intend to change our religion just to escape the penalties of this unjust law. I view this battle not just as a man-to-man type combat. There are two forces involved: the forces of good and evil. We have the God I worship versus the god of pseudoscience; the god of compulsion versus my God who gave me inalienable rights and responsibilities to protect my children.

We have been asked to voluntarily offer our healthy children as living sacrifices to a false god. The God I worship demands obedience rather than sacrifice."

"After studying the benefits and risks of vaccines, we cannot in good conscience subject them to that kind of risk," adds Donna.

The Kudabeck children were allowed to attend school in Illinois without being vaccinated because they were given an exemption based on their family's personal beliefs. But when they moved to Arkansas in 1983, they found themselves in a state that did not allow for such an objection and they began to feel as if they had come to a "different country."

"Sometimes it is hard to believe that we aren't living in a foreign country," Steve explains. "Arkansas is a beautiful state in many ways. But there are a lot of parents who feel the same way we do there, and they are scared out of their wits to stand up and do anything about it. They are afraid they will be dragged into court like us and perhaps have their children taken from them. What is happening here in Arkansas could happen in any of the states that do not allow a parent's personal belief or a philosophical objection to vaccination. There shouldn't be this kind of terror in America, but there is."

Jo Ann rests her arm, still in a cast, on the cafeteria table. Her eyes flash with defiance. "This is supposed to be the United States. If we are free, then let us be free. If we are like Russia, then tell us that our children don't belong to us, that they really belong to the state. How can the state tell us we have to feed, clothe, educate, and raise our children and pay their medical bills, but that we don't have the right to protect them from vaccine damage? If my son is damaged by the vaccines they force him to take, he will be my responsibility to care for for the rest of my life. The doctors in the Arkansas State Health Department or the CDC won't have to sit up with a brain-damaged child all night."

With the grace that comes after years of practice, Donna quickly drapes herself and her baby with a shawl and nurses him. She is a soft-spoken woman, but there is a look of urgency on her face when she talks about what is happening in Arkansas.

"The Important Information forms that parents must sign before a child is vaccinated specifically state that the parent has had a chance to read the information, have questions answered to their satisfaction, and believe they understand the benefits and risks. It then states that they 'request' that the vaccines be given to their child. 'Request' implies that you desire it, that you have been able to make a decision. Informed consent and duty to warn implies that one can refuse the shots. However, even if every parent read those Important Information forms, even if every parent was totally informed about the benefits and risks, it does them no good if they decide not to take that risk. For there is no choice other than vaccination or criminal prosecution."

Like many couples, Jo Ann and James Cook are opposites. Jo Ann is talkative and James is not. He is a man of few words, and when he is moved to speak, he is to the point: "The state won't give the vaccine unless I request it and sign a form to prove I requested it. If I don't request it, my kid can't get into school. If my kid doesn't go to school, I can be charged with truancy or child neglect, and he can be taken from me. Why should I be forced to prescribe medicine for my own child? If my child is damaged by the vaccine, the state and the drug manufacturers say, 'You requested it. We are not responsible.' "

Steve and Donna are very concerned about the "National Childhood Vaccine Injury Compensation Act" which has been introduced into Congress. If the bill passes, they don't want to see it used as an excuse to enforce mandatory vaccination.

"If the bill helps parents whose children have been injured in the past by vaccines, that is fine," says Steve. "What we don't want to see is the states using it to enforce mandatory vaccination with the justification that, if a child is injured, the parents will be paid off. Some states have not totally enforced vaccination laws, perhaps because of the fear of liability. However, with the passage of any such bill, the states will then have a remedy at law for any serious damage that occurs, thus strengthening the state's position on mandatory vaccination. Do you think money is going to take away all the pain that a parent goes through when a child is injured for life? It is not going to even start. And if states can pass laws requiring children to be vaccinated, they could in the future pass laws requiring adults to be vaccinated. There are many new vaccines being developed for us. Medicine is not an exact science. Our society has no right to legislate it. We believe the bill should contain a provision for freedom of choice in all fifty states."

Jo Ann believes that the only way doctors will be forced to inform parents about vaccine risks and reactions and the only way that drug manufacturers will be forced to produce safe vaccines is to hit them where it hurts—in the pocketbook.

"I am worried about a compensation bill that lets doctors and manufacturers off the hook on these vaccines. A doctor who administers these shots without telling a parent both sides of the story should be sued. He should lose his license. And a drug manufacturer that doesn't tell a doctor and the public the dangers of the vaccine he is producing should be sued. And legislators who pass laws that require you to take a vaccine that can damage you or your child without telling you the truth should be sued. Because that is the only thing these people understand. The only thing they understand is that you are going to sue them and how much money you are going to take from them. It is sad. But they care more about their money than they do about children's lives."

Jo Ann displays the letters she has received from the Arkansas State Health Department during her two-year battle with them, and she talks about the support she has gotten from other parents. "When the newspapers reported that Doug had been thrown out of his first-grade class, almost every parent in that class called me and told me it was fine with them if Doug attended school with their children. In fact they were mad because they said, 'The doctors told me that those shots were good. If the vaccination program is so effective, what can Doug do to my child? My child is vaccinated, he's supposed to be protected against any disease your child might get.'

"They want to make an example out of Doug so all the other parents in Arkansas will just lie down and do what they want. Because if they can take our child, they can take your child. Who gave the state that power? It is damn sure time to take that power away from doctors who have been lying to us for years about what these vaccines can do and politicians who have been backing them up," she continues as the thoughts tumble out of her almost faster than she can express them.

Jo Ann and James face months, perhaps years, of court appearances and thousands of dollars in legal fees to carry on their fight to prevent Douglas from being taken from them. They miss Doug and he misses them. Traveling hundreds of miles back and forth to Louisiana on weekends to visit Doug has put a strain on their family. Lawyer's fees have put them heavily into debt and their two-bedroom trailer is all they own.

"We take it a day at a time," says Jo Ann. "We know what we are doing is right. We know we are fighting as much to protect other children as we are fighting to protect Doug. We are prepared to take it all the way to the Supreme Court because forcing an adult or a child to be injected with vaccines that can kill or brain damage them, especially when they are medically at high risk, is a clear violation of the 14th Amendment to the Constitution which guarantees that no State shall deprive any person of life or liberty."

Steve said, "At this point it is not an issue of right or wrong, safety, or efficacy. It becomes one of basic human rights. The 1980 Compensation for Vaccine Related Injuries report indicated that those Important Information forms are handed out at the insistence of the drug companies. This 'duty to warn' was evidently started because of the lawsuits that were being brought against them when damage resulted. The point is this: is a vaccination just a simple shot, as some may say? Legally they are known as 'unavoidably dangerous products.' We are made to give our children these products by law which is enforced by police power, making them very difficult if not impossible to avoid. And parents must sign informed consent forms assuming the risk of injury.

"There are many doctors, biochemists, and other scientists who have done a great deal of research into the benefits and risks of vaccines. They have found that these biologics hold not only the possibility of immediate damage but may also harbor serious potential latent effects that can affect not only our precious children, but those of future generations as well. In view of this, does it seem reasonable that parents, who care and who do ask questions and become informed, can ultimately be accused of child abuse if they decide not to vaccinate their children? Whether it be for the risks involved as verified by a family physician, or for the sincere personal beliefs and conviction of conscience of the parent, there must be freedom of choice."

Shortly after the Kudabeck children were suspended for non-compliance with the state's immunization law, they were enrolled in an out-of-state, private Christian school to which their school records were forwarded. Steve was still charged with truancy and found guilty in municipal court. He has appealed his conviction to a higher court, where he will be representing himself.

"The Arkansas constitution says, 'The right to trial by jury shall remain inviolate and shall extend to all cases at law.' The municipal judge who convicted me of truancy and fined me $750 refused my request for a trial by jury. I appealed his conviction to a higher court but, in effect, I first had to pay $750 for the right to a trial by jury," says Steve.

The Cooks and the Kudabecks continue talking with each other, joined together by a bond born out of fighting for a common cause they know is right. When the bizarre reality of what is happening to them becomes too much, one of them tells a joke to relieve the tension.

"You have to stay alive out there. You have to be careful not to let it drive you crazy. If you don't laugh about the ridiculousness of it all once in a while, you won't be able to go the distance," says James.

The winter rain is beating against the windows of the cafeteria in the Little Rock Airport. The air is heavy and oppressive, almost too thick to breathe. A big 727 is warming up its engines as it prepares to take off. Soon it will soar up into the sky, high above the rain-soaked clouds hanging over Arkansas. They watch the passengers board with a little bit of envy in their eyes.

"We could run," Steve says quietly. "We could move to another state that allows choice. But what happens if a state that now allows a parent freedom of choice changes its laws? Do you keep on running? We all live in America and none of us are free until we are all free."

Donna has finished nursing her son. Jo Ann is still defiant. "I have five letters from doctors stating those shots could hurt my baby. This whole thing boils down to a difference of opinion between doctors, with one group of so-called medical experts in positions of power trying to discredit the medical opinion of other doctors who disagree with them. And parents are caught in the middle. If doctors can't even figure it out, how can they legislate it? What can my child do to their vaccination program that they are so scared of?"

The 727 accelerates. Its engines roar, and it barrels down the runway before effortlessly gliding up and away. The rain has stopped, and the clouds are beginning to break up. Jo Ann pauses for a moment. With the determination of a mother who knows what she must do, she adds, "They are not going to take my child from me just because some doctors want to prove they can do it. He is my son, and I am never going to stop fighting for his life."

The oppressive air at Little Rock Airport is charged with a kind of electric courage that is decidedly American. Jo Ann is right. No one said freedom was free.

18

Mandatory Vaccination: How Did It Happen?

> Law will never be strong or respected unless it has the sentiment of the people behind it. If the people of a state make bad laws, they will suffer for it. Suffering, and nothing else, will implant that sentiment of responsibility which is the first step to reform.
>
> *James Bryce*

Mandatory vaccination laws have their roots in the smallpox epidemics that killed and disfigured hundreds of millions of people throughout the world from at least the time of the Egyptian dynasties to the middle of the nineteenth century. Queen Mary II died of smallpox in England in 1694, and more than sixty million people in Europe alone died of the disease in the following century. Many societies eventually passed laws requiring those with smallpox to be quarantined or isolated from the rest of the population until they recovered.

The first attempt to prevent smallpox was a procedure developed in the Near East and imported to Europe in the eighteenth century. It consisted of infecting a small wound with pus taken from a smallpox sore and allowing the individual to develop a mild case of smallpox. Smallpox acquired in this fashion was usually very mild and rarely fatal and conferred the same immunity as a natural case of the disease.

This form of inoculation was vigorously criticized by doctors and clergymen when first introduced. In Boston, Zabdiel Boylston inoculated his only son for smallpox in 1721 and was mobbed by angry citizens denouncing his action. But as time went by, the practice became more and more accepted and was instrumental in cutting down on deaths from the disease.

335

Inoculation of this sort had one drawback. The inoculated person, while protecting himself by undergoing a mild case of smallpox, could still transmit it to others who would suffer its full fury. Therefore, the procedure was effective only if everyone in the community was inoculated; otherwise a single person might start a smallpox epidemic.

This concept of inoculated persons transmitting the very disease they have been inoculated against is as true today as in the eighteenth century. The live (Sabin) polio vaccine, given to more than 90 percent of the children in the United States, can cause polio in the vaccinated child who can then give the disease to an uninoculated person. (The killed Salk polio vaccine does not have the ability to transmit the disease.)

In fact, according to Saul Krugman, M.D., and Samuel L. Katz, M.D., authors of *Infectious Diseases of Children*, in the ten-year period between 1969 and 1978, "Approximately 242 million doses of OPV [oral polio vaccine] were distributed, and 76 cases of paralysis associated with the vaccine were reported. Eighteen cases of paralysis occurred in otherwise healthy vaccine recipients, 47 cases in healthy close contacts of vaccine recipients, and 11 cases in persons (recipients or contacts) with immune deficiency conditions."

The famous British doctor Edward Jenner introduced the practice of vaccination in 1798 by inoculating a country boy with cowpox pus and demonstrating that, when subsequently inoculated with smallpox pus, he did not come down with the disease. Since cowpox was a far milder disease in human beings, cowpox vaccination had the advantage of eliminating the problem of the inoculated person spreading smallpox to others.

Thomas Jefferson had members of his family vaccinated with Jenner's vaccine, and after that, the practice spread throughout America. While smallpox vaccination was no doubt critical in eradicating the disease, it caused its own share of death and injury. Although this is not generally known by the public, mass vaccination for smallpox was discontinued in the United States as much because the vaccine caused brain damage and death as because the disease had virtually disappeared.

The Supreme Court and *Jacobson* vs. *Massachusetts*

Laws requiring citizens to undergo smallpox vaccination were passed by individual states in the United States in the late nineteenth century.

It is against this backdrop that the U.S. Supreme Court made a historic ruling in *Jacobson* v. *Massachusetts* (1904) that set the precedent for enforcement by the states of their mandatory vaccination laws.

The Supreme Court decision went against the appeal of a man named Jacobson who was challenging a 1902 regulation adopted by the Board of Health of Cambridge, Massachusetts, requiring "all the inhabitants of the city who have not been successfully vaccinated since March, 1, 1897 to be vaccinated or revaccinated" for smallpox. The Cambridge Board of Health justified its regulation by citing a law, passed by the Massachusetts legislature, which stated that "the board of health of a city or town if, in its opinion, it is necessary for the public health or safety, shall require and enforce the vaccination and revaccination of all the inhabitants. . . ."

Jacobson claimed that he had reacted severely to a previous smallpox vaccination and believed that his system was sensitive to the toxin of the vaccination virus. His son had also reacted severely to the vaccination, and Jacobson claimed there was a hereditary factor which made him susceptible to a reaction that might harm him or endanger his life. He claimed that forcing him to be vaccinated was "an assault upon his person" and violated his constitutional rights.

Jacobson had hoped to demonstrate in the lower court that vaccination "quite often" causes injury and death, and that medicine cannot distinguish those who may be harmed from those who may not be harmed. But the Supreme Court agreed that this evidence was not admissible because the state legislature had already studied the matter and concluded not only that the vaccine does not often cause injury and death but that medicine can distinguish between those who may be harmed and those who will not be.

Convinced that doctors could predict who would be harmed by vaccination, the Supreme Court concluded, "The matured opinions of medical men everywhere, and the experience of mankind, as all must know, negative the suggestion that it is not possible in any case to determine whether vaccination is safe."

The justices went further and stated that Jacobson had not attempted to show that "he was in fact not a fit subject of vaccination at the time he was informed of the requirement of the regulation adopted by the Board of Health."

The Court also asserted that the "police power" of the states includes "such reasonable regulations established directly by legislative enactment as will protect the public health and the public safety." It went on to say that state legislatures must weigh competing medical opinions and are justified in ignoring minority opinions and accepting the view of the majority in regard to a medical procedure designed to protect the public health and safety.

The Supreme Court even went so far as to state that a lower court cannot go against the will of the legislature and redecide the medical issues once a legislature has adopted the law, except under exceptional circumstances. In fact, it said the only time that a court may reverse the intent of the legislature and nullify a law is when it conflicts with some constitutional right of the individual, and there is no general constitutional right to refuse vaccination.

The Court declared that the individual may be required to make a sacrifice for the good of society, saying, "It was the duty of the constituted authorities to keep in view the welfare, comfort, and safety of the many, and not permit the interests of the many to be subordinated to the wishes or convenience of the few."

But the justices also stated that mandatory vaccination must not be forced on a person whose physical condition would make vaccination "cruel and inhuman to the last degree. We are not to be understood as holding that the statute was intended to be applied in such a case or, if it was so intended, that the judiciary would not be competent to interfere and protect the health and life of the individual concerned. 'All laws,' this Court has said, 'should receive a sensible construction.' "

In light of what is now known about the pertussis vaccine and doctors' inability to identify high-risk children before injury or death occurs, the 1904 Supreme Court's complete confidence in the ability of the medical profession to identify those individuals who will die or be damaged by a vaccine was misplaced. The Court may also have placed too much faith in the ability of state legislators to sort through the medical advice of doctors and come up with just laws regulating such medical procedures as vaccination.

But the most significant feature of this precedent-setting decision was its implicit exemption from mandatory vaccination of any person who could demonstrate that the vaccination would probably cause severe injury to himself or his child. Today parents such as Jo Ann and James Cook, who are being forced to vaccinate their child even though he is medically at high risk of reacting severely to vaccination, have a better case for challenging mandatory vaccination laws because they are backed by a respectable minority of medical opinion as well as by evidence in the medical literature that was not available in 1904.

Jacobson v. *Massachusetts* was a landmark case because it endorsed the state's right- to pass mandatory vaccination laws and placed the burden on the individual refusing vaccination to prove—not that the law was unconstitutional—but that because of a unique health condition the vaccination could cause irreparable injury.

States Pass Laws Requiring Vaccination for School

In 1904, eleven states had compulsory vaccination laws; thirty-four did not. Not one of the states forcibly vaccinated those who did not comply with the law, while Utah and West Virginia expressly stated that vaccination could not be forced upon anyone. By 1904, Holland and Switzerland had abolished smallpox vaccination laws, and in that same year there were riots in Brazil caused by attempts to enforce smallpox vaccination.

The tetanus and diphtheria vaccines were the next to be developed, and the pertussis vaccine soon followed. In the 1950s, Jonas Salk's discovery added polio vaccine to the list. By the mid-1960s, many states had laws requiring DPT and polio vaccination, most of them ensuring compliance by making the vaccination a requirement for entry into elementary school. As new vaccines were developed, such as the ones for measles, mumps, and rubella, states automatically added these vaccines to the list of compulsory vaccinations required for school entry.

In 1964, the *Cude* v. *Arkansas* case (described in the last chapter), which was heard before the Arkansas Supreme Court, reinforced the 1904 U.S. Supreme Court decision that states have the right to enforce mandatory vaccination laws. When Archie Cude was forced to surrender his children to the state for vaccination against smallpox, despite his assertion that the procedure was against his religious beliefs, it had a chilling effect on the effort of parents fighting for the right to refuse to have their children vaccinated. (However, Arkansas and most other states now allow parents a religious exemption from vaccination if they belong to a recognized religion that officially opposes vaccination.)

The very next year, in 1965, Congress passed the Immunization Assistance Act setting up a categorical grant program to states and large metropolitan areas to provide funds and assistance in establishing immunization programs in states. This Act specified what vaccines might be purchased by states with federal funds.

The DPT vaccine, however, was not included, and it is not included today. George Hardy, M.D., an assistant director of the CDC, offered an explanation for this omission: "I think the theory of the Act was that it was going to provide assistance for those expensive new viral vaccines, and each time the Act has been amended, it has included another new live viral vaccine that is more expensive such as rubella and mumps. My assumption is that DPT was not included because it was already being given and because it was very cheap."

Under the Act, in order to get federal funds, a state must apply for them and indicate how they will be spent. The grants may pay for the purchase of any of the specified vaccines, or the state may request a CDC public health advisor to assist the state Health Department in implementing its vaccination program. Hardy explained:

"In the United States, health . . . is a state responsibility, and the immunization laws in this country are state laws. There is no federal law requiring any immunization for anything. . . . The federal immunization program gives every state money which is used for immunizations, which encourages immunizations. Every state has a public health advisor—some states more than one—at their request in lieu of cash. And those public health advisors believe in immunization as an important thing. They have worked with the state health departments. In many cases, it is the state health departments which have asked the state legislatures to adopt their immunization laws. And on the recommendation of the state health department, the state legislatures have adopted these mandatory vaccination laws. It is quite possible that the state health departments' recommendations certainly would not have been developed without the input of a person who was there and who was knowledgeable about immunization programs. But the statutes which exist are state statutes."

In the early 1970s, when Hardy worked in the Epidemic Intelligence Service (EIS) of the CDC, he was assigned to advise the state health department in Birmingham, Alabama. He described how that state developed its mandatory vaccination program.

"As I recall, we adopted an ordinance requiring immunization for school-age enterers in Birmingham-Jefferson County in about 1973 or 1974, and the state developed a statewide mandatory immunization law a year or two later. We had a requirement by local ordinance first, and the state did it later. And those were not in place before."

Commenting on CDC's role in advising state health departments on medical exemptions from vaccination, Hardy said, "The ACIP recommendations [of the CDC] are used as recommendations, as guidelines, and there is . . . always a basis for medical judgment questions. . . . The ACIP recommendations are called recommendations; they are not called laws. And that is their intent. They are intended to be recommendations to people who are responsible for administering vaccines.

"They are recommendations by a body that is supposedly knowledgeable about the use of vaccines, and this is how they would recommend that you use it. Now I am not so naive as to think that a recommendation coming from a part of the federal government doesn't carry a little bit of clout, but it is a recommendation; it is not a statute; it is not a regulation."

Hardy further clarified his point: "If a child has severe allergies, depending upon what they are, it might well be a contraindication, depending upon what they are and what the vaccine is. That is a medical decision between that parent and that child's doctor. . . . Nobody to my knowledge goes strictly according to any recommendations. Medicine is still—there is still an element of art as well as science. I think that these [medical exemptions from vaccination] are decisions that physicians make and physicians in health departments make in states. But those are judgmental decisions. I do think that is a medical decision that needs to be made in consultation with the parent, of course."

Hardy maintained that the CDC does not support removing children from parents and forcibly vaccinating them: "I think it is a very clear activity of the federal government to encourage childhood immunizations. It certainly isn't the CDC policy that children be taken from the family. There is nothing like that. . . . But these decisions are being made by the state health department."

When there is a conflict between parents who have a medical exemption written by a private physician for their child and doctors in the state health department who refuse to accept the exemption, Hardy added, "My expectation would be that the state health department would prevail. Unless the doctor, who was overruled, or the attorney for the family or both decided to challenge the state health department in court, in which case it would be decided by the state courts because it is a state statute."

Hardy supports mandatory vaccination: "Any time anyone receives a biological or any other type of medicine there is going to be some risk. And it is clear with the vaccines that there are some inherent dangers. But I think society has a responsibility to measure the benefits to society as a whole versus those risks. And society as a whole has to make a judgment . . . my personal opinion is that our society's decision at the moment is a correct one."

Hardy, however, supports the right of parents to question the wisdom of mandatory vaccination and the benefit/risk analysis of certain vaccines. "Any time in any society that people don't question decisions that are being made, then we are not a free society," he stated. "I also think that parents that have children who are damaged have a much stronger motivation than all of the rest of society to be concerned about this. But I do think that the current societal decision about risks and benefits is a correct one. That doesn't say that things don't change. In point of fact, there was a discussion a few years ago about whether or not we should continue smallpox vaccination. There are effects of smallpox vaccine that are negative . . . it took more years than I would have thought was appropriate to reach a decision to stop using smallpox vaccine, but that happened."

The Crusade to Enforce Mandatory Vaccination

When Dale Bumpers became governor of Arkansas in 1971, he and his wife, Betty, developed a mass vaccination campaign for the state. Now a U.S. Senator from Arkansas, Dale Bumpers talked in an interview about how they did it.

"First of all, this was Mrs. Bumpers' idea," he said. "She thought that it would be a very good and wise use of her time as first lady to use the influence of that position to do something really worthwhile and meaningful. She brought in the Arkansas League for Nursing, the Arkansas Nurses Association, the Arkansas Health Department, the Arkansas National Guard, the Agriculture Extension Service. . . . I asked all those people to cooperate with her. But they were more than happy to do it."

In 1978, Senator Bumpers told the U.S. Senate: "We had an immunization program in Arkansas when I was governor. We immunized virtually every child in that State against measles, mumps, rubella, in a 2-year period of time, became No. 2 in the country. . . . What did it cost us? My wife headed the program. I think I gave her $50,000 out of my emergency fund. We called in the National Guard, recruited everybody to join hands, and we immunized those children."

The health official from the CDC assigned to advise the Arkansas Department of Health "was very closely allied with Betty and was sort of orchestrating as a liaison between CDC and this program," the senator said.

One of the reasons for the vaccination crusade, Senator Bumpers noted, was because Arkansas' mandatory vaccination law "was not being enforced. It was on the books. Immunization levels would never have gotten down to that dangerously low point if those laws had been enforced."

In 1973, mass vaccination clinics were held in Arkansas. "The way we kicked it off after a lot of prepublicity was to have two massive clinics on Saturdays. I believe we immunized 300,000 children on the first Saturday," Senator Bumpers said.

The campaign was an overwhelming success. Striving for 100-percent vaccination coverage, 82 percent of the children living in Arkansas had been vaccinated with DPT after the program had been in place for only one year. When the citizens of Arkansas sent their former governor to Washington, the Bumpers decided to promote the idea of a nation-wide vaccination effort modeled after the Arkansas success story.

President and Mrs. Ford, fresh from their experience with the swine flu vaccine, apparently were not interested in the idea. But when Jimmy and Rosalyn Carter moved to the White House in 1976, the Bumpers found a more receptive audience. "When the Carters came to town, they had been friends of ours because we served as governors together. Betty went over to see Rosalyn and talked to her about it and said, 'You know this is something the President can do so that when he runs for reelection, he can say the government did it.' Because, you know, the government was in such disrepute, nobody thought the government could do anything. Betty said, 'This is one thing that the government can do effectively and beneficially.' And so Jimmy asked Secretary Califano to cooperate with Betty. Joe Califano and Betty together put the whole thing in place."

Mrs. Bumpers and Secretary Califano worked with the CDC to map out a nationwide mass-vaccination campaign. "Betty was enlisting the support of the National Governors' Conference and the governors' wives and getting an awful lot of those people on the board to help out. She was trying to get the full force of most of the governors' offices behind her because no program was going to be successful in any state if the governor or the governor's wife wasn't behind it," said the senator.

A necessary first step to ensure the success of a nationwide campaign to get every child in the United States vaccinated was to ask Congress for more money to implement the campaign. "We did increase the appropriations. One of the battles I always fought was to make sure there was the money there to buy the amount of vaccine that was going to be necessary to immunize the children in this country," said Senator Bumpers.

The Bumpers were as successful in Washington as they had been in Little Rock. Recounting the increases in federal funding for nationwide immunization programs in state public health clinics, which he successfully urged Congress to adopt, Senator Bumpers said, "When I came here, seven and a half million dollars were in the pot. . . . Jimmy Carter became President in 1976, and we got it almost double that in 1977. That's when we began the program. In 1978, it went from 14.5 million to 33 million, and in 1979, from 33 million to 46.9 million."

Senator Bumpers, a Democrat, did not have to fight hard to win approval for his nationwide immunization campaign during President Carter's term in the White House. According to him, it sailed through Congress without opposition. "We didn't have any opposition to immunizations until Ronald Reagan became President," the Senator said. "He tried to cut this one [program] back to where it would have been almost ineffective."

In 1982, the senator made a plea to Congress to restore funds to the national immunization program he and his wife had fought so long and hard to achieve. He told the Senate, "If we are really serious about holding the line on government spending and getting the most bang for the buck, these programs should be increased, not reduced."

The senator was successful in beating back President Reagan's challenge to the immunization appropriations. Praising the role the CDC played in helping to achieve by 1979 a 90-percent immunization rate throughout the United States, he added, "The Centers for Disease Control was always very actively involved in all of these programs. Dr. Foege was there most of the time . . . he's a brilliant man."

Asked whether or not he believes it is a good idea for the state of Arkansas to take children from their parents and forcibly vaccinate them even when doctors have written the children medical exemptions, the senator replied, "I do think that carried to its ultimate conclusion, if you allow enough children an exemption—and maybe there is a perfectly good medical reason for some child not being put at risk with this shot, I don't know much about how precise medicine is in making that kind of determination—but I do know that . . . if you just allowed everybody on immunizations to decide for themselves whether they were going to do it or not, medically as I understand it, you build up a pool like in polio that puts everybody at risk then. I don't think a few people ought to be allowed to put a lot at risk."

Senator Bumpers was very upset by WRC-TV's "DPT: Vaccine Roulette" and the station's 1983 update, "DPT: One Year Later." Three days after the update was shown, he addressed the Senate and concluded, "I must say that Miss Lea Thompson's motives may have been absolutely pure, but I think she did a disservice to the nation and a disservice to parents as well, who may be terribly stressed as a result of such a one-sided presentation."

Asked for a suggestion on what to do about children who are hurt by vaccines, the senator commented, "Well, that is just a continuing problem. And right now, most pharmaceutical companies require people to sign disclaimers I think before they get the shots. Maybe there ought to be some kind of national pool or something. I don't know the answer to that. . . . It is always a question of trade-offs. There is an economic theory that for every governmental action to improve some-body's economic life, you probably are harming somebody else by an equal amount. So you have to weigh and balance and make these trade-offs and that is the way it is with these immunizations."

The state of Arkansas has faithfully continued the tradition that Dale and Betty Bumpers began during their tenure in the governor's mansion. In 1983, Arkansas reportedly vaccinated 98 percent of its school children against diphtheria, tetanus, and pertussis; 98 percent against polio; 99 percent against measles; 99 percent against rubella; and 92 percent against mumps.

Congress has continued to support Senator Bumpers' effort to achieve a 100-percent vaccination rate in America. The Public Health Service grant program is doing very well. More than thirty million dollars were slotted in fiscal year 1984 to help the CDC and the states reach new goals—which include making sure that 90 percent of American children have been completely vaccinated by the age of two.

In the January 3, 1984, issue of the *Federal Register*, the CDC unveiled its current objectives, including the desire "to develop, test and implement systems for use in the States to ensure that 90 percent or more of all children complete basic immunizations by age 2." It is unclear how the CDC and the state health departments plan to ensure that all children under two years of age are vaccinated, since the controlling factor at present is school entry.

Mandatory Vaccination Laws Today

As of January 1984, only Arizona, Kentucky, Missouri, Montana, New York, Oregon, Pennsylvania, Rhode Island, and Washington did not have laws requiring pertussis vaccination as a precondition for school entry. In twenty-two states, parents can refuse to have their children vaccinated if they have a "philosophical objection" to a particular vaccination. These states include Arizona, California, Colorado, Delaware, Idaho, Indiana, Louisiana, Maine, Michigan, Minnesota, Missouri, Montana, Nebraska, North Dakota, Ohio, Oklahoma, Pennsylvania, Rhode Island, Utah, Vermont, Washington, and Wisconsin.

All states except Mississippi and West Virginia allow a religious exemption if the parents belong to a religion that objects to vaccination. All states allow a medical exemption if a parent or guardian can obtain from a licensed physician a statement that a particular vaccination would be detrimental to the child's health. Parents can have a difficult time obtaining this medical exemption, however, and in some states it is almost impossible.

Parents in many states have reported that they cannot find doctors to write their children medical exemptions; that pediatricians have threatened not to treat any child who is not vaccinated; that state health departments have refused to grant exemptions; that school boards have refused to allow unvaccinated children to attend school; and, in the case of Arkansas, that the state has attempted to take possession of their children and forcibly vaccinate them.

One of the most controversial aspects of the mandatory vaccination policy in America is the requirement in public health clinics that parents sign a "consent form" devised by the CDC before any child is vaccinated. About the DPT shot, the "consent form" states: "I have read the information on this form about diphtheria, tetanus and pertussis and DTP, DT and Td (adult tetanus) vaccines. I have had a chance to ask questions which were answered to my satisfaction. I believe I understand the benefits and risks of DTP, DT, and Td vaccines and request that the vaccine checked below be given to me or to the person named below for whom I am authorized to make this request."

Recently private pediatricians have been creating similar release forms for parents to sign before a child is vaccinated. And if parents refuse to sign such a form (which absolves the doctor of all liability if the child is injured by the vaccine), the doctor will not vaccinate. In states without a "philosophical objection" an unvaccinated child cannot attend school.

Until recently, few parents have had the courage to stand up to the medical establishment on this point. Vincent Fulginiti, M.D., testified in 1982: "In fact, in two years of using the informed consent forms in our own institution, 90 percent of the patients read the form and say, 'Doc, what do you think?' and then do whatever we suggest."

Barbara Syska was one parent who did not. In testimony before the Maryland State House of Representatives, she described how her son had been excluded from school in Maryland because he had not received a rubella shot:

"My eleven-year-old son is excluded from school for the last three and a half years because I refused to sign the informed consent form. . . . The State of Maryland does not want the responsibility for aftereffects of vaccination. A parent has to sign that form. I have the freedom not to sign it. I exercised it and my son is isolated from his peers for the last three and a half years. . . . I went to court. I was told there that I am not an expert so I could not adequately defend my case. . . . I came to this country over twenty years ago believing freedom exists here. And even if it does not, I am going to exercise my freedom to do what I consider is best for my child. Most of the dictators in the world in the past and present believe that they know what is best for their people. In Maryland we have a dictator—the Health Department."

Curiously, the United States appears to be the only major Western nation that continues to legally require that children be inoculated with the pertussis vaccine. It is not legally required in England, France, West Germany, Canada, Austria, Italy, Switzerland, Portugal, Spain, Denmark, Sweden, Belgium, Finland, Ireland, Norway, or The Netherlands. In fact, the only part of Europe where pertussis vaccination is universally imposed is in communist countries such as the Soviet Union, East Germany, Poland, and Czechoslovakia.

What is even more curious is that, while requiring parents to have their children vaccinated, the United States does not require doctors to report adverse reactions, record severe reactions in a child's permanent medical record, or keep a record of the vaccine manufacturer's name, lot, and batch number.

As one mother put it, "How can this country legally require us to have our children vaccinated but not legally require the doctors to report adverse reactions? The government and doctors keep justifying forcing our children to get the vaccines because, they say, the benefits outweigh the risks. How do they know the benefits outweigh the risks if they don't even know how many adverse reactions there are and how many of those end up in deaths and brain damage? If we are going to be told we have to get the vaccines, doctors ought to be told they have to report and record their bad side effects."

Hardy has pointed out the difficulty of enforcing mandatory reporting by doctors, even in states where the reporting of whooping cough is obligatory: "The entire reporting system in the United States is entirely voluntary. There are a few cases in which a state will pass a law saying that 'You must report this and you must report that.' But what are you going to do—go and cut off a physician's hand if he hasn't reported it? It is a voluntary system."

Yet mass vaccination in our free society is not voluntary. As parents have observed, when they do not obey the state mandatory vaccination laws, their children can be barred from school; they can also be charged with truancy and, subsequently, with child neglect, which paves the way for their children being taken from them and made wards of the state.

19

The Search for a Safer Vaccine

> We would like to enjoy reduction in disease at little or no cost.
> But this goal is difficult to achieve because the reason for im-
> munity to pertussis is obscure; hence, we have little knowledge
> of the immunizing principle of the bacterium. To accomplish
> protection we find it necessary to give the entire bacterium and
> to allow the host to sort out the effective immunologic response.
> The cost of doing this is the inclusion of all components of the
> bacterium, including the toxic ones.
>
> *Vincent Fulginiti, M.D. (1984)*

The search for a safer pertussis vaccine, at least in the United States, has been dogged by a curious lack of progress. Because the whole-cell vaccine was licensed as safe and effective and because adverse reactions were minimized by the vaccine establishment, the development of a safer vaccine has not been given a high priority.

As the FDA's Charles Manclark observed in 1976, "One of the several dilemmas facing the manufacturer or developer of a new vaccine is justifying the development and use of a new vaccine if present vaccines are judged to be safe and effective. In addition, pertussis vaccine is a relatively low-profit item, and the cost of developing and field testing it would be very high." But despite these problems, he commented in 1981 that "most pertussis vaccines are whole-cell preparations that were developed before many of the recent advances in immunology, biochemistry, and genetics, and the development of an improved vaccine is a desirable goal that should be pursued."

In 1983, however, Dr. William Jordan, of the NIAID (National Institute of Allergy and Infectious Disease), played down the pressing need for a safer pertussis vaccine. The NIAID is the body within the National Institutes of Health responsible for federal vaccine research grants to scientists and private research laboratories. Jordan stated:

"We all would like to have a less reactogenic vaccine, because the pertussis vaccine is associated with a low incidence of adverse reactions. I would emphasize, however, that the current vaccine is regarded as safe and effective and is recommended for its use, except for a few contraindications. . . . In September of 1982, when the Institute set its priorities, included among the top five priorities was an improved pertussis vaccine. I must say, it was not the first of those five, because there is an effective vaccine to prevent pertussis. We selected some other diseases, such as meningitis in neonatal children, gonorrhea, some severe respiratory diseases, but we put pertussis within the first five for an improved vaccine."

As discussed in Chapter 16, it has been known for more than twenty years that the vaccine is not being adequately tested for safety, because the FDA's mouse toxicity test apparently bears little relationship to adverse reactions in children. The vaccine has continued to cause deaths and neurological damage even though it is passing FDA potency and toxicity tests. Why, then, have few steps been taken by the government and manufacturers to improve or replace it?

The reasons given by the FDA and vaccine manufacturers for this curious failure may be divided into four categories: scientific, manufacturing, financial, and ethical/legal. Before these are discussed, however, it is useful to take a look at the history of the two attempts that have been made to purify the vaccine and make it substantially less toxic.

The First Attempt To Reduce Reactivity

As discussed in Chapter 3, the whole-cell pertussis vaccine is primitive and crude, but the production process is simple and inexpensive. The first commercially successful attempt to reduce toxicity by "splitting" the whole cell and attempting to extract and separate the toxic components from the protective ones was the creation of Trisolgen in the 1960s by the Eli Lilly Company (see Chapter 16).

When Wyeth financed a study in 1981, conducted by the University of Texas Health Science Center, comparing the reactivity of their version of the Lilly Trisolgen vaccine with current whole-cell vaccines, the result showed the extracted vaccine to be less reactive. Philip Brunell, who was a principal author of the study, told the 1982 FDA Symposium that "the adverse reactions were generally higher overall with the whole cell pertussis antigen. There was a much higher incidence of systemic reactions with the whole cell pertussis antigen."

When the study was published in 1983, the authors concluded: "Although the whole cell, aluminum phosphate containing antigen is the most commonly used in the United States, it is clearly the most reactogenic in terms of common reactions. . . . this study suggests that the combination of whole cell and aluminum phosphate, which is currently used in the United States, is probably not the optimal formulation for pertussis vaccine."

If the extracted vaccine was really less reactive, why didn't Wyeth manufacture it? When interviewed in early 1984, M. Z. Bierly of Wyeth Laboratories stated, "The Office of Biologics was not interested in this vaccine, because it would take a lot of highfalutin' statistical workup to demonstrate that it was any better than the existing one. Thus we have not applied for a license to manufacture the Trisolgen vaccine."

At the time that Lilly was manufacturing Trisolgen, a product insert explained that Trisolgen was created "by an extraction procedure which permits the cellular debris of the pertussis organism to be discarded." But scientists evidently did not know precisely what was in it; as recently as 1982, the Wyeth Laboratories scientist responsible for work on the extract vaccine stated at the FDA Symposium, "We have only really begun to attempt to characterize these vaccines with respect to the various factors [in them]."

Bierly reiterated that sentiment in a 1984 interview, "Nobody really knew what was in Trisolgen. The extraction process was such that you never really knew what was being extracted."

A Delicate Boundary Between Toxicity and Efficacy

The inability to characterize the pertussis bacterium has haunted scientists trying to develop a safer pertussis vaccine (see the discussion in Chapter 3). The difficulty centers around defining precisely which components of the whole pertussis cell are toxic and which stimulate immunity. The prevailing theory seems to be that they are one and the same, and that the real problem lies in inactivating this toxin sufficiently to render the vaccine harmless but still protective against whooping cough.

Scientists have identified certain components in the pertussis bacterium as extremely dangerous: the endotoxin (a bacterial lipopolysaccharide); dermonecrotic or heat-labile toxin; tracheal cytotoxin; and LPF (also known as HSF, IAP, pertussigen, and pertussis toxin).

Although more such toxins may be identified in the future, scientists believe that, of the four already known, only LPF is immunogenic (protective). There is a general consensus that the endotoxin, dermonecrotic toxin, and tracheal cytotoxin play no role in immunogenicity and should be removed or inactivated completely in a purified vaccine.

LPF is one of the most toxic substances in nature, a true bacterial exotoxin with an enormous range of effects on the living organism. One of its effects is to stop the recycling of lymphocytes (white blood cells), resulting in an apparent increase in their number. This is why it is called "lymphocytosis-promoting factor (LPF)."

LPF can also apparently make the brain tissue more porous. In a common laboratory experiment, LPF is added to a solution of nerve tissue and injected into sensitized mice to cause brain inflammation. This has been known since 1955. Without the LPF, the brain inflammation would not occur. Does this mean that LPF has a direct action on brain tissue? The answer is that it probably does.

As is the case with many biochemical substances, scientists have only a limited understanding of their effects upon the body. LPF is no different and FDA's John Robbins commented in 1982: "The physiologic role of the LPF for Bordetella pertussis is not yet known. The mechanism of its biologic and toxic activity in the host on a molecular level also is not known."

Despite this lack of understanding, many scientists now believe that LPF is the key to a better vaccine; their goal is to strike a delicate balance between toxicity and efficacy by inactivating or "toxoiding" just the right amount of LPF to make a more purified, safer pertussis vaccine that is still protective. A new vaccine of this type is called the "acellular" vaccine.

But, here again, there are many unknowns. Manclark wrote in 1981, "The boundary between vaccine toxicity and potency is not well defined, and the situation is further complicated by the technical limitations of laboratory methods of defining these parameters. . . . the main difficulty is that the bases for vaccine potency and toxicity are not known."

Researchers in the Soviet Union and Yugoslavia tried for years to isolate a component of the B. pertussis that would be nontoxic but still give protection. They were unsuccessful, and Manclark noted, "It may be unwise to attempt to find less toxic strains for vaccine production, since the factors producing toxicity, e.g., LPF, may be the most potent immunogens."

Louis Sauer urged in the 1930s that the toxins be left in the vaccine rather than washed out. He held that it was the toxins which made the vaccine protective. When Sweden attempted to reduce the toxicity of its vaccine in the late 1960s and early 1970s to lessen the incidence of adverse reactions, the vaccine proved ineffective and was eventually withdrawn.

How nontoxic should a vaccine be, and still be protective? Japanese scientists, who have developed a purified "acellular" pertussis vaccine, apparently are not completely toxoiding it. Japanese scientists at the 1982 FDA Symposium were asked by Charles Manclark, "Ideally, a vaccine should be completely toxoided, don't you think?" Dr. Yuji Sato, who developed the new vaccine, answered, "I don't think so." He appears to have suggested that the Japanese vaccine still had some LPF activity.

Manclark stated in a 1983 interview, "Essentially toxoidization has been an empirical procedure in the past, with formalin and the like. . . . If we knew how to do toxoidization properly, we could probably use much less material, much smaller doses."

If 100-percent toxoidization is what is needed, and if that cannot ever be accomplished without rendering the vaccine ineffective, adverse reactions may occur even with an improved pertussis vaccine. There is little doubt, however, that reactions would occur at a much lower rate, given the 90-percent reduction in endotoxin content and the marked reduction in exotoxin (i.e., LPF, pertussis toxin) in the acellular vaccine.

Apparently, scientists have known for some time that a less toxic pertussis vaccine could be made by using this separation and toxoiding process, a point which will be discussed later in this chapter. Of course, compared to the simplicity of manufacturing the whole-cell vaccine, the production of an acellular vaccine is complex. It is also more expensive. But it is not impossible, as the Japanese have proved with their development and use since 1981 of an acellular vaccine that is reputed to be safer than the whole-cell vaccine being used by the rest of the world.

The Japanese Acellular Vaccine

Japan's experience with whooping cough and the pertussis vaccine is a good illustration of how one nation had the foresight to respond with sensitivity and intelligence to a crisis involving public acceptance of mass immunization programs. Instead of denying the problem, Japan chose to deal with it.

After World War II, when Japan was under U.S. occupation, the Preventive Vaccination Law of 1948 was enacted making it a legal requirement for children to be inoculated with pertussis vaccine. Vaccination was begun at three to six months of age. (The reason that this vaccination schedule was used, according to a Japanese scientist attending the 1982 Symposium, was because "it was adopted by the order of the American occupational army in 1948.")

As the vaccine became widely used, whooping cough cases rapidly declined. By 1967, there was less than one case of pertussis per 100,000 people. The government, however, acknowledged that vaccines, particularly smallpox and DPT vaccines, could cause damage. In 1970, a bill to compensate persons injured by vaccines was enacted.

In 1975, two babies died suddenly after receiving DPT shots. The Japanese government quickly responded to public concern about the safety of the vaccine. By order of the Minister of Health, the pertussis component was temporarily removed from the DPT shot. Later that year, however, DPT shots were once again available for use with the recommendation that DPT vaccination begin at twenty-four months of age or older. Another Japanese scientist at the FDA Symposium remarked, "Subsequently, the number of serious adverse reactions became very rare. However, coverage rate of DPT vaccine declined rapidly in the following years."

He pointed out that Japan's response to this crisis was to find a solution: "In order to achieve satisfactory performance of the national program of pertussis vaccination, it was considered to develop a new and less toxic pertussis vaccine made of the purest possible protective antigens."

The result of this high priority search for a safer vaccine was that Dr. Yuji Sato, who had once worked at NIH with American pertussis vaccine researchers, developed an acellular vaccine by using separation and toxoiding procedures to render the vaccine less toxic. Between 1978 and 1981, the new vaccine was clinically tested on about 5,000 children.

Results of these clinical trials and details about the manufacturing techniques used to produce the acellular vaccine were published in January 1984, by Drs. Sato, M. Kimura, and H. Fukumi in *The Lancet*. They stated that laboratory tests "clearly show that component [acellular] vaccine is as effective as conventional whole-cell vaccine and that it is one-tenth as toxic as judged by tests for histamine sensitisation, leucocytosis promotion, and endotoxicity."

Results of the clinical trials showed that "the incidence of fever with component vaccine is only 10 percent of that with whole-cell vaccine, and it did not produce febrile fits [convulsions]. The incidence of local side-effects was also 75–80 percent less than that with whole-cell vaccine."

The Japanese scientists also reported that the new vaccine appears to be as effective as the whole-cell vaccine because "among the children who were exposed to infection from a member of the household, pertussis developed in 82.8 percent of those unvaccinated, 14.3 percent of those who received whole-cell vaccine, and 11.1 percent of those who received component vaccine."

When these laboratory and clinical test results became known to Japanese scientists in 1981, they were eager to plunge ahead and use the apparently safer acellular vaccine that Sato developed in order to quickly restore public confidence in mass immunization programs and, particularly, to stop the rise in whooping cough cases. Kimura stated at the 1982 FDA Symposium that the excellent results of the clinical trials "and the epidemic situation of pertussis after discontinuance of regular DPT immunization made the Ministry of Health and Welfare approve the new vaccine in August, 1981."

In August 1981, the government also organized the national disease surveillance system, which included 2,000 pediatricians whose job it was to report the number of their infectious disease cases and vaccine reactions every week to the government in order to generate statistical data. Kimura reported to the 1982 Symposium that "Since 1981 about one million doses of the new vaccine have been injected on a nationwide scale without serious adverse reactions."

The question remains, if Japan has been using a safer vaccine since 1981, why hasn't the United States? Sato once worked for the NIH with Manclark, Robbins, and other FDA scientists who have been conducting research on a purified vaccine for more than a decade.

In an exchange between one Japanese scientist and Manclark at the 1982 Symposium, Manclark asked why the Japanese government decided to go ahead and use the new acellular vaccine in 1981. The Japanese scientist replied, "The situation from 1975 was quite difficult for physicians because of the adverse reactions which became a big problem in Japan, not only in Japan but also in other countries of the world. And there is one motivation for the change."

Manclark commented, "Well, what I think you are saying is that you had to do something because the previous vaccine was not being accepted, and you had disease, so some change needed to be made, and it added pressure to the system."

Here again, one reason American children are still being injured by the whole-cell vaccine appears to be because there has been no public recognition in the United States of the extent of vaccine injuries. Why? Because government health officials and members of the medical establishment have been denying there is a serious problem for more than four decades and American parents have believed them.

Money: The Bottom Line

Production of the acellular vaccine involves all the difficulties associated with the whole-cell vaccine in addition to new problems resulting from the extraction procedure. It is very difficult to make, as many manufacturers have found out. Cameron said in 1982, "I don't know how many people realize the practicalities of making an extract vaccine. . . . Licensees have dropped like flies in the United States."

Most notably, the acellular vaccine will be more expensive to produce than the inexpensive whole-cell vaccine. As John Cameron pointed out in 1982: "As far as vaccines are concerned at this moment in terms of production, pure and simple production, you couldn't make a cheaper vaccine than Bordetella pertussis. . . . It is simply a whole culture which has been washed, nothing else."

The added expense of manufacturing an acellular vaccine appears to have been a major reason why a purified vaccine has yet to be used in the United States. Another particpant at the 1982 Symposium revealed that manufacturers have known for some time a safer pertussis vaccine could be produced. The catch is that it would involve throwing away 90 percent of their product:

"Sure, you can produce a much less toxic product in very low yields, and anyone who has worked on pertussis knows this, you can get a little bit out—maybe 10 percent which is active—and you throw the rest away. . . . Now what you are saying to me as a producer is, you must increase your production another fourfold or fivefold. Now, with the enormous amount of vaccine that is required, this is going to pose certain practical problems to many manufacturers."

As with any radically new vaccine, the manufacturer will be running an expensive risk. The vaccine may not consistently pass FDA tests, it may cause side effects, or it may not be accepted by the public or the medical profession. William Jordan commented at the 1982 FDA Symposium that the manufacturers are reluctant to invest money in a new vaccine without assurance of a wide and stable market: "Who is going to be bold enough to invest industrial dollars with the risk of little or no return so that those who want to test vaccines will have products to test?'"

Frank Perkins of the WHO agreed: "I know the manufacturers are not going to put a lot of money and effort and investment into a vaccine that is not going to be marketed."

If the vaccine was going to be sold only in the United States, this increased production cost might not be a significant factor. But the vaccines are also being produced for the Third World countries, paid for by these countries themselves or by the WHO. As a result, there is great reluctance to abandon the present inexpensive vaccine in favor of a more expensive one. Perkins stated (1982) that the WHO "buys for 57 cents the total immunization vaccines for a child, three doses of polio at 4 cents a dose, three doses of DPT at between 10 cents and 12 cents a dose, and measles costs us in 20-dose vials 10 cents a dose. . . . there is no way in which you are going to beat these prices with a new vaccine."

Developing countries spend, on the average, one dollar per capita per year on public health. Perkins asked his colleagues attending the 1982 FDA Symposium: "How can you put the price of your vaccine, total vaccine package deal, beyond 57 cents, when they only spend a dollar? . . ."

Dennis Stainer, of Connaught Laboratories, commented: "I know that you shouldn't bring money into the argument among scientists, but I think we have to. What we are really faced with I think now is going from a vaccine which costs literally cents to produce to one which I believe is going to cost dollars to produce. . . . And I wonder whether the major users of the vaccines, which are chiefly the developing nations, where most of the vaccine is going to be used, I wonder are they prepared to pay the cost? I think it is all very well for the Canadians and for the U.S. and for Europe, they can afford it. But are we going to put ourselves in a position where we are going to have two vaccines, one for the wealthy and one for the rest? Because I don't think any of us want that. We want one vaccine. But I think we have to be very realistic in terms of how much this is going to cost."

Today the problem of liability for vaccine producers and the doctors who administer vaccines dominates any public discussion of the mass vaccination issue. When Senator Paula Hawkins introduced the National Childhood Vaccine-Injury Compensation Act in 1983, she stated, "One by one, U.S. vaccine manufacturers have decided that this business is not commercially attractive and have dropped out. Why? Rising costs and inadequate prices have been a significant factor in the decision to withdraw from the vaccine markets, but a major vulnerability is the unresolved public policy problem of liability for unavoidable injury in mass immunization programs. The specter of high and uncertain damage awards contributes to driving manufacturers out of vaccine production."

Some have left the business because, according to one company president, 50 percent of all liability claims were attributable to vaccines which represented less than 10 percent of the company's entire business. Connaught raised the price of a fifteen-dose vial of the DPT vaccine in June 1983, from $4.67 to $42.00, claiming that the only alternative was to stop making it.

When Wyeth Laboratories suddenly and dramatically withdrew from the pertussis vaccine market on June 13, 1984, a little more than one month after the May 3 Senate Hearings on the vaccine compensation bill, its press release declared: "This decision was dictated by dramatic increases in the cost of participating in this market." At the same time, Lederle also raised its price for a fifteen-dose vial of DPT vaccine to $42.00.

The cost of settling DPT vaccine damage suits appears to have taken its toll. In fact, Wyeth and other manufacturers as well as the AMA have been complaining to Congress for years that they do not want to continue bearing the cost of these suits. They are fighting against the National Childhood Vaccine Injury Compensation Act, which allows a parent the right to choose either federal compensation or a lawsuit, because they want a compensation bill prohibiting lawsuits against manufacturers or physicians for vaccine-related deaths and injuries (see Chapter 21).

Testing Problems: Scientific, Practical, and Ethical

Testing a new vaccine will present a major public-relations problem for United States health authorities. As Charles Manclark observed in 1981: "Clinical trials of a new vaccine will be complicated by serious ethical, legal, and logistic problems, since it would be very difficult to justify injecting children with a new vaccine when safe, effective vaccines are already available."

Paradoxically, while stubbornly clinging to the justification that there is a safe and effective pertussis vaccine already on the market, vaccine researchers simultaneously express a singular lack of faith in the tests used to proclaim the vaccine "safe and effective." Again and again, problems with existing tests for safety and potency appear to block an improved pertussis vaccine in the United States and Europe.

At the 1982 FDA Symposium, A. H. Griffith talked about the limitations of the mouse potency test and how it affects future clinical trials on a new vaccine:

"It is extremely difficult to embark on a major clinical trial in children in a very sensitive area when we, as clinicians, are not quite certain whether our assessment of potency, the tests carried out, is a reliable one, when we have a suspicion that this varies between laboratory and laboratory; when the same laboratory carries out the same tests and it is not reproducible, and so on. And as clinicians with a responsibility of persuading parents to get their children vaccinated with a new vaccine, and going on a large program, are we doing good by changing from a vaccine which is effective and . . . relatively safe?"

In this context, scientists are struggling with the ethical question of how to run a controlled experiment using the purified acellular vaccine, which will necessarily pass more stringent safety tests, while continuing to administer the cruder, more toxic whole-cell vaccine to the rest of the population. John Cameron warned scientists at the 1982 FDA Symposium:

"As far as the whole cell vaccine is concerned, the only standard it has to meet is efficacy in the mouse protection test and passing the mouse weight gain test. That is all. Nobody is talking about LPF content; nobody is talking about LPF activity, or anything like that, although we are talking about this in relation to the purified antigen . . . if this data is put before an ethical committee, how will they respond? I don't think they would be necessarily as sympathetic as this audience."

John Robbins answered simply, "Well, I would like to give a personal opinion, I think it is unethical not to try the new vaccine."

Another Symposium participant agreed: "We have a product that has established its usefulness, but it would be, I think, as was said earlier, quite unethical to ignore the scientific advances that make it possible to refine that product. . . ."

A U.S. Test of Acellular Vaccine?

American health authorities appear to believe that Japan bypassed many of the preliminary tests before licensing the acellular vaccine for public use. Manclark stated in a 1983 interview, "The Japanese have started giving an acellular vaccine to their people without doing all the necessary previous testing which we would have to do. . . . We are, of course, very happy that they did it."

Unless this country decides to rely upon Japan's experience with the acellular vaccine as proof of safety and efficacy in order to license it in the United States, some kind of controlled clinical trial will have to be held. Most health officials do not believe that this can be done in the United States.

Even though there are thought to be about 30,000 to 40,000 cases of whooping cough in the United States annually instead of the 1,000 to 3,000 cases actually reported, this is still not a large enough group for a meaningful test of vaccine efficacy. A group of two million American babies would be required and there would probably be no more than one thousand cases of whooping cough in the group.

In a Third World country like Kenya, however, the same statistical outcome could be achieved with a sample size of only 360. In Brazil, where the incidence of whooping cough is 10 percent of what it is in Kenya, a sample of 10,000 would suffice.

But testing in these countries runs up against many scientific obstacles. According to Manclark, in a country like Bangladesh, where there is a lot of whooping cough, many infants have already been exposed and have acquired pertussis antibodies. Even a weak trial vaccine will act powerfully on them because they are already partially immune. But that same vaccine might not have the same effect on a population of unexposed American children.

Politically, this kind of vaccine testing also has its risks, making American scientists vulnerable to charges of exploiting underprivileged Third World populations. Yet under the best of circumstances, it is hard to perform research on American babies.

Daniel Levitt, M.D., of the Guthrie Research Institute, stated in an interview, "It is hard to do studies on the immune system of an infant because you can't get the infant population on which to do the study. How am I going to get a group of normal two-month-olds—what parents are going to sign contracts to let me take 10 or 20 cc. of blood —maybe two thirds of an ounce—and repeat it at intervals? What parent is going to allow you to do that?"

American researchers have sometimes solved that problem by running clinical studies on the whole-cell vaccine in the minority inner-city populations of America's larger metropolitan areas.

Parke-Davis's Quadrigen trials in the 1960s were performed among a primarily black inner-city Detroit infant population. This type of trial is still being run today. In 1979, 91 healthy full-term newborn infants in the Harbor/UCLA Medical Center Nursery were enrolled in a pertussis vaccine study, of which 62 percent were Spanish-surnamed, 23 percent were white, 10 percent were black and 5 percent were Asian. Forty-five of these infants were injected with a full dose of pertussis vaccine and given oral polio vaccine at discharge from the newborn nursery. The mean age of the babies at the time of inoculation was 3.5 days.

In a letter to Edward Ornitz, M.D., chairman of the Human Subject Protection Committee (HSPC) at UCLA Medical Center, Kevin Geraghty, M.D., pointed out that two infants mentioned in the UCLA-FDA study "Final Report" appear to have received their first DPT shot at Harbor/UCLA Medical Center while newborns. The first infant is described as follows: "This two month old black female received her second DPT at the Harbor General Hospital on 18 October, 1979. On 22 October, 1979, the child was found dead in bed by her father." Another child, who was part of the non-prospective portion of the UCLA-FDA study, also appears to have been injected with DPT vaccine while a newborn. The record states: "This two month old white male received his second DPT in his left buttock at 1115 hours on 17 October, 1978. The first DPT was given at three days of age with no reaction."

Geraghty asked, "In general, we wish to know if these children were *not* enrolled in a research project at UCLA or its affiliated hospitals, why were they given DPT shortly after birth and while in the newborn nurseries? We would appreciate copies of English and Spanish consents for what appears to us to be a most extraordinarily unorthodox practice." He also asked why these two deaths were not reported in the published version of the UCLA-FDA study.

Ornitz replied, "the issues you raise are not within the purview of the HSPC, but seem to concentrate on the interpretation of scientific findings." He did not answer Geraghty's specific question about the routine vaccination of newborns with DPT at Harbor/UCLA Medical Center.

Joseph W. St. Geme, M.D., was a principal author of the study published in 1984 in *Pediatrics* under the title "Immunologic Response to Early and Routine DTP Immunization in Infants." He wrote to Geraghty in September 1983, "We have discontinued the routine DPT-OPV immunizations of newborn infants in our hospital because of the concern about immunological tolerance to pertussis antigens."

If vaccinating babies within a few days of their birth appears to be "extraordinarily unorthodox," so does the practice of injecting children with seven different vaccines at once. A 1980–81 FDA internal Project Report details a government project entitled "A study of the simultaneous administration of Measles, Mumps, and Rubella vaccine: Diphtheria and Tetanus Toxoids and Pertussis Vaccine and Oral Polio Vaccine."

The setting for the study, which appears to be a joint effort between the FDA and CDC, is inner-city Baltimore. The Project Report states its objectives: "In spite of the effectiveness of the vaccines, certain children remain unprotected or inadequately protected against the immunizable diseases because of failure to deliver the vaccine at the appropriate time. Present pediatric practice calls for five physician visits between the ages of 6 and 18 months. A major reason for the last two visits, which occur at 15 and 18 months, is the administration of MMR and DTP plus OPV, respectively. Administration of these vaccines at one time could eliminate the need for one of the visits. Furthermore, the knowledge that these vaccines can be given simultaneously would allow physicians the opportunity to make up deficiencies in immunization status noted during a visit."

The Project Report goes on to justify the study: "Firsthand knowledge of the practice of combining MMR, DTP, and OPV is important to the Bureau's mission to assure that these biologics are both safe and effective when used in the clinic."

Even though both of these studies obtained parental permission for the children involved, it is questionable whether the parents fully understood the magnitude of the risk their children were running. This is especially true for those parents whose native language is not English and whose education would not permit them to be fully cognizant of the ramifications of injecting their newborns with pertussis vaccine or injecting their toddler with seven bacterial and viral vaccines all at once.

What Is the United States Doing?

What progress has been made since the 1982 FDA Symposium when Japanese scientists announced their success with the development and use of acellular vaccine?

Wyeth Laboratories was very interested in this new vaccine. Bierly stated in an interview: "The Japanese vaccine is a much better defined product. The Japanese extraction process is much better, and you have a good idea of what is coming out."

The company began negotiations with Takeda, Ltd., of Japan to manufacture the vaccine and run clinical trials. Initially Takeda was unwilling to grant a license out of concern over liability issues, but it subsequently permitted Wyeth to undertake the trials. In a October 20, 1983, letter to Senator Paula Hawkins, Richard Bogash, Ph.D., president of Wyeth, said, "The initial studies will be in small groups of about thirty healthy children between the ages of four and seven to be followed sequentially by 18-month old children, and then 6, 4 and 2-month old infants. . . . At the conclusion of these studies, which will probably take about eighteen months, we will have tried the vaccine on a population of several hundred children and should have obtained valuable data on immunogenicity and local and systemic adverse effects commensurate with the study population."

After Wyeth's sudden withdrawal from the pertussis vaccine market in June 1984, the fate of their acellular vaccine clinical trials is unclear.

In February 1984, the National Institute of Allergy and Infectious Disease (NIAID) awarded a three-year, $486,674 grant to the Michigan Public Health Department to produce an improved pertussis vaccine. Dr. David Klein, of NIH, was quoted in the *Washington Post* as saying, "We want to eliminate 95 percent of the garbage that has nothing to do with protection but does contribute to adverse reactions."

Shortly after the grant was announced, Dr. John Mitchell, chief of the Biological Products Program of the Michigan Department of Public Health, said in an interview, "We started research on a new acellular vaccine here in Michigan about two years ago. It is a manufacturing process that is different from the Japanese acellular vaccine. The Japanese vaccine is not very good. They really don't know what is in it."

Mitchell went on to say that the Michigan Public Health Department was chosen by NIAID for the grant because the department "has been producing whooping cough vaccine since the early 1940s." He added, "According to the contract, the single pertussis component should be available by the end of 1985. The NIAID estimates that clinical trials may take from five to seven years and would probably be conducted in the Third World since there is so little whooping cough in the United States."

An Alternative to Acellular Vaccine: Passive Immunization

One alternative to the acellular vaccine which the FDA is exploring is "passive immunization," i.e., vaccinating a pregnant woman so she passes her antibodies to the baby she is carrying. There has been research on passive immunization since at least 1938.

Manclark, who has been working on such a vaccine for some years, stated in a 1983 interview: "The real problem is the newborn child, who is very susceptible to pertussis. The existing vaccine doesn't do them any good, since they are not immunologically developed enough to benefit from it. The only way to reach them would be to immunize the mothers and have passive immunity conveyed from the mother to the infant in the uterus. We know that this is possible."

However, politically it may be difficult to convince American mothers to be injected with pertussis bacteria while they are carrying a baby.

Fears of possible neurological damage to mother and unborn child will no doubt surface with the suggestion of introducing this kind of vaccine.

An Oral Pertussis Vaccine

For unexplained reasons, one interesting line of research into development of a safer pertussis vaccine has been entirely ignored in the United States. This is the use of an oral vaccine which has been developed and applied in several European countries, especially Austria.

Professors Wilhelm Falk and K. Rosanelli of Graz University Clinic in Graz, Austria, administered an oral pertussis vaccine to 6,700 babies from early 1980 to the end of 1982 and closely monitored them to see if they developed reactions or pertussis.

Out of the 6,700 children vaccinated, nine developed pertussis, including three children more than one year old. In a control group of 1,200 unvaccinated infants, five acquired pertussis. Clearly the incidence of whooping cough is very low in Graz, even in the absence of vaccination, but the doctors are convinced of the efficacy of their vaccine. Their study indicates that without the oral vaccine, there would have been 28 cases of whooping cough among the 6,700 newborns. They wrote, in a communication to the authors, "We are convinced that oral vaccine is at least as good as the parenteral vaccine, and that protection can be achieved at a considerably earlier time, which we think is an important point."

The oral vaccine is a killed vaccine made of Phase I-B pertussis bacteria inactivated by heat. It is given in the form of drops, starting on the second day of life: 6 drops per day (0.5 ml) for four days. An antibody reaction can be measured serologically in these babies, but Falk and Rosanelli find an increase in levels of T-cells also, meaning that the vaccination may also induce cellular immunity to pertussis. This may indicate that the oral vaccine prevents the pertussis bacteria from getting an initial foothold on the mucous membranes. The oral vaccine can be administered to older children as well.

Just as important is the fact that the oral vaccine appears to be free of adverse reactions. All the babies in the study were seen in the University Clinic four to six weeks after vaccination, where mothers were questioned about side effects. They subsequently were enrolled in the pediatric clinic of the University Hospital, where pediatricians were alerted to the possible occurrence of any side effects, especially seizures and brain damage. Falk and Rosanelli wrote, "there was no seizure seen in any of the . . . newborns; all the babies were followed for at least one year."

The Vienna Serum Therapy Institute is presently producing the oral pertussis vaccine which is being given in several other hospitals in Austria. Falk and Rosanelli submitted an article on their oral vaccine to the *Journal of Pediatrics* but, said Falk, "We were told that it could not be recommended for publication because the children were not selected in random fashion and it was felt that the data were not clear enough to allow a conclusion about the effectiveness of the vaccine."

The Child's Vulnerability vs. Vaccine Quality

If the specific vulnerability of each child is found to be an inescapable ingredient in adverse reactions regardless of the nature of the pertussis vaccine or the tests used to measure it, a certain number of babies will always be damaged by it. Coinciding with the search for a safer vaccine, therefore, should be a priority program of identifying high risk children. To date the FDA has expressed little interest in this, as is evidenced by its lack of follow-up on the UCLA-FDA study's eighteen children who reacted neurologically to the vaccine (see Chapter 16).

The FDA's Petricciani expressed just this sentiment at an FDA public meeting in 1983: "The real question is, even though there may be a new test for neurotoxicity, how can one use that to extrapolate to the individuals receiving the vaccine, and is it possible to use that as a predictor for those individuals receiving the vaccine that might be at high risk? And those are two different things. There is no question but that we should be looking at newer ways to assess neurotoxicity, but just by virtue of doing that is no guarantee that in any individual case there won't be a severe reaction."

20

Benefits and Risks: Costs to Our Society

> All our knowledge brings us nearer to our ignorance.
> *T. S. Eliot*

Whenever anyone questions the wisdom of mandatory pertussis vaccination, the medical establishment immediately responds that the vaccine, whatever its defects, saves more lives and prevents more damage than it causes. E. A. Mortimer and P. K. Jones maintained this in 1978: "Even accepting the highest estimates of encephalopathy due to pertussis vaccine and the most modest estimates of benefits from the vaccine, there is clearly more benefit than risk from the vaccine on the basis [of] the experience of the United States."

In 1982, Harry Meyer of the FDA said the same: "I think if one were to back away and look at the question of pertussis vaccine from a distance today, after so much discussion, one would clearly say that the overwhelming consensus is that the whole cell pertussis vaccines are safe and effective biologics in the sense that the benefits of their use far exceed whatever risks there are."

Two official attempts have been made by the government to analyze the benefits and risks of the pertussis vaccine. Jeffrey Koplan and his colleagues at the Centers for Disease Control (CDC) and the Harvard Medical School tried to put a dollar value on a benefit/risk analysis of the pertussis vaccine. They published "Pertussis Vaccine—An Analysis of Benefits, Risks, and Costs," in 1979 in the *New England Journal of Medicine*. In June 1984, Alan Hinman, M.D., also of the CDC, and Koplan coauthored "Pertussis and Pertussis Vaccine: Reanalysis of

Benefits, Risks, and Costs," which was published in the *Journal of the American Medical Association.*

Both analyses came to the same conclusion: the benefits of pertussis vaccination far outweigh the risks.

The tone of confidence in these analyses suggests that the data used to reach this conclusion were comprehensive and reliable and were based upon accurate information on the incidence of death and permanent neurological damage from whooping cough as well as the incidence of death and permanent damage from the pertussis vaccine in the United States today.

In truth, nearly all of the data are incomplete and, where they do exist, are often inconsistent. This situation exists because the vaccine has been administered for decades without any particular effort being made to provide statistical justification for its use.

As it is, there is little reason to have confidence in official estimates of vaccine reactions, not only because the reaction reporting system is flawed and inadequate, but also because these estimates are used to justify an existing mass vaccination policy. Nor is there any reason for confidence in official estimates of the incidence of whooping cough, because the government itself admits that it is generally underreported (although it may be overreported when publicity about vaccine reactions is prevalent or disease surveillance is increased).

Thus, the following benefit/risk analysis involves as many unverifiable assumptions as those made by the CDC. It accepts some of the CDC's assumptions and rejects others. Both analyses necessarily suffer from the absence of reliable data on whooping cough and vaccine reactions in the United States.

Whooping Cough Today

Even the number of pertussis cases in the United States today is not known. From 1,000 to 3,000 cases are reported every year, but Alan Hinman, M.D., stated at a 1983 FDA "Open Meeting on Pertussis and Pertussis Vaccines" that "it is possible that the degree of underreporting in this country might be as great as only one-fifteenth to one-twentieth of the total cases occurring."

In any case, the Hinman-Koplan 1984 reanalysis concludes there are 34,048 cases of whooping cough in the United States every year.

Whooping Cough Complications Today

The CDC's William Foege testified at 1982 U.S. Senate hearings that "brain damage probably occurs in one of every 10,000 cases of pertussis. Death occurs in approximately one in every 1,000 cases, although the ratio of deaths to recorded numbers of cases reported varies in different countries."

This estimate is accepted by Hinman and Koplan, who also rely upon a study of 8,000 cases of whooping cough in the United Kingdom (1974–1975) to conclude that in the United States, there are forty-four deaths and three cases of permanent neurological damage from whooping cough each year. This estimate of neurological damage seems realistic, but the estimate of deaths seems exaggerated. These 1974–1975 British data yield a death rate of 1.29/1000 cases; however, British data from 1982 yield a death rate of only .22/1000 cases—one sixth of the Hinman-Koplan figure; and a 1981 British analysis by Robinson and coworkers concluded that the 1978 death rate was even lower—.18/1000 cases.

Based on these recent British death rates and allowing for a margin of error, the present analysis will assume a mortality rate in the United States today of .29/1000. When applied to the CDC estimated pertussis incidence of 34,048, this yields ten deaths per year from whooping cough, which is essentially the number reported to the CDC every year. (It stands to reason that any whooping cough death is more likely to be reported to the CDC than an otherwise uneventful case of the disease.)

Whooping Cough Incidence and Mortality Without Mass Vaccination

The 1979 CDC analysis concludes that, in the absence of a vaccination program, the incidence of whooping cough would be 71 times greater than it is today; the death rate would be 25 times greater; and the incidence of permanent injury would be 27 times greater. According to this formula, there would be 2,417,000 cases of whooping cough, 1,100 deaths, and 81 cases of permanent neurological damage were there no mass pertussis vaccination program in the United States today.

In 1984, the CDC revised these estimates downward. Koplan and Hinman predicted that there would be 356,566 cases· of whooping cough, 457 deaths, and 29 cases of permanent neurological damage if there were no mass pertussis vaccination program in this country today.

This means that the CDC assumes that, of the U.S. population of 236 million, 1 person in 662 would become sick with pertussis in the absence of a vaccination program.

This figure seems far too high since the incidence of whooping cough between 1922 and 1945 (when vaccination started to be used on a small scale) approached this high-water mark in only eight years (1926, 1927, 1929, 1932, 1934, 1937, 1938, and 1941). It is hardly credible that the annual incidence of whooping cough would increase to the worst levels of the pre-war decades in light of the vastly improved nutrition, sanitation, and medical care in the U.S. today.

The 1984 analysis is also unrealistic in assuming that vaccine coverage would decline to zero in the absence of a mandatory vaccination program. A more realistic assumption is based on the situation of England today, where about one third of the population accepts the vaccine even after widespread publicity about adverse reactions.

The future whooping cough incidence with about one-third vaccination coverage can be estimated by examining a period in American history when coverage was one third. No data are available to determine the year in which one-third coverage was reached, but probably no more than one third of the infant population was being vaccinated in the years 1945–1949, when the program was just beginning.

Between 1945 and 1949 (according to an FDA estimate) average whooping cough incidence was one person in 1,455. If applied to the present United States population of 236 million, this would mean an outbreak of 162,200 cases of whooping cough, considerably less than the CDC's 1984 estimate of 356,566 cases.

The Hinman-Koplan 1984 estimate of 457 deaths from pertussis also seems overestimated, being an extrapolation from the British 1974–1975 figures. Even if adjusted for the lowered estimate of whooping cough incidence (162,200 cases), i.e., 208 deaths, this figure would still be high, since it is based on data which do not conform with Britain's most recent experience.

Britain reported 14 deaths out of 65,000 cases of whooping cough in 1982, or 1 death in 4,642 cases. If 162,200 cases occurred in the U.S., there would be 35 deaths in the U.S. by this projection.

Because the future whooping cough mortality in the United States might be marginally higher than in England today, the figure of

.29/1000 discussed earlier will be applied, which yields a mortality of 47 deaths. For the CDC to maintain that the United States would have a mortality rate almost five times greater than Britain is to assume that there is a much lower standard of medical care and competence in the United States than in Britain.

And if the Hinman-Koplan estimate of permanent neurological damage from whooping cough is reduced in proportion to a reduced estimate of disease incidence, the resulting figure is 13 cases of permanent neurological damage per year.

Incidence of Complications from the Pertussis Vaccine

The pertussis vaccine causes acute neurological reactions, of which a certain proportion will result in long-term damage. Precisely what proportion of these acute reactions lead to long-term damage should be known with some precision in order to perform a benefit/risk analysis of the vaccine.

Medicine generally accepts the premise that for every three cases of whooping cough encephalitis, one case will result in long-term damage. This 3:1 ratio was accepted by the 1979 CDC analysis as well as the 1984 reanalysis. Until the National Childhood Encephalopathy Study (NCES) was published in 1981, it was not known if this same ratio held for severe neurological complications of pertussis vaccination.

The NCES was a study of all cases of acute neurological illnesses in British children from two to thirty-six months of age who were admitted to hospitals between 1976 and 1979. A proportion of these infants had been vaccinated shortly before the neurological illnesses occurred. When their vaccination histories were examined, it was concluded that 1 in 110,000 vaccinations caused an acute neurological reaction while 1 in 310,000 vaccinations caused permanent neurological damage. Therefore, acute and long-term reactions of the vaccine were found to be in the same 3:1 ratio as acute and long-term complications of whooping cough itself.

However, the NCES had a very narrow definition of an acute neurological reaction. For example, it excluded those infants who suffered a convulsion lasting less than thirty minutes or were not hospitalized. In a letter to the *British Medical Journal* in 1981, Ehrengut vigorously criticized the NCES for this exclusion.

"The NCES excludes cases with convulsions lasting less than 30 minutes. This exclusion is unjustifiable, as we can show from the records of cases receiving compensation from the West German Health Authority for 100% disability occurring after pertussis vaccination. Out of 35 cases receiving awards for this reason, there are six which had encephalopathy without convulsions. The other 29 cases all had convulsions but in 22 these were of less than 30 minutes' duration. . . . the majority of children with severe brain damage have been missed by incorrect elimination of those who had fits lasting less than 30 minutes. From my personal experience of 25 years as a medical referee, I can say, in addition, that 20% of convulsions following various vaccinations are missed because patients are not admitted to hospitals."

There are other reasons why the incidence of vaccine reactions found in the NCES cannot be mechanically applied to American conditions. Britain uses a different vaccine manufactured to a different opacity standard (see Chapter 16) which may be causing fewer reactions; British physicians have a list of contraindications which excludes categories of high-risk children not excluded in the United States; and finally, British physicians typically vaccinate babies beginning at six months of age, not at six weeks to two months of age as in the United States. All these factors mean that the incidence of vaccine reactions in Britain is probably lower than in the United States.

It is inappropriate, therefore, to base a calculation of the incidence of complications due to the vaccine in the United States on figures from the NCES. Nevertheless, there seems to be no reason to reject the 3:1 ratio between neurological reactions and long-term damage, as revealed by the NCES data.

The principal source of information on pertussis vaccine reactions in the U.S. is the UCLA-FDA study discussed in Chapter 14, which found that there were 9 cases of convulsions, 9 cases of collapse, and either 17 or 22 cases of high-pitched screaming (encephalitic crying) within forty-eight hours of a DPT shot. The Chapter 14 discussion concluded that 7,000 infants were enrolled in the UCLA-FDA Study. With this information, it can be estimated that 1 in 778 children have convulsions; 1 in 778 have collapse; and 1 in 318 (22 in 7,000) have high-pitched screaming within forty-eight hours of a DPT shot.

If this incidence of vaccine reactions is extrapolated to the total U.S. infant population undergoing vaccination every year, i.e., 3.3 million, it yields the following totals: 4,248 children with convulsions; 4,248 with collapse; and 10,377 with high-pitched screaming within forty-eight hours of a DPT shot.

This means (again on the assumption that 7,000 infants participated in the UCLA-FDA study) that 18,873 American infants suffer these acute neurological reactions within forty-eight hours of a DPT shot every year.

Somewhat surprisingly, the 1984 Hinman-Koplan reanalysis came up with a much higher figure, also based on the UCLA-FDA study. Since each American child must receive five shots, these authors apparently assumed that, for purposes of statistical extrapolation, the number of children in the UCLA study must be taken as equivalent to one fifth of the 15,752 shots administered, i.e., 3,114. This would lead to their conclusion that, of the 3.3 million children vaccinated every year in the U.S., 8,484 have convulsions, 8,484 undergo collapse, and 16,038 have high-pitched screaming, for an annual total of 33,006 cases of acute neurological reactions occurring within forty-eight hours of a DPT shot.

Assistant Secretary of Health Edward Brandt, Jr., M.D., testifying on May 3, 1984, before the U.S. Senate Committee on Labor and Human Resources, rounded these figures off to 9,000 cases of convulsions, 9,000 cases of collapse, and 17,000 cases of high-pitched screaming for a total of 35,000 acute neurological reactions occurring within forty-eight hours of a DPT shot among America's children every year.

The higher estimate given by the Hinman-Koplan reanalysis, as rounded off by Brandt, seems more accurate because the UCLA-FDA study arbitrarily used a forty-eight-hour cut-off period for reactions. Yet acute neurological reactions may occur days and even weeks after a DPT shot. The NCES study found that there is a statistically significant relationship between the DPT shot and neurological events occurring up to seven days later. Therefore, the UCLA-FDA study may have missed an unknown number of acute neurological reactions which should have been added to its reaction incidence data.

But the most significant question that must be answered is how many of these 35,000 cases of acute neurological reactions result in long-term damage? Here the Hinman-Koplan 1984 reanalysis ignored the UCLA-FDA figures entirely, and for its estimate of long-term damage accepted the more favorable NCES figure of 1 in 310,000 shots, which yields 51 cases of long-term damage.

This is an incorrect procedure, as discussed above, because of the different vaccines and conditions in Britain as compared to the United States. There is no reason to assume that the overall incidence of vaccine reactions would be the same in the two countries.

However, the 3:1 ratio between acute neurological complications and long-term damage historically accepted by medical science and reinforced by the NCES experience can reasonably be accepted. If that ratio is applied to HEW Secretary Brandt's estimate of 35,000 acute neurological reactions per year, 11,666 children may be expected to manifest long-term damage every year as a result of DPT vaccination.

Not all of these long-term consequences will be uncontrollable seizure disorders or severe mental retardation. There will be a spectrum of residual defects ranging from severe damage to learning disabilities, hyperactivity, behavioral problems, and chronic systemic illness.

The Hinman-Koplan reanalysis does not address the possibility that the vaccine can cause death. In Chapter 14, there is a discussion of the two infants in the UCLA-FDA study who died within four days of being vaccinated with DPT. Again assuming that there were 7,000 infants in the study and that both of these SIDS-labeled deaths were actually related to DPT shots, the conclusion would be that 1 infant in 3,500, or 943 out of 3.3 million in the United States, die from the vaccine every year. (Taking Hinman and Koplan's apparent assumption that there were 3,114 children in the study, 1 infant in 1,557 may be expected to die from the vaccine or, at the national level, 2,119 infants every year.)

Since more than 7,000 infants die of what is diagnosed as SIDS every year, it could be concluded that as many as 13 percent are actually due to the DPT shot but are misdiagnosed as SIDS.

This conclusion is supported by an independent study conducted by Baraff and others and published in 1983 in the *Journal of Infectious Diseases*. The authors investigated all 382 cases of SIDS reported by the Los Angeles County Coroner's Office from January 1, 1979, to August 23, 1980. They were able to contact the families of 145 of these infants and found that 53 of the babies had recently received the DPT shot.

When they plotted the time of death of these 53 infants in relation to the date of immunization, they found a significant clustering within one day and one week of immunization. Specifically, 17 had been immunized within one week of death and, of these, 6 within 24 hours of death. They reported, "This distribution is skewed toward the time of immunization, with significantly more than the expected number of deaths occurring within one day and one week of vaccination, suggesting a temporal association between DPT and SIDS."

Therefore, the authors found that 17 out of 145 cases of SIDS or 12 percent of the SIDS cases investigated in Los Angeles County were associated with the DPT shot. This is close to the 13-percent figure yielded by the two SIDS cases in the UCLA-FDA study and is added reason for further investigation into this issue.

It is also worthwhile mentioning Geraghty's investigation of SIDS deaths in Contra Costa County, California, discussed in Chapter 9. He found that three out of the ten deaths recorded during the first six months of 1983 had the typical clinical histories of infants who reacted to the vaccine and then died some days later. All three died within four days of the first DPT shot, two within twenty-four hours of the shot. All three manifested one or more neurological symptoms such as excessive somnolence, unresponsiveness, or high-pitched screaming after the DPT shot. All were classified as SIDS.

If random selection of a single American county could find 30 percent of the SIDS deaths reported there in a six-month period to be related to the DPT shot, it is probable that many more cases exist throughout the country and could be identified.

Therefore, the annual toll from the pertussis vaccine might be as high as 943 deaths and 11,666 cases of long-term damage.

Vaccine Damage in Perspective

The general perception is that whooping cough causes large numbers of deaths and injuries while the pertussis vaccine is nearly risk-free. Thus, at first glance, these higher estimates of vaccine-induced death and damage seem inconceivable. When looked at in perspective, however, they are quite realistic.

About 7,000 apparently healthy infants die in the United States every year from unexplained causes. It is not an exaggeration to hypothesize that 13 percent of them are dying from the neurotoxic effects of the pertussis vaccine administered beginning at the age of six to eight weeks. The actual figure may be higher.

The long-term damage estimate here must be viewed with the understanding that it includes a variety of conditions ranging from minimal brain dysfunction and hyperactivity to uncontrollable seizure disorders and mental retardation. Every year in America, 126,000 infants are diagnosed as mentally retarded "from birth," with 60,000 to 90,000 of them considered to be "severely and profoundly retarded." That 5 or 6 percent of these infants, or perhaps a larger proportion, could be mentally retarded due to the effects of the pertussis vaccine is by no means improbable and merits investigation.

Every year 20,000 infants are diagnosed as having epilepsy or some other seizure disorder "from birth." That a proportion of these could be victims of the pertussis vaccine is also not improbable. Few of the infants, after all, are actually diagnosed at birth. They are diagnosed as "epileptic" or "severely and profoundly retarded" when they are six, eight, or twelve months old or older (see the case of Sherry in Chapter 4). By that time, the great majority have received one, two, or three DPT shots.

Between 15 and 20 percent of American schoolchildren are considered to be learning-disabled with minimal brain dysfunction. That several thousand of the 35,000 children who react neurologically to the DPT shot each year could be manifesting long-term effects of the vaccine in the form of hyperactivity, dyslexia, auditory processing deficit, or other types of learning disabilities, is well within the limits of rational belief.

Furthermore, it is probable that a portion of the children who react to the pertussis vaccine every year may recover without apparent neurological damage, but may continue to be chronically ill with severe allergies, continuous bouts of upper respiratory tract infection, and otitis media, which impose additional financial burdens upon parents and society.

The Human Cost to Society of Mass Pertussis Vaccination

The human cost of a mass pertussis vaccination program in the United States may be determined by comparing the death and disability from both the disease and the vaccine, at the present 95-percent vaccination coverage, with estimates of death and disability if vaccination became voluntary and coverage dropped to about one third.

	At 95% coverage	At 33⅓% coverage
Whooping cough morbidity	34,048	162,000
Mortality	10	47
Long-term damage	3	13
Vaccination morbidity (acute)	35,000	11,666
Mortality	943	314
Long-term damage	11,666	3,888

According to these figures, if the pertussis vaccination program were made voluntary and coverage declined to one third of all infants, the incidence of whooping cough would rise almost five times to 162,200 cases, but there would be a far lower combined incidence of morbidity and mortality from the disease and the vaccine. Morbidity, mortality, and long-term damage from the vaccine would drop to one third of their present levels, which would more than offset the morbidity, mortality, and long-term damage from the increased incidence of the disease.

Total mortality at 95-percent coverage would be 10 deaths from the disease and 943 from the vaccine for a total of 953. Total long-term damage would be 3 from the disease and 11,666 from the vaccine for a total of 11,669.

At 33⅓-percent vaccination coverage, these figures would drop to 47 deaths from the disease and 314 from the vaccine, for a total of 361 deaths. Long-term damage would fall to 13 from the disease and 3,888 from the vaccine for a total of 3,901.

The difference between the two sets of figures is 592 deaths (953 less 361) and 7,768 cases of permanent neurological damage each year (11,669 less 3,901). These 592 deaths and 7,768 cases of permanent neurological damage are the cost to society in human life and suffering of the mass pertussis vaccination program.

If these projections are correct, total elimination of the current whole-cell pertussis vaccine program would increase the incidence of death and disability from the disease, but that from the vaccine would disappear. This would make the disparity between the cost of vaccinating and of not vaccinating even greater.

The Dollar Cost to Society of the Pertussis Vaccine

This analysis indicates that universal vaccination produces 592 more deaths and 7,768 more cases of long-term damage than would one-third coverage. Melissa Patterson, of Albuquerque, New Mexico, an expert on the economic aspects of liability, has provided figures with which to estimate the financial cost to society of these 592 deaths and 7,768 cases of long-term damage.

According to Patterson, it is assumed that an infant who dies would otherwise have lived to the age of seventy. The value of the infant's life is estimated as the sum of money that would have to be invested today at the prevailing rate of interest to yield the value of the infant's wages during his or her working life. This amount of money is called the "present value" of that life, and the assumption is that it would be invested at ten percent. The amount of such an award today is just under $150,000.

Under these assumptions, the dollar cost of 592 additional infant deaths each year would be $88,800,000.

The "present value" is much higher for an infant who does not die but is severely damaged and requires institutional care. According to Patterson, the courts customarily evaluate such awards in two parts: (1) the "present value" of the sum needed to maintain the child to age 18; and (2) the "present value" of the sum which would have to be invested today to maintain the child from the age of eighteen to the end of his life, with estimated life expectancy still being seventy years.

Before the age of eighteen there are two possibilities: (1) that the infant will be cared for at home; and (2) that the infant will be maintained in an institution.

Beyond the age of eighteen there are four possibilities: (1) the adult can live alone in society and fend for himself, even if unemployable; (2) he can live in a group home for the handicapped, with little or no supervision; (3) he can live in a public nursing home or hospital; and (4) he can live in a private nursing home or have private nursing care.

The breakdown of costs is as follows:

1. Up to age eighteen, cared for at home: present value is $35,316; cared for in an institution: $445,550.

2. Age eighteen to seventy, living alone: present value is $45,900; living in a home for the handicapped: $75,822; living in a publicly

supported nursing home: $699,990; living in a private nursing home or having private nursing care: $1,796,475.

While these figures seem extremely high, they are the ones which are frequently used as the basis for vaccine-damage awards or settlements in litigation today. Therefore, the present value of a vaccine-damaged child who is incapable of holding a job can be computed from the various combinations of the preceding figures. For example:

At home to age 18 and then in a home for the handicapped:
$35,316 + $75,822 = $111,138
At home to age 18 and then in private nursing home or with private nursing care:
$35,316 + $1,796,475 = $1,831,791
In an institution to age 18 and then in a private nursing home or with private nursing care:
$445,550 + $1,796,475 = $2,242,025

Since it is not known today what proportion of the permanently damaged children suffer more severe disabilities and what proportion suffer less severe ones, it is impossible to calculate the total financial cost to America with any accuracy. But depending upon the way in which children are allocated to the various categories, the cost can be estimated at from $1 billion to $3 billion per year.

Added to this is the cost of special education programs in the public school systems for vaccine-damaged children whose range of handicap extends from severe and profound retardation to learning disabilities.

The Sixth Annual Report to Congress on the Implementation of P.L. 94-142 (The Education for All Handicapped Children Act) stated that during 1982–83 more than four million handicapped children were served under that Act. In 1983, the total federal tax allocation to fund state public schools charged with providing special education for these handicapped children totaled more than $931 million.

Out of the four million children served under P.L. 94-142, more than 70 percent or some 2,844,000 children were learning-disabled or speech-impaired. How many of these children can trace their problems back to the pertussis vaccine? According to data provided by one public school system in Maryland, the cost of educating a learning-disabled child is about twice the cost of educating a normal child through high school.

At the kindergarten level, it costs the county $6,000 per year to educate the learning-disabled child against $2,189 for a normal one. Much of this cost is due to a lower child-to-teacher ratio in learning disabled classes (10:1) versus the child-to-teacher ratio (27:1) in the average classroom. From grades one to six, the difference is between $6,000 and $3,438; in junior high it is between $6,000 and $3,660; in high school it is between $6,000 and $3,486.

Moderately or severely handicapped children cost the county $7,360 per year to educate from kindergarten through high school. Part of this cost is for special transportation of severely and profoundly handicapped children to and from school as well as to maintain a seven-to-one ratio of children per teacher.

Balanced against the above costs of vaccine damage is the cost of the estimated additional 128,200 cases of whooping cough (162,200 less the 34,000 assumed occurring under the current vaccination program).

In the United States about 60 percent of whooping cough cases are hospitalized and the average stay reported, for instance, during the Maryland 1982 "epidemic" was just over eight days. The cost of such a hospital stay could be as high as $4,000 or more when intensive care units and extra nursing are included. Assuming that 60 percent of the above 128,200 cases are hospitalized for an average cost of $5,000 per case, the total amount expended would be only $385 millon. This hardly compares with the estimated dollar (and human) costs of the mass vaccination program.

Moreover, there is probably no need for such a high level of hospitalization. This 60 percent figure more than likely reflects the preference of American physicans for treating patients in the hospital rather than making house calls. In England, only ten percent of whooping cough cases have been hospitalized in recent years, while in West Germany the figure is 3.1 percent.

Regardless of the hospitalization costs, few parents would not be willing to shoulder this expense rather than expose their child to measurable risk of mental retardation or epilepsy. Calculating the cost of the mass-vaccination program in dollars alone misses the point that this is a human equation.

Summary

To summarize these projections, if pertussis vaccination coverage were to decline to one third of all children in the United States instead of the present 95-percent coverage, then the number of whooping cough cases would rise from the present 34,000 cases to 162,200 cases. But there would be 592 fewer deaths and 7,768 fewer cases of long-term damage each year from both whooping cough and vaccination.

The cost of the vaccination program is calculated by comparing the cost of an additional 128,200 cases of whooping cough (162,200 less 34,000) with the cost of the excess of 592 deaths and 7,768 cases of long-term damage. While the hospitalization of 60 percent of these 128,200 cases would amount to $385 million, the cost of the deaths from vaccine and the vaccine-damaged children whose lifelong care must be borne by parents and society can be estimated at between $1 billion and $3 billion.

If the mass pertussis vaccination program were eliminated entirely, the incidence of death and long-term damage from the disease would rise somewhat, while that from the vaccine would disappear. Since this analysis concludes that the contribution to death and disability from the vaccine is greater than from the disease, the resulting disparity between vaccinating and not vaccinating is magnified.

The cost of vaccine-damaged children is being paid today, not directly but indirectly: these as yet unrecognized children and adults fill an unknown portion of the 273,000 beds in American psychiatric hospitals, 416,757 beds in nursing homes, and 46,264 beds in long-term residential care facilities.

Additional thousands of severely damaged children are being cared for at home by their parents. Thousands more are not profoundly brain damaged but have learning disabilities, behavioral disorders, severe allergies, and chronic illnesses. Who is to say what proportion of these millions are part of the pertussis vaccine harvest? No one yet knows the answer.

Thus, this benefit/risk analysis has explored not only the possibility but also the probability that pertussis vaccine damage in the United States is far greater than is accepted by the official estimates upon which the CDC's benefit/risk analysis are based. Like all other benefit/risk analyses of the pertussis vaccine, it is hampered by the shortage of reliable data on the incidence of whooping cough and of reactions to the pertussis vaccine. The truth may lie somewhere between the unrealistically low official figures and the high figures yielded by this chapter's analysis. It is also possible that the true figures are even more devastating.

21

What Parents Can Do

Enough, if something from our hands have power
To live, and act, and serve the future hour.
William Wordsworth

Shortly after "DPT: Vaccine Roulette" first was shown in Washington, D.C., in April 1982, a group of parents in the area banded together, as mentioned in previous chapters, and formed the national organization known as Dissatisfied Parents Together (DPT). This nonprofit, educational, and charitable foundation has distributed information on the pertussis vaccine to more than five thousand parents across the nation and has collected data on many hundreds of cases of vaccine damage.

DPT's major goals are to educate parents, doctors, and community leaders about the pertussis vaccine and to encourage both government agencies and physicians to conduct research that will identify high-risk children and develop a safer vaccine. The group also assists parents by providing information about legal and medical professionals who are knowledgeable about the pertussis vaccine.

DPT provided information to legislators in Maryland for the bill that was signed into law by Governor Harry Hughes in 1984 requiring doctors to report vaccine reactions; provide parents with written information about vaccine reactions; record vaccine reactions in the child's permanent medical record; and record the name of the vaccine manufacturer, batch and lot number in a permanent record. The group also participated in discussions with the American Academy of Pediatrics, out of which came recommendations that served as the basis for the National Childhood Vaccine-Injury Compensation Act. The bill, which provides financial support for vaccine-damaged children and embodies information, reporting, and recordkeeping requirements contained in the Maryland bill, was introduced by Senators Paula Hawkins (R-Florida) and Orrin Hatch (R-Utah) into Congress on November 17, 1983. It was introduced into the House by Congressman Henry Waxman (D-Calif.) and others on June 7, 1984.

Japan, England, Switzerland, West Germany, France, and Denmark have compensation programs to provide financial assistance to persons who are injured by vaccines even though none of these countries legally requires pertussis vaccination. California, which allows parents a philosophical objection to vaccination, also has a compensation system for vaccine-damaged children, but it is limited to paying out a maximum of $25,000. England's compensation system pays about the same amount to vaccine-injured children and, of the approximately 2,800 claims that have been submitted by parents, only about one quarter or 700 have been accepted by doctors sitting on the compensation review board and paid by the government.

The National Childhood Vaccine-Injury Compensation Act gives the parents of vaccine-damaged children an alternative to suing the doctor and/or drug manufacturer. The bill, however, protects parents' right to sue the doctor and drug company for a child's vaccine injuries. It gives parents a choice: they may sue or ask for compensation under the Act. They cannot do both; and should parents asking for compensation for their injured child be turned down by the compensation system, they are barred from going to court. Similarly, if the parents lose their case in court, they cannot seek compensation under the federal system.

The Act proposes a no-fault system, which would be financed by a surcharge on childhood vaccines. It would be open to parents with a child who has been seriously injured by DPT, MMR, polio, or other childhood vaccines, regardless of how long ago the injury occurred. The bill also requires private doctors and public health clinics to provide written information to parents on vaccine risks and contraindications before any vaccine is given.

In addition, the bill requires doctors and clinics to keep records of the manufacturer and lot number of all vaccines given, to record serious reactions on patients' charts, and to report serious reactions to the CDC. The bill defines reactions and specifies time periods within which a reaction must occur for a child's injury to be compensated through the system. Furthermore, the reaction must have resulted in significant and permanent damage for compensation to be granted.

The proposed bill has been both praised and criticized. Those who praise it stress the need for financial support for children who have been mentally and physically injured by vaccines, particularly in cases where the parents do not have the funds or emotional stability to withstand years of litigation. They point out that the bill not only gives financial support to these children but also will help prevent further damage by requiring doctors to report reactions and enter them in patients' medical records.

Other parents fear that the bill will only give more power to states to enforce existing mandatory vaccination laws under the justification that parents will now be financially reimbursed for injuries sustained by their children. These parents maintain that no amount of money can justify forcing parents to risk brain damaging their children with an unsafe vaccine.

Critics of the bill do not like the idea of a compensation act that will be financed by federal funds and will remove even partial liability from doctors and/or drug manufacturers. They also fear that the bill may be amended in the future to make it an exclusive remedy and prevent parents from suing doctors or manufacturers, thereby eliminating the liability of those doctors who administer vaccines despite contraindications, as well as those drug manufacturers who produce vaccines that may be unsafe without adequate testing or warnings to doctors and parents about risks and contraindications.

Compensation for Vaccine Damage

It appears that the fear of an "exclusive remedy" compensation bill is well founded. At May 3, 1984, hearings before the Senate Labor and Human Resources Committee called by Senator Hawkins, vaccine manufacturers joined with the American Medical Association in urging that the Hawkins-Hatch bill be modified to eliminate the right to sue doctors or manufacturers. Representatives from DPT vaccine manufacturers Wyeth, Connaught, and Lederle declined to testify in person at the hearing. However, Richard Bogash, Ph.D., president of Wyeth, pointed out in written testimony that drug companies are particularly concerned about protecting themselves from liability because they want to introduce new vaccines on the market and are afraid of lawsuits involving these future vaccines:

"To preserve the immunization system and to extend it to other disease states, a singular legislative remedy is now required, one which covers all participants—including manufacturers, distributors, and the people responsible for the administration of the vaccine. . . . We feel very strongly that the legislative remedy finally chosen must cover all participants of what is now a very effective immunization chain. Otherwise this chain could be broken at any point from the development of new vaccine through the continuing availability of current vaccines, to the very point of advice, counsel and administration of vaccine. For these reasons we submit that to be effective any Federal compensation program for vaccine injury must be an exclusive, mandatory remedy."

John E. Lyons, president of Merck Sharp & Dohme, the sole provider of MMR (measles, mumps and rubella) vaccine in the United States, justified the need for an exclusive remedy compensation system: "Although most vaccines are extraordinarily safe, they can be associated with adverse reactions in a small percentage of the people who use them. Most of these reactions are minor and self-limiting. But some very rare reactions can be harmful, even fatal. Seldom, if ever, is anyone at fault when these unfortunate incidents occur."

Lyons went on to assert that "A workable compensation system should serve three objectives beyond its primary purpose of helping the victims of adverse reactions: first, it should increase the willingness of the public to participate in immunization programs; second, it should help assure the continued willingness of physicians and other health care professionals to conduct immunization programs; and third, it should encourage manufacturers to provide vaccine not only for existing programs, but also to devote substantial resources to the discovery and development of new vaccines."

Alan Nelson, M.D., of the American Medical Association, testified in agreement with the vaccine manufacturers and expressed support for the mandatory state vaccination laws: "The AMA encourages and supports state mandated childhood vaccination requirements and continued research into the development of new and improved vaccines. . . . States mandate such immunization because of the epidemiologic fact of 'herd immunity,' i.e., all of society benefits from vaccination against communicable diseases—not just the vaccine recipient.

"The problem confronted in the context of vaccine administration is that an injury may result even where no one has committed a negligent act. . . . we advocate solutions that will continue to encourage parents to have their children immunized. . . . [The AMA] supports state or federal legislation that will hold physicians and manufacturers harmless for any vaccine-related injury not caused by physician or manufacturer negligence."

Perhaps one of the biggest dangers of an "exclusive remedy" federal compensation system is that children whose reactions did not occur within the time periods, or whose type of damage is not specified in the guidelines used to award compensation, would be left to cope throughout their lives without any hope of financial support.

For example, if the guidelines consider only those children whose convulsions occurred within twenty-four hours of a shot, then all other children suffering convulsions would be excluded. If the guidelines do not recognize a particular health problem such as infantile spasms as a vaccine-related injury, then no children who reacted with infantile spasms and are now brain damaged will ever receive financial support either through the federal compensation system or the courts.

When Dissatisfied Parents Together (DPT) and the American Academy of Pediatrics (AAP) were formulating recommendations for the Hawkins-Hatch bill, they finally agreed upon a vaccine-injury compensation table defining time periods and types of damage to be compensated, even though DPT wanted broader guidelines and the AAP wanted narrower guidelines. This table has been criticized by the AMA and vaccine manufacturers, who want to have more control over the guidelines used to decide which children are to be compensated under the federal system.

The report of the AMA's Ad Hoc Commission on Vaccine Injury Compensation stated, "The Commission recommends that the compensable events not be defined in the legislation, but be defined wholly by expert advisors."

The Michigan Department of Health also disliked the vaccine injury table devised by the AAP and DPT and stated they wanted to "provide input on the determination of recognized reactions and the time period within which the reactions are to occur for compensation to be provided to a petitioner."

The question here is who should decide which vaccine-damaged children will receive compensation—doctors, scientists, vaccine manufacturers, lawyers, legislators, or parents? It is apparent that some have an interest in defining vaccine damage in the narrowest terms so that its scope appears minimal and few children are compensated. Others have an interest in defining vaccine damage in terms not to exclude children who are prevented by lifelong vaccine-related injuries from becoming self-supporting members of society.

No matter who ultimately decides which vaccine-damaged children are compensated, the result will be a federal system that excludes certain categories of vaccine-damaged children. Their only recourse will be to exercise their constitutional right to seek redress in the court system. Free access to the court system is particularly relevant for childhood vaccine injuries because, unlike DES or Thalidomide or Benedectin, vaccines have been mandated for many years and more vaccines are being developed for mass, mandatory use by children.

Interestingly, manufacturers made two exceptions to the ban on lawsuits in cases of vaccine injury. Wyeth stated, "We support the continuation of manufacturer liability for any vaccine not meeting government standards."

Merck Sharpe & Dohme agreed, adding, "When a manufacturer fails to produce a vaccine in accordance with government standards or a health care provider fails to administer the vaccine in accordance with medical standards, the tort system should be open for an injured party to recover. But to accomplish the objectives of fair compensation, the tort system should be eliminated from any other type of action."

The manufacturers are putting the onus back on the federal government, which sets vaccine safety and efficacy standards to which the manufacturers must adhere. If the standards, such as the mouse toxicity and potency tests, are defective (and both the government and the manufacturers know they are), then who should pay for vaccine injuries —the government (i.e., the taxpayer) or the manufacturers? Or should they more properly share the responsibility as the Hawkins-Hatch bill proposes?

Dr. J. Anthony Morris explains why he believes a federal compensation system will do more harm than good: "This idea came from the idea that you bring people into an army and you say to them, 'Look, we are going to have to fight to save our country and we will expect a few casualties and a few deaths and if you should be hit or injured, we will take care of you. And if you are killed, we will take care of your family. Because you have been a soldier in our battle to save our country.'

"This is the same rationale that is being used in the fight against infectious diseases. In saving a million people, we might have 100 that will die from the vaccine or 1,000 that will be injured for the rest of their lives. Therefore, if this occurs, the greater good justifies taking care of these people. That sounds fine. The philosophy is great. But we will now put the physician in the same position that a general finds himself in when he wants to take a hill. You get a doctor or a public health service official who wants to save the world from pertussis. So he says, well, the greater good is that we are going to save millions of kids from getting pertussis and we expect 1,000 kids to be damaged but the government will take care of them.

"This is a dangerous precedent. It means that the doctor is free now to do with children as a general does with soldiers. If he is responsible for his actions, he is going to think a long time before he gives a vaccine to a child who shouldn't get it. The person who should be responsible for damaging a child with a vaccine is the person who made it, the person who approved it for public use, and the person who injected it into the child. Compensation is a beautiful idea, but in the real world it will do more harm than good."

Gordon Stewart, M.D., who has worked with parents of vaccine-damaged children in both Scotland and England and who has observed their fight to win awards under Britain's compensation system (which allows parents to obtain government compensation plus sue doctors or the drug manufacturer), said,

"It is premature to let the pharmaceutical companies off the hook. They are trying by every means to avoid squaring up to the issue that they are really liable for hundreds of millions of dollars in damages. What they are trying to do is to get the taxpayer to take on that burden. The government is being misled because the people advising them are virtually all on the side of the pharmaceutical companies.

"What you should have is a system that allows a parent to get government compensation and to sue the pharmaceutical company. This is the way it is set up in England, West Germany and other countries. And you have to make sure that your government compensation system contains a right to appeal because most of the parents will be turned down. That is what happened in Britain. Two thirds of them are turned down. But when they go to an independent government tribunal for an appeal, they are awarded compensation."

Jeff Schwartz, president of Dissatisfied Parents Together, spoke about the Hawkins-Hatch bill and how it will help parents of vaccine-damaged children. He defended the bill's provision allowing parents to choose the option of federal compensation or the option of suing the doctor or manufacturer:

"We reject the idea of the exclusive remedy compensation bill supported by the AMA and the manufacturers. Parents must be allowed to have the choice of whether to go through the federal system or through the court system. The Hawkins bill protects the rights of parents to do that. And it does a lot more. We need this bill because it will create strong incentives for the government and manufacturers to produce safer vaccines and for doctors to administer vaccines properly. It will create a better informed public so parents will know enough to tell a doctor, 'No, my child isn't getting the shot' if the doctor is not observing contraindications. It will help create an accurate reporting system so we can truly assess the dimensions of adverse reactions. Above all, it is a fair, quick, and relatively painless system of compensation for children and families who have suffered from vaccine damage in the past.

"It will help parents, for example, whose doctors were negligent but are inadequately insured and who would only get perhaps $100,000 from a doctor's insurance policy if they went to court. $100,000 can't begin to support a severely damaged child for the rest of his life. Compensation under this system in that case would be much more just because it provides for adequate lifetime care. The bill is not perfect, but it is so much better than the ignorance and lack of justice that we have now. Our society has failed to accept responsibility for the risks of vaccination. This is the first piece of legislation that forces a national debate on the risks and benefits of our national immunization program."

DPT was originally formed for the sole purpose of disseminating information about the pertussis vaccine. But the group has recently widened its scope to include other vaccines. Parents of MMR (measles-mumps-rubella) vaccine-damaged children are beginning to contact the group. One mother of a MMR-damaged child has become a DPT chapter leader in Florida, home of Senator Paula Hawkins, one of the bill's cosponsors. Wendy Scholl is working in her state to win support for the bill. She believes it will help children, like her own daughter, Stacy.

At a Congressional hearing in July 1983, Wendy testified that Stacy had almost died and was left partially paralyzed after a measles vaccine shot. She talked about how beautiful her sixteen-month-old daughter was until "eight days after her measles shot" when she discovered that Stacy was running a temperature of 102 degrees. The next day Stacy broke out in a rash, and the following day Wendy found her in her crib "panting, eyes affixed and a pool of blood on the sheet where her mouth was." The doctors diagnosed "post-vaccinal encephalitis," and Stacy is now paralyzed on her left side.

Wendy, who has been waiting six years for her case to be brought to trial, said, "I feel that if the Government . . . has committed itself to taking on the responsibility of enforcing vaccine programs prior to a child's entrance to school, then it is just logical that they must take the responsibility of coming up with a compensation program for any injured party as a result of their enforced commitment. I do not think that is wrong. I think it is just."

Wendy added, "I have been through hell. I still feel the vaccine program is a good idea, but only if we are presented good vaccines, good vaccine programs, and the truth about all information involved. If we cannot be honest with the parents and the public, then I think we have lost a whole lot of integrity as far as the medical profession is concerned and any other agency involved with regulating vaccines."

Wendy has met with officials from the Florida Health Department to develop a state adverse-reaction reporting system that will truly monitor vaccine reactions within the state in order to generate accurate reaction statistics. She has appeared on radio and television talk shows in her state to inform parents about adverse reactions, contraindications, and all the other information that DPT has available for parents. She has also worked with DPT national headquarters in Washington, D.C., to help parents of vaccine-damaged children network with each other for emotional support.

There are other parents like Wendy who are forming DPT chapters throughout the country and helping parents network with each other. Kathi Williams, DPT director, stresses that parents of healthy children, as well as those with damaged children, are becoming involved in the movement: "Our organization is a blend of parents with terribly damaged children as well as parents of healthy children, who know how lucky they are that their children were not hurt. It is a sad reality that mothers of vaccine injured children have to spend a significant amount of their day coping with the extra responsibilities of raising brain damaged children. Our group simply could not function unless we also had parents with children who escaped vaccine damage. We all need each other if we are going to change vaccine policy in this country."

DPT is also gathering data on cases of vaccine damage. Parents who wish to add their child's severe reaction and resulting permanent injury to the group's data bank may submit a description of the reaction to DPT national headquarters. The group, which is primarily operated by volunteers, requests that parents include their telephone number with area code as well as a $3.00 tax-deductible contribution, so that the group may forward a parent information packet in response to all inquiries. Those who would like to join and receive the organization's newsletter in addition to the parent information packet may do so by sending $20 (tax-deductible) annual dues to DPT, 128 Branch Road, Vienna, Virginia 22180.

Preventing Vaccine Damage

Before a child is vaccinated, there are several precautions parents can take to minimize the possibility of vaccine damage.

1. Ask the doctor to give the child a careful physical examination before each shot. This should include taking his temperature and making a thorough examination of the child's throat and ears to check that no infection is present. Parents should report any illness, however slight, that the child has had in the previous month, as well as any viral or bacterial infections that members of the family may currently have.

In general, the American medical profession agrees that children with a fever should not be vaccinated; but there is also growing concern among doctors about vaccinating a child who has been recently ill or currently has any signs of illness, including a cold, and especially an upper-respiratory infection, diarrhea, or ear infection. The optimum time to give a child vaccine is when the child is healthy.

2. The examining physician should take a detailed medical history of the child and his family before the first vaccination. Parents should mention if their child or anyone in the family has a history of convulsions or neurologic disease. As mentioned previously, most European countries consider that if a child or his immediate family has a history of seizures or other neurologic disease, the pertussis vaccine should not

be given. This is a particularly important contraindication to discuss with the doctor.

3. Parents should be sure to tell the doctor if the child or his family has a history of severe allergies or immune deficiency diseases. It is also important to mention if there is a history of severe reactions to the DPT shot in the family.

4. If it is not the child's first DPT shot, parents should notify the doctor of any reactions the child may have had to each of his earlier shots, including a severe local reaction such as extreme swelling, redness, or pain at the site of the injection. Of course, a severe reaction to a previous pertussis vaccination contraindicates another shot of pertussis vaccine.

5. If a baby has a problem with breathing which could predispose to sudden infant death syndrome (SIDS), parents may want to discuss with the doctor the comparative risks of administering pertussis vaccine before the child stops having breathing problems. If a baby is born prematurely or is significantly underweight, parents may want to discuss delaying the shot until the baby reaches the normal weight for his age group.

6. Parents who decide their child should receive the DPT vaccine, but who would like to delay the first shot until the baby is six months of age or older, should discuss with the doctor the benefits and risks of deferring the shot.

7. If parents and the doctor decide a child should receive only the DT vaccine (that is, diphtheria-tetanus vaccine without the pertussis component), they should make sure they look at the vial of vaccine before it is administered. As DT vaccine is infrequently given in doctors' offices, it is easy for mistakes to occur. Parents should know there is nothing wrong with asking a doctor or nurse who is about to administer the shot if they may read the label on the vial before the shot is given. At the same time, parents should ask the doctor to write down the vaccine manufacturer's name, lot, and batch number in the child's medical record. This should be done for *any* vaccine a child receives.

8. If a child has a moderate or severe reaction, parents can ask the child's doctor to report it to the CDC (and MSIFI) and to the state health department.

9. Finally, parents should know their legal rights and obligations concerning pertussis vaccination. Laws and regulations vary from state to state, and even within counties of some states. Before a child re-

ceives the pertussis vaccine, parents may wish to ask their state or county health department the following questions:

> Is vaccination for pertussis legally required to enroll my child in school? If so, how many shots are required? What flexibility does the law provide if I want to defer pertussis vaccination until my child is two years old or older? What is the legal consequence if my child does not get the required number of shots before he or she enters school?
>
> Does the law say that a child does not have to be vaccinated if the parents have a "personal conviction" or "philosophical objection," i.e., if parents believe vaccination is not in the child's best interest? Does the law provide an exemption on the grounds of religious conviction?
>
> What is the legal definition in my state or county of a "medical exemption" to the pertussis vaccine? What do I have to do to obtain a medical exemption for my child? What latitude is given to the physician's judgment as to whether or not the pertussis vaccine is medically contraindicated for a particular child?

In most states, if a child has a severe reaction to a previous DPT shot and parents do not want him to receive more pertussis vaccine, they can legally refuse to allow the child to have the pertussis vaccine injection. If a doctor or anyone else encourages parents to have a child vaccinated in the face of a previous severe reaction, parents should feel free to consult another doctor for a second opinion. If they cannot find a doctor who they feel is sufficiently sensitive to their concerns, they may consider consulting a lawyer in order to prevent the child from being vaccinated and possibly permanently injured.

It is important to remember that, whatever mandatory vaccination laws your state may have on its books, it is the parents who are ultimately responsible for their child's health and well-being. The choice of whether to have a child vaccinated is an informed decision parents must make in consultation with one or more doctors and after a careful weighing of the benefits and risks involved. If at any time parents believe that vaccination could cause serious harm to their child, either because the child has had a previous severe reaction or is medically at risk for another reason, they must think carefully before being pressured by private doctors, school officials, or state health officials into allowing the vaccination. If damage does occur, it is the parents who will be left to deal with the consequences.

Better Educational and Rehabilitation Programs for Vaccine-damaged Children

One of the biggest problems that needs to be addressed by counties and states throughout the nation is what to do about educating and caring for vaccine-damaged children. Many parents have reported that the public school system, rehabilitation services, and availability of residential home placements do not meet the unique needs of vaccine-damaged children.

Part of this problem may be due to the fact that, because medical science has not studied vaccine damage in any depth, it has not defined the vaccine-damage syndrome. In 1979 the Panel on Review of Bacterial Vaccines and Toxoids observed: "At present there are virtually no standards set for what constitutes untoward reactions to vaccines except for their most severe and dire complications." Without a definition of the syndrome, which will result in proper identification of the child who suffers from it, it is impossible to tailor special education and therapy programs for what many are beginning to call "DPT kids." One of the most frequently mentioned features of the syndrome, however, is that the vaccine-damaged child can understand more than he can communicate verbally or physically (see Chapter 7).

This particular feature of the neurological damage caused by the vaccine, together with the vaccine's ability to cause medication-resistant seizures, may help differentiate DPT kids from children who are mentally and physically handicapped from other causes. The pertussis vaccine-damaged child, who has medication-resistant seizures and an ability to understand more than he can verbally or physically communicate, is often difficult to place in existing special education programs.

In most states, handicapped children are evaluated by public schools and placed in classes for the physically handicapped, mildly mentally handicapped, moderately mentally handicapped, severely to profoundly mentally handicapped, or multiply handicapped. Federal law PL 94-142 guarantees that handicapped children will receive public education in the least restrictive environment, but most school systems do not have the funding to sort out children by their particular disabilities and gear an education program to help them achieve their highest potential. So handicapped children with unique problems are all lumped into the same categories. In some school systems, there is marked resistance to even diagnosing a child as learning disabled or mentally handicapped because more money will then have to be spent to educate him (see Chapter 15).

The biggest hurdle faced by parents of a vaccine-damaged child is what to do with the child after age twenty-one (eighteen in some states) who is no longer eligible for public education. At that point, parents may have to keep their fully grown child at home. If both parents work, they will have to find a full-time sitter willing to care for a handicapped adult who may need to be fed, who may not be able to go to the bathroom alone, who may have trouble walking and suffer violent seizures.

The problem of providing care for mentally retarded or developmentally delayed young adults is widespread throughout the nation. In 1983, *The New York Times* quoted Lieutenant Governor Alfred B. Del-Bello as having said, "Virtually all our resources are placed in the facilities for pre-21-year-olds while the post-21-year-olds are, for the most part, neglected or abandoned."

Some states have sheltered workshops or job-training programs for handicapped adults. In sheltered workshops, the adults may work on projects for which they get paid, such as clipping off pieces of cardboard from a box that has been cut incorrectly at a box-manufacturing plant. Or, if less severely handicapped, they may be able to participate in a job-training program in preparation for work in the wider community.

As one parent put it, "My child could sit in a sheltered workshop and get paid seven cents an hour to pull film off of reels. She might even be able to learn how to sweep floors in a job-training program. But she would probably continue to sweep floors in the job-training program for the rest of her life because, until someone in the community wants to hire her, there is no place for her to go."

Not only is there no place for grown DPT kids to go in the daytime, there is no place for them to go at night, except to their parents' home. There are far too few group homes for the handicapped in America. The concept of setting up group homes in the community to care for handicapped adults is a trend that is growing, but it is not growing fast enough. Homes for severely and profoundly retarded adults, those with violent seizures or behavior problems, are pathetically few.

Most states have private, nonprofit agencies that receive state funds to operate group homes, which usually house from three to six handicapped individuals plus trained professional supervisors. Rent is paid to the home by the handicapped residents through the SSI benefits that they receive.

In Maryland, for example, the Montgomery County Association for Retarded Citizens (MCARC) operates twenty-four group homes for approximately 120 handicapped adults, as well as a number of supervised independent apartments for high-functioning handicapped adults. There is a waiting list of about three hundred, and applicants must wait an average of five years for an opening. Three of the twenty-four group homes house twelve severe and profoundly handicapped individuals. Alice McGee, of MCARC, describes the situation facing parents who are trying to place their child:

"I know one father with a severely retarded, blind son, who just cannot find an opening in a group home for his son. He is thinking about getting together with other parents of severely retarded children and trying to form his own group home. We have three homes for the severely damaged but a long waiting list. And there is no question that, throughout the United States, many group home programs will not even take the more severely damaged, such as those who have constant seizures or are in diapers or cannot walk. If a parent can't find a group home, the only alternative is to either keep the child at home or place him in an institution."

What about institutions? There are two kinds of institutions for the mentally retarded: those run by the state with public funds and those run by private organizations on money paid by parents. A trend is that full-time state institutions are beginning to be reserved for the severely mentally ill with significant behavior problems, rather than simply the mentally retarded. However, most institutions still care for severe and profoundly retarded children and adults. Parents who must place their grown children in state institutions turn over the child's SSI check and sometimes contribute other funds to the state for the care of their child.

Private institutions can cost from $26,000 to $50,000 per year. The parent who is fortunate enough to be able to afford a private full-time care facility may also have to place a large amount of money in trust for the child as security. Some of the better private institutions have waiting lists just like those of group homes.

Unfortunately, full-time institutions for the mentally and physically handicapped vary dramatically in quality from state to state. And no matter how good a full-time facility is, parents are always traumatized when faced with the bitter reality that their fully grown child will someday end up in an institution after care in the home is no longer possible. Many come to the conclusion that they must now place their child in a full-time institution simply because he must learn to adjust to the world he must live in for the rest of his life. But they are torn by guilt and the knowledge that nobody in that institution will ever love him or care for him the way they do.

What is needed is a more sensitive public education system that will recognize the special needs of vaccine-damaged children and more group homes that will accommodate their growing numbers. The bitter struggle Harriet and her family (see Chapter 15) have undergone to obtain special education for her vaccine-damaged children in the Arkansas public school system is just one example of the need to educate our society about recognizing its responsibility to handicapped children. Vaccine damage does not just affect a single child; its impact is felt by the whole family. For every child permanently injured by vaccination, there is a set of parents whose lives are permanently and traumatically changed.

Careers can be altered or ended. A family's financial stability can be so disrupted that it causes bankruptcy as parents try to meet the skyrocketing medical bills. Dreams are shattered. For some, the future stretches out as one long nightmare filled with hospitals, neurologists, physical therapists, anticonvulsant medications that don't work, fights with insensitive school systems, futile searches for baby-sitters, and the certain knowledge that their child will never be able to function on his or her own and will be dependent upon them for as long as they live.

Some will say that life is not fair and that many children are born each year with birth defects and that others are injured in accidents or crippled by diseases and that vaccine-injured children are no different. It is true that our society has not responded adequately to the general issue of helping the handicapped reach their fullest potential. But vaccine-damaged children are unique in that their injuries occurred as a result of our society's failure to properly test and monitor a biological that is legally required by most states in our nation. The lack of adequate social services to meet the needs of vaccine-damaged children and their parents is just one more example of how our society has allowed children to be injured and then left them and their parents to cope with the devastating result of those injuries.

Passage of a federal compensation system will not remedy the injustices of the past unless state and county governments respond with increased funding for special education programs, group homes, sheltered workshops, and job training to make the lives of vaccine-damaged children and the lives of their parents more bearable.

The Need for an Educated Public

As the public becomes more educated about infectious diseases and vaccines, it becomes easier to interpret the political and economic implications of publicity surrounding this issue. In May 1984, the *Washington Post* reported that the CDC awarded a $250,000 grant to Baltimore, Baltimore County, and the states of Wisconsin and Colorado to study ways to improve the reporting and diagnosis of whooping cough. With new emphasis on reporting and diagnosis, there will undoubtedly be an increase in whooping cough statistics, particularly in these three states.

As CDC officials have said, whooping cough may be underreported in the United States by as much as ten or twenty times. Increased surveillance will yield pertussis cases that until now have remained undiagnosed and unreported. When there is a publicized report of a rise in whooping cough cases in a community, parents may contact their state health department and ask for verification of the vaccination status of all reported victims plus substantiation that the reported cases were laboratory tested and confirmed as whooping cough.

There may also be more media reports about the prevalence and seriousness of other infectious diseases, particularly those for which vaccines have been developed for future mass-vaccination programs.

Soon after publicity surrounding the May 3, 1984, congressional hearings on the Hawkins-Hatch bill, Merck Sharpe & Dohme announced that it had developed a chicken pox vaccine that was found to be safe and effective in nearly 1,000 children. The May 31, 1984, *Washington Post* reported that "Government estimates suggest that there are about 4,500 hospitalizations and 100 deaths related to chicken pox each year." Robert E. Weibel, M.D., the pediatrician who headed the study, was quoted by the paper as saying, "I do foresee this being used on all children as a routine immunization." Merck, Sharpe & Dohme plans two more years of testing the chicken pox vaccine, however, to evaluate long-term risks which may include the later development of shingles and other illnesses.

A few weeks later, there were press reports about a conference attended by federal and state health officials in Minneapolis at which it was announced that the incidence of hepatitis and H-flu meningitis was increasing among day-care children. They reported that between 40 and 50 percent of the nation's 10,000 annual cases of Hemophilus influenzae B or "H-flu" meningitis occur in children attending day-care centers, and that 10 to 15 percent of the 25,000 annual cases of hepatitis A are related to transmission of the disease in day-care centers. As mentioned in Chapter 16, a vaccine for "H-flu" meningitis is being developed by vaccine manufacturers and it has been suggested that this vaccine be combined with the DPT shot. Speakers at the conference reportedly urged mandatory immunizations for day-care children.

Parents who are interested in obtaining more information following publicity about increases in cases of infectious diseases should contact their state health departments, the vaccine manufacturer mentioned, or the CDC in Atlanta for documentation of the facts contained in the report.

Legal Help

Some parents of severely vaccine-damaged children need legal help to assist them in deciding whether or not to undertake a lawsuit to obtain financial support for their child's uncertain future. Parents should be aware that the course of litigation is not easy and there is no guarantee of success. A lawsuit can be costly and take many years. A major vaccination case can cost $75,000 to $100,000 in out-of-pocket expenses, not even counting the lawyer's time. However, in individual circumstances, a lawsuit may be necessary and advisable. The most important part of entering into litigation is to find the right lawyer.

A lawyer should be chosen as carefully as a doctor is chosen. Credentials and record for winning cases should be investigated. The method and amount of payment should be established in advance. A group of lawyers specializing in DPT vaccine cases has been formed within the American Trial Lawyers Association. Consulting lawyers with good backgrounds in product liability or medical malpractice cases is one place to start.

A handful of DPT vaccine cases have been settled in the past twenty years. In 1982, *Holcomb* v. *United States & Richardson-Merrell*, on behalf of a child who reacted with excessive screaming after a DPT shot, was given a second and third shot at a military health clinic, and suffered post-pertussis encephalopathy, was settled out of court for $600,000.

In 1982, *Wilson* v. *United States* was settled on behalf of a child who was given repeated DPT shots at military health clinics despite convulsions and other neurological reactions, and who, as a result, was severely mentally retarded. After a three-week trial, the judge entered a verdict for the child of approximately $2.5 million. While the case was on appeal, a settlement was reached which is designed to pay some $17 million over the remainder of the child's life through a tax-free annuity. Also included was $875,000 cash for the boy, his mother, and their attorney, and $466,000 cash for the mother's own claim.

There have been settlements against physicians who administered the DPT shots in the face of contraindications. In 1984, *Thom* v. *Allen* was settled on behalf of parents whose child was given a third DPT shot despite a history of convulsions following previous DPT shots. The child has a continuing seizure disorder. This malpractice suit was settled for approximately $5.5 million.

There have also been some settlements against the manufacturers of DPT vaccine. For example, in 1982, *Kindrex* v. *Merrell-National Laboratories*, on behalf of a child who developed encephalopathy after receiving a fourth DPT shot given by public health nurses in a state-run clinic, was settled for $175,000 cash and $1,000 a month for the rest of the child's life.

In 1984, a DPT case against a manufacturer was finally brought to trial. The Idaho jury in *Toner* v. *Lederle* found that the manufacturer was negligent in the manufacture of the DPT vaccine administered to a child, and the jury awarded $1.14 million to the child and his parents. The manufacturer is appealing, but this case marks the first trial jury verdict against a manufacturer.

Taking Action

Those interested in working to change present vaccine policies have several options. Dissatisfied Parents Together (DPT), whose address is listed at the beginning of this chapter, can identify sources of information in a number of states.

Contacting local radio, television, and newspapers is another step concerned citizens can take. Local call-in radio shows and television talk shows or letters to the editor of the local newspaper are all possibilities. The national television networks—ABC, NBC, CBS, and PBS—or local cable news networks can be encouraged to cover the DPT issue.

Meetings with state representatives and senators and your U.S. representatives and senators may also be arranged. Those opposing an "exclusive remedy" compensation system can call or write their congressional representatives. Petitions can also be an effective means of communicating concerns and goals to elected representatives.

Another approach is meeting or corresponding with the doctor in charge of the state chapter of the AAP or AMA or other physician groups, as well as the director of the state health department, to find ways to help disseminate information to physicians about adverse reactions and contraindications to the pertussis vaccine. Speaking and giving information to parent groups such as childbirth education classes, church groups, and the PTA is another means of making parents more aware that they can help prevent unnecessary vaccine damage by becoming educated about high-risk children and contraindications.

Parents of a vaccine-damaged child have many organizations to contact in addition to Dissatisfied Parents Together. The Epilepsy Foundation of America, Association for Retarded Citizens, United Cerebral Palsy Foundation, National Sudden Infant Death Foundation, Feingold Association, Association for Children with Learning Disabilities, Orton Dyslexia Society, and others are concerned with health conditions that may be related to the pertussis vaccine. Some have state chapters.

Finally, the decision whether or not to have a child vaccinated should be made only after parents become informed about the particular vaccine to be given, consider state laws, and hold discussions with one or more physicians.

22

Conclusion

> This is no time to speak of the hopes of the future, or the
> broader world which lies beyond our struggles and our victory.
> We have to win that world for our children. We have to win it
> by our sacrifices. We have not won it yet. The crisis is upon us.
> *Winston Churchill*

The pertussis vaccine story is not over. Every week, more than
57,000 American children are taken into pediatricians' offices and
public health clinics to be vaccinated. Mothers cradle newborn babies
in their laps before they receive their first DPT shot. Toddlers due for
a booster shot wiggle away when they see the needle. Five-year-olds
about to enter kindergarten close their eyes and try to be brave. Some
of these children are healthy; some are sick; some have a history of
convulsions; some have reacted to a previous shot. Each one of them
is taking a risk whose dimensions are still unknown. Most of them
will escape injury; some will not.

Jackie was one who did not. "I think of Jackie when I hear the
phrase, 'A mind is a terrible thing to waste,' " said Jackie's mother.
"Jackie's older sister is a nurse, her other sister an attorney. But Jackie
is now twenty-one years old and living in an institution because she
was severely injured by the pertussis vaccine. What might Jackie and
all of our other vaccine-damaged children have contributed to our
society? How many potential geniuses have been cut down without a
choice?"

After the mothers of vaccine-damaged children tell about their
convulsive, mentally retarded, physically handicapped, and learning-
disabled children, many parents still think, "It won't happen to my

child." Or will it? The pertussis vaccine does not discriminate. Until the medical profession defines the high-risk child, all parents take a chance.

Scientists and physicians in positions of authority in the Food and Drug Administration, Centers for Disease Control, American Academy of Pediatrics, American Medical Association, and drug companies have known about the dangers of the pertussis vaccine since at least 1948, when Byers and Moll published their study in *Pediatrics*. They have had more than thirty-five years to adequately inform parents and pediatricians about these dangers, more than thirty-five years in which to evaluate the "risks" by investigating the number and severity of adverse reactions. Instead, they have turned away and minimized them.

Drug manufacturers and the FDA have known since at least the early 1960s that the FDA's mouse toxicity test bears little relation to adverse reactions in children. Knowing the vaccine was not being properly evaluated for toxicity, they continued to inject it into more than sixty million children during the following twenty years. The result is that America's children are being required to take a vaccine that is inadequately tested for safety.

After the UCLA-FDA study in 1979 showed a high incidence of serious neurological reactions and even death, the FDA, CDC, and leaders of the medical establishment did not respond by immediately investigating high-risk children and revising the vaccine's contraindications. Their response was to continue business as usual and make the same dangerous claim they have made for the past thirty-five years: that it is safe for virtually every child to receive the pertussis vaccine.

In their dogged pursuit of a 100-percent vaccination rate, policymakers in the government and the medical establishment have encouraged state legislatures to require all children to get five doses of pertussis vaccine before being allowed to attend school. Practicing physicians, following their lead, have often refused to provide exemptions for children who suffered serious reactions to previous shots, or whose parents object to the vaccine.

Without the truly informed consent of the American public, these vaccine policymakers determined that it was necessary and morally acceptable to sacrifice an unknown number of children for the theoretical well-being of the rest of the society. And then vaccine-damaged children and their parents were left to fend for themselves. Perhaps it was easy to do that when one assumed somebody else's child would be sacrificed. Again and again, mothers of vaccine-damaged children have said, "When it happens to your child, the risks are 100 percent."

Despite the fact that a Japanese scientist, who once worked on pertussis vaccine research at the NIH, has developed a purified pertussis vaccine which has been used in Japan since 1981, the United States has yet to make it available to the American public. The Japanese have reported their vaccine to be less than one tenth as toxic as the vaccine given our children—with a dramatic reduction in local, systemic, and neurological reactions. What reasons can the FDA, CDC, and vaccine manufacturers give to explain why Japan can do it and we can't?

Do the same officials who have expressed the opinion among themselves that it would be "unethical" not to try the acellular vaccine prefer to wait, for political and economic reasons, for a more favorable climate in which to introduce it to America? Do they await an America in the midst of a whooping cough epidemic, real or false; an America in which private vaccine manufacturers refuse to make the whole-cell vaccine with the justification that they cannot continue to bear the cost of "frivolous lawsuits" due to publicity surrounding reports such as this book; and an America in which a misinformed Congress is pushed into passing an "exclusive remedy" vaccine-injury compensation bill?

It is this kind of political posturing, bureaucratic inertia, and lack of concern that has outraged the parents of America. It touches at the very heart of what is wrong with American medicine today. We have been taught to trust and believe in our scientists and doctors, to believe they are among the brightest and best in our society. We have willingly given them our respect and we have accorded them wealth, prestige, and power. And we have given them the right to tell us what to do with our children, because we always believed they knew what was best. We have treated them as gods, forgetting they are our fathers and mothers, wives and husbands, sons and daughters. They are us, with all the frailty and ignorance and susceptibility to temptation that is implicit in being human.

Mothers and fathers in cities and towns across America are entering libraries and reading medical literature, not only on the pertussis vaccine, but on all the vaccines and drugs that doctors prescribe. They are educating themselves about medicine, and in the process finding that it is by no means beyond comprehension. It is becoming clear that their learning may save children's lives.

This is a revolution that has been a long time coming, a necessary first step in making medical decisions truly a shared responsibility between parents and doctors. As parents become educated and understand that medicine is not an exact science, that doctors of equal competence may disagree with each other, and that what is touted as safe today may be condemned as dangerous tomorrow, they realize medicine cannot and should not be legislated.

The pertussis vaccine story is a prime example of what is wrong with the 1904 Supreme Court decision which removed the individual's right to refuse to be injected with a vaccine, a decision justified by the rationalization that the welfare of society must supersede that of the individual. The nine very human men who made that decision eighty years ago believed in the infallibility of medical science and the ability of doctors to determine before inoculation which individuals will be harmed by a vaccine. As the pertussis vaccine story makes painfully evident, they were mistaken.

The legal standard generally applied to vaccines defines them as "unavoidably unsafe products" that are "quite incapable of being made safe for their intended and ordinary use." That being the case, it is time to reclaim the right to choose whether vaccinations are appropriate for us or our children. Like every other product sold in the free-enterprise system of a democratic society, a vaccine should be allowed to withstand the marketplace test of consumer demand.

And like other commercial products sold in a free society, vaccines should not be treated with special consideration by eliminating the legal responsibiliy of those who make and administer them. The attempt by the AMA and drug manufacturers to pass a compensation bill abolishing a parent's right to due process of law is alarming. The passage of an "exclusive remedy" compensation bill would remove liability from manufacturers for unsafe vaccines and make it easier for the government to mandate new vaccines.

We do not want to see our children die or become brain damaged from a disease that can be prevented by a product involving negligible risk. Most parents who question the benefit/risk calculations of the present pertussis vaccine faithfully have their children receive polio and diphtheria-tetanus vaccines, for example, because they accept the benefit/risk calculations of those vaccines.

The truth is that if a product is overwhelmingly safe and effective, it will not need legislation for mass acceptance. And conversely, if it proves to be questionable, legislation is the only way to ensure mass acceptance. This is most poignantly illustrated in totalitarian societies where powerful bureaucrats routinely decide what is good for the rest of the population. As parents in a democratic society, we are responsible for protecting the rights and well-being of our children, and the choice of whether or not to inject them with a drug or vaccine should remain with us.

There should be no misunderstanding about the responsibility that comes with freedom. The government and physicians have led parents to believe for thirty-five years that vaccines are virtually free of serious risks. That is not true. And it is also not true that pertussis is risk-free, even in its current apparently milder form. If parents choose to take their chances with the natural disease instead of the vaccine as parents have in England, there will be more whooping cough in this country and some children will die from it. That is a reality which must be faced as honestly as we face the reality of vaccine damage.

It is important to remember, however, that despite the frightening ads that appear on British television and radio warning parents to vaccinate, nearly two thirds of British parents have apparently decided natural whooping cough is preferable to the whole-cell pertussis vaccine. They have the ability to stop their seven-year-old whooping cough "epidemic" at any time—all they have to do is have their children vaccinated. The same is true for parents in Sweden and West Germany, where whooping cough has been experienced by many children since these countries stopped using the whole-cell vaccine on a mass basis more than ten years ago.

Another reality that has been too long ignored is that although vaccines have been credited with saving millions of lives, the bottom line is that they are big business. The research and administration of vaccines employs tens of thousands of people in drug companies, private research laboratories, universities, state health departments, public health clinics, the FDA, the CDC, hospitals, and doctors' offices. States obtain federal immunization grants to implement mass vaccination programs and to hire additional personnel in their health departments.

The CDC estimates that 151 million doses of eight major vaccines were distributed in the United States in 1981, which generated more than $300 million for the drug industry. Federal budget appropriations for childhood vaccines rose from $6.2 million in 1975 to more than $46 million in 1979. And the fact that at least seven childhood vaccines are legally required for admission to school assures drug manufacturers a stable, ready-made market. Will the vaccines now being tested for chicken pox, meningitis, hepatitis, influenza, gonorrhea, herpes, and pneumonia be added to the present list of seven vaccines now required for our children to enter school?

If even half the vaccines being developed today are used by the general public tomorrow, drug manufacturers will realize profits of many millions of dollars. And just as we are told to give our children the pertussis vaccine today "for the greater good of society," we may be told to give them the herpes vaccine tomorrow "for the greater good of society." But what guarantee do we have that adequate tests for safety and toxicity will be developed and adverse reactions will not be suppressed with other vaccines as has been done with the pertussis vaccine?

Gordon Stewart said, "If the Centers for Disease Control has its way, Americans and their children are going to become human pin cushions." Polio, diphtheria, and tetanus vaccines are the only ones used as universally in Western Europe as in the United States. In America, all of our children are routinely injected with four doses of DPT vaccine (containing 12 antigens), one dose of MMR vaccine (3 antigens), and four doses of oral polio (12 antigens), for a total of 27 different antigens by the time they are eighteen months old. And we are racing to develop more vaccines for everything from croup to tooth decay.

What are we doing to ourselves and our children? The answer is, we do not know. Just as doctors and scientists have not understood the effects of the pertussis bacterium and the pertussis vaccine, they do not know the long-term effects of challenging our immune systems with so many bacterial and viral antigens about which little is known. Just as we have polluted our environment with man-made chemicals, we may well be polluting ourselves with a myriad of man-made vaccines in our quest to eradicate all disease and infection from the earth.

In her exploration of the ways that Americans have polluted the air, water, and earth with synthetic chemicals, Rachel Carson concluded in *Silent Spring* that "The choice, after all, is ours to make. If, having endured much, we have at least asserted our 'right to know,' and if, knowing, we have concluded that we are being asked to take senseless and frightening risks, then we should no longer accept the counsel of those who tell us we must fill our world with poisonous chemicals; we should look about and see what other course is open to us."

One mother of a vaccine-damaged child drew a parallel to what Rachel Carson has observed. She spoke of her son, who cannot speak. "What makes me so mad is that it could have been avoided. I thought I was being a good parent to give him that shot. If I had known about the risks, if I had been given an option, I might have taken my chances with the natural disease. I don't know. But I do know that God gave me a perfect child. I was so happy when he was born. He was so beautiful, with ten toes and ten fingers. God gave me a perfect child and man, with his own ways, damaged God's perfect work."

That is what this story is all about—parents grieving for their children, who were healthy and now are broken, many with futures too bleak to comprehend. As mothers, we miraculously conceive our babies and carry them for nine months while we eat the right foods and read books about how to be a good mother. As fathers, we attend childbirth classes so we can help mothers withstand the pain of giving birth without anesthetics that might harm our child. As mothers, we breastfeed to give our babies the best start in life, and we sit up nights rocking them to sleep so they will feel safe. As parents, we work long hours and make sacrifices of every kind to make their future secure.

We give everything we have to our children. They are part of us. We love them more than we love ourselves and more than we ever thought we could love anyone else. We hope for them and want them to lead productive, fulfilled lives. There is nothing we would not do for them and nothing we would not risk for them. They are our children. And they will have our grandchildren. We fight with all our strength and all our love to protect them from harm. The time has come to educate ourselves about vaccines.

Bibliography

I. Books and Articles

Adams, R. D., and Victor, M. 1981. *Principles of neurology.* 2nd ed. New York: McGraw-Hill.

Adler, S. P. 1982. The effects and side effects of vaccines. *Virginia Medical* 109: 410–11.

Alexander, E. R. 1984. Inactivated poliomyelitis vaccination. *Journal of the American Medical Association* 251(20): 2710–12.

Ambrosch, F., and Wiedermann, G. 1979. Changes of risk and benefit in immunization against pertussis and tuberculosis. *International Symposium on Immunization*, Brussels, 1978. *Developments in Biological Standardization* 43: 85–90. Basel. S. Karger.

American Academy of Pediatrics. 1982. Committee on Infectious Diseases. *Red Book* update. *Pediatrics* 70(5): 819–20.

———. 1955. *Report of the Committee on the Control of Infectious Diseases.* 11th ed.

———. 1957. *Report of the Committee on the Control of Infectious Diseases.* 12th ed.

———. 1961. *Report of the Committee on the Control of Infectious Diseases.* 13th ed.

———. 1966. *Report of the Committee on the Control of Infectious Diseases.* 15th ed.

———. 1970. *Report of the Committee on Infectious Diseases.* 16th ed.

———. 1974. *Report of the Committee on Infectious Diseases.* 17th ed.

———. 1977. *Report of the Committee on Infectious Diseases.* 18th ed.

———. 1982. *Report of the Committee on Infectious Diseases.* 19th ed.

American Medical Association. 1980. *AMA drug evaluations.* 4th ed. Chicago.

———. 1983. *AMA drug evaluations.* 5th ed. Chicago.

———. 1984. *Report of Ad Hoc Commission on Vaccine Injury Compensation.*

409

Amiel-Tison, C. 1973. Neurologic disorders in neonates associated with abnormalities of pregnancy and birth. *Current Problems of Pediatrics* 3(2): 3–37.

Anderson, I., and Morris, D. 1950. Encephalopathy after combined diphtheria-pertussis inoculation. *Lancet* (March 25), 537–9.

Anderson, R., and May, R. 1982. The logic of vaccination. *New Scientist* (November 18), 410–15.

Annell, A. L. 1953. Pertussis in infancy: A cause of behavioral disorders in children. *Acta Societatis Medicorum Upsaliensis LVIII*, Supp. 1.

Ash, D. 1982. Whooping cough immunization. *Medical Journal of Australia* (May 1), 369–70.

Baird, H., and Borofsky, L. G. 1957. Infantile myoclonic spasms. *Journal of Pediatrics* 50: 332–39.

Bannister, R. 1978. *Brain's clinical neurology.* 5th ed. New York and Toronto: Oxford University Press.

Baraff, L. J., Ablon, W. J., and Weiss, R. C. 1983. Possible temporal association between diphtheria-tetanus toxoid-pertussis vaccination and sudden infant death syndrome. *Pediatric Infectious Disease* 2(1): 7–11.

—————, and Cherry, J. D. 1978. Nature and rates of adverse reactions associated with pertussis immunization. In Manclark, C. R., and Hill, J. C., eds. *International Symposium on Pertussis*, 291–96 (see ref.).

—————, Cody, C. L., and Cherry, J. D. 1984. DPT-associated reactions: An analysis by injection site, prior reactions, and dose. *Pediatrics* 73(1): 31–36.

—————, Leake, R. D., Burstyn, D. G., Payne, T., Cody, C. L., Manclark, C. R., and St. Geme, J. W. 1984. Immunologic response to early and routine DTP immunization in infants. *Pediatrics* 73(1): 37–42.

Barrett, C. D., Jr. Timm, E. A., Molner, J. G., Wilner, B. I., Anderson, C. P., and Carnes, H. E. 1958. Multiple antigen for immunization against poliomyelitis, diphtheria, pertussis, and tetanus. *Journal of the American Medical Association* 167(9): 1103–7.

—————, McLean, W., Jr., Molner, J. G., Timm, E. A., and Weiss, C. F., 1962. Multiple antigen immunization of infants against poliomyelitis, diphtheria, pertussis, and tetanus. *Pediatrics* 30: 720–36.

Barkin, R. M., and Pichichero, M. E. 1979. Diphtheria-pertussis-tetanus vaccine: Reactogenicity of commercial products. *Pediatrics* 63(2): 256–60.

Barrie, H. 1983. Campaign of Terror. *American Journal of Diseases of Children* 137: 922–23.

Bassili, W. R., and Stewart, G. T. 1976. Epidemiological evaluation of immunization and other factors in the control of whooping cough. *Lancet* (February 28), 471–73.

Beckwith, J. B. 1973. The sudden infant death syndrome. *Current Problems in Pediatrics* 3(8): 3–36.

Beeson, P. B., and McDermott, W. 1975. *Textbook of medicine.* 14th ed. Philadelphia: W. B. Saunders.

Behrman, R. E., and Vaughan, V. C. 1983. *Nelson's textbook of pediatrics.* Philadelphia: W. B. Saunders.

Bellman, M. H., Ross, E. M., and Miller, D. L. 1983. Infantile spasms and pertussis immunization. *Lancet* (May 7), 1031–34.

Berg, J. M. 1958. Neurological complications of pertussis immunization. *British Medical Journal* (July 5), 24–27.

Bernier, R. H., Frank, J. A., and Nolan, T. F. 1981. Abscesses complicating DTP vaccination. *American Journal of Diseases of Children* 135: 826–28.

————, ————, Dondero, T. J., and Turner, P. 1982. Diphtheria-tetanus toxoids-pertussis vaccination and sudden infant deaths in Tennessee. *Journal of Pediatrics* 101(5): 419–21.

Bradford, W. L., Day, E., and Martin, F. 1949. Humoral antibody formation in infants aged one to three months injected with a triple (diphtheria-tetanus-pertussis) alum-precipitated antigen. *Pediatrics* 4(6): 711–17.

Broder, J. 1980. Parents of three children sue state over faulty vaccine. *Detroit News* (November 24).

Brody, M. 1947. Neurologic complications following the administration of pertussis vaccine. *Brooklyn Hospital Journal* 5: 107–13.

Broome, C. V., and Fraser, D. W. 1981. Pertussis in the United States, 1979: A look at vaccine efficacy. *Journal of Infectious Diseases* 144(2): 187–90.

————, Fraser, D. W., and English, W. J. 1978. Pertussis—Diagnostic methods and surveillance. In Manclark and Hill (see ref.).

————, Preblud, S. R., Bruner, B., McGowan, J. E., Hayes, P. S., Harris, P. R., Elsea, W., and Fraser, D. W. 1981. Epidemiology of pertussis, Atlanta, 1977. *Journal of Pediatrics* 98(3): 362–67.

Brunell, P. 1983. Impact of litigation on immunization of children. *Pediatrics* 72(6): 822–23.

Buchanan, D. 1946. Convulsions in infancy and childhood. *Medical Clinics of North America* 30: 163–71.

Byers, R. K., and Moll, F. C. 1948. Encephalopathies following prophylactic pertussis vaccination. *Pediatrics* 1(4): 437–56.

————, and Rizzo, N. D. 1950. A follow-up study of pertussis in infancy. *New England Journal of Medicine* 242(23): 887–91.

Cameron, J. 1978. Pertussis vaccine: Control testing problems. In Manclark and Hill (see ref.).

————. 1980. The potency of whooping cough (pertussis) vaccines in Canada. *Journal of Biological Standardization* 8: 297–302.

————. 1982. Whooping cough: Infection and disease. *Lancet* (June 5), 1301.

Carlos-Ponce, J. 1951. Sindrome convulsivo mortal consecutivo al uso profilactico de vacuna antipertussis antidifterica. *Archivos Argentinos de Pediatria* 35: 232–33.

Cavanagh, N. P. C., Brett, E. M., Marshall, W. C., and Wilson, J. 1981. The possible adjuvant role of bordetella pertussis and pertussis vaccine in causing severe encephalopathic illness: A presentation of three case histories. *Neuropediatrics* 12(4): 374–81.

Champsaur, H., Bottazzo, G.-F., Bertrams, J., Assan, R., and Bach, C. 1982.

Virologic, immunologic, and genetic factors in insulin-dependent diabetes mellitus. *Journal of Pediatrics* 100(1): 15–20.

Charles, D., and Finland, M. 1973. *Obstetric and perinatal infections.* Philadelphia: Lea and Febiger.

Charlton, M. H. 1975. Infantile spasms. In M. H. Charlton, ed., *Myoclonic seizures.* Amsterdam: Excerpta Medica/American Elsevier.

Cherry, J. 1984. The epidemiology of pertussis and pertussis immunization in the United Kingdom and the United States: A comparative survey. *Current Problems in Pediatrics* 14: 2.

Chiarello, R. A. 1982. Antibody titers after DPT immunization. *Hospital Practice* (April), 17.

Christensen, C. N. 1963. More risky to give or not to give? *American Journal of Diseases of Children* 105: 417.

Clements, S. D., and Peters, J. E. 1981. Syndromes of minimal brain dysfunction. In P. Black, ed., *Brain dusfunction in children: Etiology, diagnosis, and management.* New York: Raven Press.

Cockburn, W. C. 1951. Whooping-cough immunization. *Practitioner* 167: 232–36.

Cockrell, J. L. 1982. Vaccine reactions: The challenge to pediatricians. *Virginia Medical* (June), 380–81.

Cody, C. L., Baraff, L. J., Cherry, J. D., Marcy, S. M., and Manclark, C. R. 1981. Nature and rates of adverse reactions associated with DTP and DT immunizations in infants and children. *Pediatrics* 68(5): 650–60.

Cohen, S. M., and Wheeler, M. W. 1946. Pertussis vaccine prepared with phase-I cultures grown in fluid medium. *American Journal of Public Health* 36: 371–76.

Connaught Laboratories, Inc. 1980. Diphtheria and tetanus toxoids and pertussis vaccine absorbed USP (package insert) (rev. July).

Connor, I. M. 1982. Neurological reactions to pertussis vaccination. *Archives of Disease in Childhood* 57: 240–43.

Connor, J. S., and Speers, J. F. 1963. A comparison between undesirable reactions to extracted pertussis antigen and to whole-cell antigen in DPT combinations. *Journal of the Iowa Medical Society* 53: 340–43.

Cook, R. 1978. Pertussis in developing countries: Possibilities and problems of control through immunization. In Manclark and Hill (see ref.).

Cooke, J. V., Holowach, J., Atkins, J. E., Jr., and Powers, J. R. 1948. Antibody formation in early infancy against diphtheria and tetanus toxoids. *Journal of Pediatrics* 33(2): 141–46.

Dick, G. W. A. 1967. Reactions to the pertussis component of quadruple and triple vaccines. *International Symposium on Combined Vaccines,* Marburg. *Symposia Series in Immunobiological Standardization* 7: 21–28. Basel and New York: Karger.

————. 1974. Convulsive disorders in young children. *Proceedings of the Royal Society of Medicine* 67: 371–2.

————. 1978. The whooping cough vaccine controversy. In A. Voller and H. Friedman, eds., *New trends and developments in vaccines*. Baltimore: University Park Press.

————. 1981. Letter to the editor. *British Medical Journal* 282: 2051.

Dobbing, J. 1968. Effects of experimental undernutrition on development of the nervous system. In N. S. Scrimshaw, and J. E. Gordon, eds., *Malnutrition, learning, and behavior*. Cambridge: MIT Press.

Ebrahim, S. 1981. Letter to the editor. *British Medical Journal* 282: 1871.

Ehrengut, W. 1974(a). Kann die pertussis-schutzimpfung noch empfohlen werden? *Deutsche medizinische Wochenschrift* 99(45): 2307–10.

————. 1974(b). Ueber convulsive reaktionen nach pertussis-schutzimpfung. *Deutsche medizinische Wochenschrift* 99(45): 2273–79.

————. 1977. Neurale komplikationen nach pertussis-schutzimpfung. *Monatsschriftfuer Kinderheilkkunde* 125: 908–11.

————. 1978. Whooping cough vaccination. *Lancet* (February 18), 370–71.

————. 1980. Laesst sich die reserve gegenueber der pertussis-schutzimpfung begruenden? *Paediatrische Praxis* 23: 3–13.

————. 1981. Die parenterale pertussis-impfung schaden-nutzen relation. *Monatschrift Kinderheilk* 129: 67–69.

————. 1981(a). Pertussis vaccine. *British Medical Journal* 283: 494.

————. 1981(b). Impfschutz und kinderkrankheiten in der anamnese von Hamburger schulanfaengern. *Hamburger Aerzteblatt* 2: 40–42.

————, and Sturm H. 1975. Pertussis und ihre komplikationen—Eine analyse der krankenhausaufnamen in Hamburg 1950 bis 1970. *Immunitaet und Infektion* 3(6): 169–77.

Eldering, G. 1971. Symposium on pertussis immunization in honor of Dr. Pearl Kendrick in her eightieth year: Historical notes on pertussis immunization. *Health Laboratory Science* 8: 200–205.

Ellenberg, J. H. 1984. The age of onset of seizures in young children. *Neurology* (NY) 34(5): 637–41.

————, and Nelson, K. B. 1978. Febrile seizures and later intellectual performance. *Archives of Neurology* 35: 17–21.

Emery, J. L. 1981. Letter to the editor. *British Medical Journal* 282: 2052.

Falk, W., Hoefler, K.-H., Rosanelli, K., and Kurz, R. 1981. Gegenwart und zukunft der oralen pertussis-schutzimpfung. *Fortschritte der Medizin* 99(34): 1363–66.

Felton, H. M., and Willard, C. W. 1944. Current status of prophylaxis by hemophilus pertussis vaccine. *Journal of the American Medical Association* 126(5): 294–99.

Fenichel, G. M. 1983. The pertussis vaccine controversy: The danger of case reports. *Archives of Neurology* 40: 193–94.

Fine, P., and Clarkson, J. 1982. The recurrence of whooping cough: Possible implications for assessment of vaccine efficacy. *Lancet* (March 20), 666–69.

Forrester, R. M. 1963. Immunization against whooping cough. *British Medical Journal* (July 24), 232.

Frankel, H. H. 1979. Potential effects of temperature on killed vaccines. *New England Journal of Medicine* 301(3): 159.

Friedman, E., and Pampiglione, G. 1971. Prognostic implications of electro-encephalographic findings of hypsarrhythmia in first year of life. *British Medical Journal* (November 6), 323–24.

Froggatt, P., Lynas, M. A., and MacKenzie, G. 1971. Epidemiology of sudden unexpected death in infants ("cot death") in Northern Ireland. *British Journal of Preventive and Social Medicine* 25: 119–34.

Fukuyama, Y., Tomori, Y., and Sugitate, M. 1977. Critical evaluation of the role of immunization as an etiological factor of infantile spasms. *Neuro-paediatrie* 8(3): 224–37.

Fulginiti, V. R. 1976. Pertussis vaccine—Does it work? Is it safe? *Current Problems in Pediatrics* 6: 3–35.

————. 1982. Pertussis. In V. A. Fulginiti, ed., *Immunization in clinical practice*. Philadelphia: J. B. Lippincott.

————. 1983(a). A new pertussis vaccine: Hope for the future? *Journal of Infectious Diseases* 148(1): 146–47.

————. 1983(b). Sudden infant death syndrome, Diphtheria-tetanus toxoid-pertussis vaccination and visits to the doctor: Chance association or cause and effect? *Pediatric Infectious Diseases* 2(1): 5–6.

————. 1983(c). Letter from the editor. *American Journal of Diseases of Children* 137: 923.

————. 1984. Pertussis disease, vaccine, and controversy. *Journal of the American Medical Association* 251(2): 251.

Further contributions to the pertussis vaccine debate. 1981. *Lancet* (May 16), 1113–14.

Garty, B. Z., Drucker, M. M., and Nitzan, M. 1981. Etiology of pertussis syndrome. *Pediatrics* 68(1): 148–49.

Gastaut, H., Roger, J., Soulayrol, R., and Pinsard, N. 1964. *L'Encephalopathie myoclonique infantile avec hypsarythmie*. Paris: Masson.

————, Roger, J., Soulayrol, R., Salamon, G., Regis, H., and Lob, H. 1965. Encephalopathie myoclonique infantile avec hypsarythmie (syndrome de west) et sclerose tubereuse de Bourneville. *Journal of the Neurological Sciences* 2: 140–58.

Geschwind, N. 1982. Why Orton was right. *Annals of Dyslexia* 32: 13–30.

————, and Behan P. 1982. Left-handedness association with immune diseases, migraine, and developmental learning disorder. *Proceedings of the National Academy of Sciences* 79: 5097–100.

Gibbs, E. L., Fleming, M. M., and Gibbs, F. A. 1954. Diagnosis and prognosis of hypsarrhythmia and infantile spasms. *Pediatrics* 13: 66–72.

Gibbs, F. A., and Gibbs, E. L. 1952. *Atlas of Electroencephalopathy*, vol. 2: *Epilepsy*. Cambridge, Mass.: Addison-Wesley.

Globus, J. H., and Kohn, J. L. 1949. Encephalopathy following pertussis vaccine prophylaxis. *Journal of the American Medical Association* 141(8): 507–9.

Gomez, M. R., and Klass, D. W. 1972. Seizures and other paroxysmal disorders in infants and children. *Current Problems in Pediatrics* 2(6): 3–27.

Gonzalez, E. R. 1982. TV report on DPT galvanizes U.S. pediatricians. *Journal of the American Medical Association* 248(1): 12–23.

Grady, G. W., and Wetterlow, L. H. 1978. Pertussis vaccine: Reasonable doubt? *New England Journal of Medicine* 298(17): 966–67.

Granstroem, M., Granstroem, G., Lindfors, A., and Askeloef, P. 1982. Serologic diagnosis of whooping cough by an enzyme-linked immunosorbent assay using fimbrial hemagglutinin as antigen. *Journal of Infectious Diseases* 146(6): 741–45.

Griffith, A. H. 1978. Reactions after pertussis vaccine: A manufacturer's experiences and difficulties since 1964. *British Medical Journal* (April 1), 809–15.

————. 1981. Vaccination against whooping cough. *Journal of Biological Standardization* 9: 475–82.

————. 1982. ABC of 1 to 7: Whooping cough. *British Medical Journal* 284: 1263.

————, and Freestone, D. S. 1981. Letter to the editor. *British Medical Journal* (June 20).

Halpern, S. R., and Halpern, D. 1955. Reactions from DPT immunization and its relationship to allergic children. *Journal of Pediatrics* 47: 60–67.

Hannik, C. A. 1969. Major reactions after DPT-polio vaccination in the Netherlands. *International Symposium on Pertussis*, Bilthoven. *Symposium Series on Immunobiological Standardization* 13: 161–70. Basel, München, New York: Karger.

————, and Cohen, H. 1978. Changes in plasma insulin concentration and temperature of infants after pertussis vaccination. *International Symposium on Pertussis*, 297–99 (see ref.).

Harrison, H. R., and Fulginiti, V. A. 1980. Bacterial immunizations. *American Journal of Diseases of Children* 134: 184–93.

Hauser, W. A. 1981. The natural history of febrile seizures. In K. B. Nelson and J. H. Ellenberg, eds., *Febrile Seizures*. New York: Raven Press.

Hennessen, W., and Quast, U. 1979. Adverse reactions after pertussis vaccination. *International Symposium on Immunization: Benefit vs. Risk Factors*, Brussels. *Developments in Biological Standardization* 43: 95–100. Basel: Karger.

Hinman, A. R., and Koplan, J. 1984. Pertussis and pertussis vaccine: Reanalysis of benefits, risks, and costs. *Journal of the American Medical Association* 251(23): 3109–13.

Hirtz, D. G., Nelson, K. B., and Ellenberg, J. H. 1982. Seizures following childhood immunizations. *Journal of Pediatrics* 102(1): 14–18.

————, ————, and ————. 1984. The risk of recurrence of nonfebrile seizures in children. *Neurology* 34: 637–41.

Hoefler, K. H., Binder, B., and Koch, M. 1977. Vergleich der wirksamkeit von parenteraler und enteraler pertussis-immunisierung bei kaninchen. *Wiener klinische Wochenschrift* 89: 386–89.

Hoekelman, R. A., ed. 1978. *Principles of pediatrics.* New York: McGraw-Hill.

Hoffman, H. J., Hunter, J. C., and Hasselmeyer, E. G. 1982. SIDS and DTP. In *Seventeenth Immunization Conference Proceedings,* CDC (May), 79–88. Washington, D.C.: GPO.

Hooker, J. M. 1981. A laboratory study of the toxicity of some diphtheria-tetanus-pertussis vaccines. *Journal of Biological Standardization* 9: 493–506.

Hopper, J. M. 1961. Illness after whooping cough vaccination. *Medical Officer* (October 20), 241–44.

Hull, D. 1981. Interpretation of the contraindications to whooping cough vaccination. *British Medical Journal* (November 7), 1231–33.

Idiosyncrasy to whooping-cough vaccine. 1949. *British Medical Journal* (December 24), 1478.

Illingworth, R. 1955. Sudden mental deterioration with convulsions in infancy. *Archives of Disease in Childhood* 30: 529–37.

―――――. 1980. Contraindications to immunization. *British Medical Journal* (July 19), 229.

Immunization in the practice of pediatrics. 4. Immunization procedures. 1951. *Pediatrics* 7: 126–30.

Is it safe? 1981. *British Journal of Hospital Medicine* (July), 5.

Isaacson, P., and Stone, A. 1971. Allergic reactions associated with viral vaccines. *Progress in Medical Virology* 13: 239–70.

Jacob, J., and Manning, F. 1979. Increased intracranial pressure after diphtheria, tetanus and pertussis immunization. *American Journal of Diseases of Children* 133: 217–18.

Jeavons, P. M., and Bower, B. D. 1964. *Infantile spasms: A review of the literature and a study of 112 cases.* London: Spastics Society.

―――――, Harper, J. R., and Bower, B. D. 1970. Long-term prognosis in infantile spasms: A follow-up report on 112 cases. *Developmental Medicine and Child Neurology* 12: 413–21.

Kahn, E., and Cohen, L. M. 1934. Organic drivenness: A brain-stem syndrome and an experience. *New England Journal of Medicine* 14: 748–56.

Kalokerinos, A. 1981. *Every second child.* New Canaan, Conn.: Keats.

Kanai, K. 1980. Japan's experience in pertussis epidemiology and vaccination in the past thirty years. *Japanese Journal of Medical Science and Biology* 33: 107–43.

Kanner, L. 1942–1943. Autistic disturbances of affective contact. *The Nervous Child* 2(1): 217–50.

―――――. 1949. Problems of nosology and psychodynamics of early infantile autism. *American Journal of Orthopsychiatry* 19: 416–26.

Kavee, R. 1979. Babies tested for sudden death syndrome. *The New York Times* (November 18), XXI: 6.

Keller, M. A., Aftandelians, R., and Connor, J. D. 1980. Etiology of pertussis syndrome. *Pediatrics* 66(1): 50–55.

Kendrick, P. 1942. Use of alum-treated pertussis vaccine, and of alum-precipitated combined pertussis vaccine and diphtheria toxoid, for active immunization. *American Journal of Public Health* 32: 615–26.

————. 1943. A field study of alum-precipitated combined pertussis vaccine and diphtheria toxoid for active immunization. *American Journal of Hygiene* 38: 193–202.

————, and Eldering, G. 1936. Progress report on pertussis immunization. *American Journal of Public Health* 26: 8–12.

————, and ————. 1939. A study in active immunization against pertussis. *American Journal of Hygiene* 29: 133–53.

Köng, E. 1953. Zur pertussisimpfung und ihre gegenindikationen. *Helvetica Pediatrica Acta* 8: 90–98.

Kolata, G. 1983. Math genius may have hormonal basis. *Science* 222: 4630.

Koplan, J. P., Schoenbaum, S. C., Weinstein, M. C., and Fraser, D. W. 1979. Pertussis vaccine—An analysis of benefits, risks, and costs. *New England Journal of Medicine* 301(17): 906–11.

Kringelbach, J., and Senstius, J. 1966. Hypsarrhytmia efter triplevakcination. *Nordisk Medicin* 76(9): 1435–36.

Krugman, S., and Katz, S. L. 1977. Childhood immunization procedures. *Journal of the American Medical Association* 237(20): 2228–30.

————, and ————. 1981. *Infectious diseases of children.* 7th ed. St. Louis: C. V. Mosby.

Kulenkampff, M., Schwartzman, J. S., and Wilson, J. 1974. Neurological complications of pertussis inoculation. *Archives of Disease in Childhood* 49: 46–49.

Kurt, T. L., Yeager, A. S., Guenette, S., and Dunlop, S. 1972. Spread of pertussis by hospital staff. *Journal of the American Medical Association* 221 (3): 264–67.

Lapin, J. 1943. *Whooping cough.* Springfield, Ill., and Baltimore, Md.: Charles C. Thomas.

Lederle Laboratories Division, American Cyanamid Co. 1980. Diphtheria and tetanus toxoids and pertussis vaccine adsorbed: Tri-Immunol (package insert. rev. February).

Leslie, P. H., and Gardner, A. D. 1931. The phases of hemophilus pertussis. *Journal of Hygiene* 31: 423–34.

Leviton, A., and Cowan, L. D. 1981. Methodological issues in the epidemiology of seizure disorders in children. *Epidemiologic Reviews* 3: 67–86.

Lewis, J. S. 1982. DTP vaccine—Worth the risk? *TRIAL* (August), 23–29.

Linnemann, C. C., Jr., Perlstein, P. H., Ramundo, N., Minton, S. D., and Englender, G. S. 1975. Use of pertussis vaccine in an epidemic involving hospital staff. *Lancet* (September 20), 540–43.

Linthicum, D. S., Munoz, J. J., and Blaskett, A. 1982. Acute experimental autoimmune encephalomyelitis in mice. *Cellular Immunology* 73: 299–310.

Livingston, S. 1954. *The diagnosis and treatment of convulsive disorders in children.* Springfield, Ill. Charles C. Thomas.

Low, N. L. 1955. Electroencephalographic studies following pertussis immunization. *Journal of Pediatrics* 47: 35–39.

Lurie, L. A., and Levy, S. 1942. Personality changes and behavior disorders of children following pertussis. *Journal of the American Medical Association* 120(12): 890–94.

MacNeil-Lehrer Report: DPT Danger. 1983. Transcript no. 2042 (July 26).

Madsen, T. 1925. Whooping cough: Its bacteriology, diagnosis, prevention, and treatment. *Boston Medical and Surgical Journal* 192(2): 50–60.

————. 1933. Vaccination against whooping cough. *Journal of the American Medical Association* 101(3): 187–88.

Mahler, H. 1979. La sante des enfants du monde. *Afrique Medicale* 18: 716.

Manclark, C. R. 1976. The current status of pertussis vaccine: An overview. *Advances in Applied Microbiology* 20: 1–7. New York: Academic Press.

————. 1981. Pertussis vaccine research. *WHO Bulletin* 59(1): 9–15.

Manclark, C. R., and Hill, J. C., eds. 1978. *International Symposium on Pertussis,* National Institutes of Health, Bethesda, Md. Washington, D.C.: GPO.

Maurer, H., Hoefler, K. H., Hilbe, W., and Huber, E. G. 1979. Erste ergebnisse mit oraler keuchhustenimpfung bei jungen saeuglingen. *Wiener Klinische Wochenschrift* 91(21): 717–18.

Medical Research Council, Whooping Cough Immunization Committee. 1956. Vaccination against whooping cough: Relation between protection in children and results of laboratory tests. *British Medical Journal* (August 25), 454–62.

————. 1959. Vaccination against whooping cough: The final report. *British Medical Journal* (April 18), 994–1000.

Melchior, J. C. 1969. Infantile spasms and vaccinations. *Ugeskrift for Laeger* 131: 17.

————. 1971. Infantile spasms and immunization in the first year of life. *Neuropaediatrie* 3(1): 3–10.

————. 1977. Infantile spasms and early immunization against whooping cough. *Archives of Disease in Childhood* 52: 134–37.

Melin, K. A. 1953. Pertussis immunization in children with convulsive disorders. *Journal of Pediatrics* 43(6): 652–54.

Menkes, J. H. 1980. *Textbook of child neurology.* Philadelphia: Lea and Febiger.

Menolaschino, F. J., and Egger, M. L. 1978. *Medical dimensions of mental retardation.* Lincoln: University of Nebraska Press.

Merritt, H. H. 1979. *A textbook of neurology.* 6th ed. Philadelphia: Lea and Febiger.

Miller, D. L., Alderslade, R., and Ross, E. M. 1982. Whooping cough and whooping cough vaccine: The risks and benefits debate. *Epidemiologic Reviews* 4: 1–24.

————, Ross, E. M., Alderslade, R., Bellman, M. H., and Rawson, N. S. B. 1981. Pertussis immunization and serious acute neurological illness in children. *British Medical Journal* 282: 1595–99.

—————, and Ross, E. M. 1982. ABC of 1 to 7: Whooping cough. *British Medical Journal* 284: 1874.

Miller, H. 1956. Discussion on the neurological complications of the acute specific fevers. *Proceedings of the Royal Society of Medicine* 49: 139–46.

Miller, H. J., and Stanton, J. B. 1954. Neurologic sequelae of prophylactic inoculation. *Quarterly Journal of Medicine* NS 23(89): 1–27.

Miller, J. J., Faber, H. K., Ryan, M. L., Silberberg, R. J., and Lew, E. 1949. Immunization against pertussis during the first four months of life. *Pediatrics* 4: 468–78.

Millichap, J. G. 1976. The hyperactive child. *Practitioner* 217: 61–65.

Mizrahi, A., Hertman, I., Klingberg, M. A., and Kohn, A., eds. 1980. New developments with human and veterinary vaccines. *25th OHOLO Biological Conference*, Zichron Ya'acov, Israel. Israel Institute for Biological Research, Ness-Ziona, Israel. New York: Alan R. Liss.

Money, J., ed. 1966. *The disabled reader: Education of the dyslexic child.* Baltimore: Johns Hopkins University Press.

Morley, D., Woodland, M., and Martin, W. J. 1966. Whooping cough in Nigerian children. *Tropical and Geographical Medicine* 18: 169–82.

Morris, J. A., and Hoffman, J. C. 1983. Letter to the editor. *MD State Medical Journal* (January), 19–20.

Mortimer, E. A., Jr. 1980. Pertussis immunization: Problems, perspectives, prospects. *Hospital Practice* (October), 103–18.

—————, and Jones, P. K. 1978. Pertussis vaccine in the United States: The benefit-risk ratio. In Manclark and Hill (see ref.).

Murphy, M. D., Rasnack, J., Dickson, H. D., Dietch, M., and Brunell, P. A. 1983. Evaluation of the pertussis components of diphtheria-tetanus-pertussis vaccine. *Pediatrics* 71(2): 200–205.

Nelson, J. D. 1978. The changing epidemiology of pertussis in young infants. *American Journal of the Diseases of Children* 132: 371–73.

Nelson, K., and Ellenberg, J. 1976. Predictors of epilepsy in children who have experienced febrile seizures. *New England Journal of Medicine* 295: 1029–33.

Nelson, W. E. 1959. *Textbook of pediatrics.* 7th ed. Philadelphia: W. B. Saunders.

The new vaccines: More uses . . . safer products . . . fresh competition. 1982. *Chemical Week* (November 24).

Noah, N. D. 1976. Attack rates of notified whooping cough in immunized and unimmunized children. *British Medical Journal* (January 17), 128–29.

Oda, M., Izumiya, K., Sato, Y., and Hirayama, M. 1983. Transplacental and transcolostral immunity to pertussis in a mouse model using acellular pertussis vaccine. *Journal of Infectious Diseases* 148(1): 138–45.

Olshin, I. J. 1982. Infectious disease vaccines: Primary care update and review. 1982. *Modern Medicine* (January), 122–25.

Omokoku, B., and Castells, S. 1981. Post-DPT inoculation cervical lymphadenitis in children. *New York State Journal of Medicine* (October), 1667–68.

Pampiglione, G., and Pugh, E. 1975. Infantile spasms and subsequent appearance of tuberous sclerosis syndrome. *Lancet* (November 22), 1046.

Pan American Health Organization. World Health Organization. 1971. *International Conference on the Application of Vaccines Against Viral, Rickettsial, and Bacterial Diseases of Man.* Washington, D.C.: Pan American Health Organization.

Pertussis vaccine. 1981. *British Medical Journal* (May 16), 1563.

Pertussis vaccine and encephalopathy. 1950. *British Medical Journal* (January 14), 110–111.

Physicians' desk reference. 1979. Oradell, N.J.: Medical Economics.

Pittman, M. 1954. Variability of the potency of pertussis vaccine in relation to the number of bacteria. *Journal of Pediatrics* 45: 57–69.

————. 1970. Bordetella pertussis—Bacterial and host factors in the pathogenesis and prevention of whooping cough. In S. Mudd, ed., *Infectious agents and host reactions.* Philadelphia: W. B. Saunders, 239–70.

————. 1979. Pertussis toxin: The cause of the harmful effects and prolonged immunity of whooping cough. A hypothesis. *Reviews of Infectious Diseases* 1(3): 401–412.

————. and Cox, C. B. 1965. Pertussis vaccine testing for freedom-from-toxicity. *Applied Microbiology* 13(3): 447–56.

Pollock, T. M., and Morris, J. 1983. A 7-year survey of disorders attributed to vaccination in North West Thames region. *Lancet* (April 2), 753–57.

Provenzano, R. W., Wetterlow, L. H., and Ipsen, J. 1959. Pertussis immunization in pediatric practice and in public health. *New England Journal of Medicine* 261(10): 473–78.

Robbins, J. B. 1978. Critique of the meeting. In Manclark and Hill (see ref.).

————, Hill, J. C., and Sadoff, J. C. 1982. *Bacterial vaccines.* Seminars in Infectious Diseases, vol. 4. New York: Thieme-Straton.

Robinson, D. A., Mandal, B. K., Ironside, A. G., and Dunbar, F. M. 1981. Whooping cough—A study of severity in hospital cases. *Archives of Disease in Childhood* 56: 687–91.

Robinson, R. J. 1981. The whooping cough controversy. *Archives of Disease in Childhood* 56: 577–80.

Rosanelli, K., Falk, W., Hoefler, K. H., and Seibert, H. 1979. Orale pertussisimmunisierung beim neugeborenen. *Wiener klinische Wochenschrift* 91: 720–22.

Sako, W. 1947. Studies on pertussis immunization. *Journal of Pediatrics* 30: 29–40.

————, Treuting, W. L., Witt, D. B., and Nichamin, S. J. Early immunization against pertussis with alum precipitated vaccine. *Journal of the American Medical Association* 127(7): 379–84.

Salk, J. E. 1984. Considerations in the preparation and use of poliomyelitis virus vaccine. *Journal of the American Medical Association* 251(20): 2700–2709.

Sato, Y., Kimura, M., and Fukumi, H. 1984. Development of a pertussis component vaccine in Japan. *Lancet* (January 21), 122–126.

Sauer, L. 1933(a). Whooping cough: A study in immunization. *Journal of the American Medical Association* 199(4): 239–41.

———. 1933(b). Immunization with bacillus pertussis vaccine. *Journal of the American Medical Association* 101(19): 1449–51.

———. 1935. The known and unknown of bacillus pertussis vaccine. *American Journal of Public Health* 25: 1226–30.

———. 1937. Municipal control of whooping cough. *Journal of the American Medical Association* 109(7): 487–88.

———. 1946. Whooping cough: Prevention and treatment. *Medical Clinics of North America* 30: 45–59.

———. 1959. Earlier poliomyelitis immunization with quadruple antigen. *Quarterly Bulletin of the Northwestern University Medical School* 33: 259–61.

Schain, R. J. 1977. *Neurology of childhood learning disorders.* 2nd ed. Baltimore: Williams and Wilkins.

Shannon, D. C., and Kelly, D. H. 1982. SIDS and Near-SIDS. *New England Journal of Medicine* 306(17): 959–1028.

Shaw, E. B. 1982. Pertussis vaccine: Still an open question? *Pediatrics* 69(3): 386–87.

Should the child with convulsive disorders be immunized against pertussis?" 1953. *Journal of Pediatrics* 43: 746–50.

Singer, J. E., Westphal, M., and Niswander, K. 1968. Relationship of weight gain during pregnancy to birth weight and infant growth and development in the first year of life. *Obstetrics and Gynecology* 31(3): 417–23.

Steinman, L., Sriram, S., Adelman, N. E., Zamvil, S., McDevitt, H. O., and Urich, H. 1982. Murine model for pertussis vaccine encephalopathy: Linkage to H-2. *Nature* 299: 738–40.

Steinschneider, A., Weinstein, S. L., and Diamond, E. 1982. The sudden infant death syndrome and apnea/obstruction during neonatal sleep and feeding. *Pediatrics* 70(6): 858–63.

Stetler, H. C. 1982. Monitoring system for illness following immunization (MSIFI): Strengths and weaknesses of the system. *Seventeenth Immunization Conference Proceedings*, CDC (May), 95–98. Washington, D.C.: GPO.

Stewart, G. T. 1977. Vaccination against whooping cough: Efficacy vs. risks. *Lancet* (January 29), 234–37.

———. 1978. Pertussis vaccine: The United Kingdom's experience. In Manclark and Hill (see ref.).

———. 1979. Whooping cough in Hertfordshire. *Lancet* (September 1), 472–74.

———. 1979. Toxicity of pertussis vaccine: Frequency and probability of reactions. *Journal of Epidemiology and Community Health* 33(2): 150–56.

———. 1979. Letter to the editor. *Lancet* (August 18), 354–355.

———. 1981. Whooping cough in relation to other childhood infections in 1977–1979 in the United Kingdom. *Journal of Epidemiology and Community Health* 35: 139–45.

————. 1980. Benefits and risks of pertussis vaccine. *New England Journal of Medicine* 303(17): 1004.

————. 1982. ABC of 1 to 7: Whooping cough. *British Medical Journal* 284: 1263.

————. 1983. Reactions to pertussis vaccine. *Lancet* (May 28), 1217.

————, and Wilson, J. 1981. Pertussis vaccine and acute neurological disease in children. *British Medical Journal* (June 13), 1968–69.

Stickl, H., Schweier, P., and Van Thiel, D. 1976. Preliminary results with an oral application of killed pertussis bacteria in newborn infants. Fourteenth Congress of the International Association of Biological Standardization, 1975. *Developments in Biological Standardization* 33: 54–56.

Stott, N., and Davis, R. H. 1981. Pertussis vaccine and pseudo whooping cough. *British Medical Journal* 282: 1871.

Ström, J. 1960. Is universal vaccination against pertussis always justified? *British Medical Journal* (October 22), 1184–86.

————. 1967(a). Social development and declining incidence of some common epidemic diseases in children: A study of the incidence in different age groups in Stockholm. *Acta Pediatrica Scandinavica* 56: 159–63.

————. 1967(b). Further experience of reactions, especially of a cerebral nature, in conjunction with triple vaccination: A study based on vaccinations in Sweden, 1959–1965. *British Medical Journal* 4: 320–23.

————. 1969. Reactions of a cerebral nature in conjunction with triple vaccination in Sweden. *International Symposium on Pertussis*, Bilthoven, 1969. *Symposium Series on Immunobiological Standardization* 13: 157–60.

Stuart-Harris, C. H. 1978. Experiences of pertussis in the United Kingdom. In Manclark and Hill (see ref.).

————. 1981. Pertussis vaccine. *British Medical Journal* 283: 494.

Suggestion of a SIDS-DTP link is challenged. 1982. *Medical World News* (June 7), 136–37.

Sutherland, J. A. 1953. Encephalopathy following diphtheria-pertussis inoculation. *Archives of Disease in Childhood* 28: 149–50.

Taranger, J. 1982. Mild clinical course of pertussis in Sweden. *Lancet* (June 12), 1360.

Taylor, E. M., and Emery, J. L. 1982. Immunization and cot deaths. *Lancet* (September 25), 721.

Taylor, F. M. 1952. Myoclonic seizures in infancy and childhood. *Texas State Journal of Medicine* 48: 647–49.

Thrupp, L. D. 1958. Immunization of infants with poliomyelitis vaccine. *Journal of the American Medical Association* 166(2): 160–61.

Toenz, O., and Baic, S. 1980. Zerebrale kramnfanfaelle nach pertussisimpfung. *Schweizerische medizinische Wochenschrift* 110: 1965–70.

Toomey, J. A. 1949. Reactions to pertussis vaccine. *Journal of the American Medical Association* 139(7): 448–50.

Torch, W. C. 1982. Diphtheria-pertussis-tetanus (DPT) immunization: A potential cause of the sudden infant death syndrome (SIDS). American

Academy of Neurology, 34th Annual Meeting, April 25–May 1. *Neurology* 32(4): pt. 2.

Trollfors, B., and Rabo, E. 1981. Whooping cough in adults. *British Medical Journal* (September 12), 696–97.

Tsuboi, T. 1977. Genetic aspects of febrile convulsions. *Human Genetics* 38: 169–73.

Ueoka, K. 1979. Clinical and electroencephalographic study in febrile convulsions, with special reference to follow-up study. *Brain and Development* 1(3): 196.

Vaccination against whooping cough. 1981. *Lancet* (May 23), 1138–39.

Valman, H. B. 1980. Contraindications to immunization. *British Medical Journal* (May 3), 1138–39.

————. 1982. ABC of 1 to 7: Whooping cough. *British Medical Journal* 284, 886–87.

Vazquez, H. J., and Turner, M. 1951. Epilepsia en flexión generalizada. *Archivos Argentinos de Pediatría* 35: 111–41.

Vinken, P. J., and Bruyn, G. W. 1974. *Handbook of clinical neurology. Volume 15: The epilepsies.* Amsterdam and New York: North Holland Publishing Company.

Wade, N. 1972(a). Division of Biologics Standards: In the matter of J. Anthony Morris. *Science* 175(4024): 861–66.

————. 1972(b). Division of Biologics Standards: Scientific management questioned. *Science* 175(4025): 966–70.

————. 1972(c). DBS: Officials confused over powers. *Science* 175(4026): 1089.

————. 1972(d). Division of Biologics Standards: The boat that never rocked. *Science* 175(4027): 1225–30.

————. 1972(e). DBS: Agency contravenes its own regulations. *Science* 175(4030): 34–35.

Weihl, C., Riley, H. D., and Lapin, J. H. 1963. Extracted pertussis antigen: A clinical appraisal. *American Journal of Diseases of Children* 106: 124–29.

Werne J., and Garrow, I. 1946. Fatal anaphylactic shock occurrence in identical twins following second injection of diphtheria toxoid and pertussis antigen. *Journal of the American Medical Association* 131(9): 730–35.

White, R., Finberg, L., and Tramer, A. 1964. The modern morbidity of pertussis in infants. *Pediatrics* 33(5): 705–10.

Whooping cough vaccination. 1975. *British Medical Journal* (October 25), 186–87.

Wilson, G. S. 1967. *The hazards of immunization.* London: Athlone Press.

Williams, W. O. 1981. Whooping cough in adults. *British Medical Journal* 283: 1122.

Wingerson, L., and Bloom, M. 1982. Did vaccine get smeared on national television? *Medical World News* (June 7), 30–32.

Wyeth Laboratories. 1979. Diphtheria and tetanus toxoids and pertussis vaccine adsorbed (product insert) (rev.).

Yannet, H. 1951. The treatment and prognosis of convulsive disorders in children. *Bulletin of the New York Academy of Medicine* 27: 466–74.

————, Deamer, W. C., and Barba, P. S. 1949. American Academy of Pediatrics, Inc. Round Table Discussion. Convulsive Disorders in Children. *Pediatrics* 4(5): 677–80.

Year Book of Pediatrics, 1957–1958. Chicago: Year Book Medical Publishers.

II. Public Documents

GREAT BRITAIN

Department of Health and Social Security. 1981. *Whooping Cough: Reports from the Committee on Safety of Medicines and the Joint Committee on Vaccination and Immunization.* London: Her Majesty's Stationery Office.

UNITED STATES: FEDERAL GOVERNMENT

(a) EXECUTIVE BRANCH

Comptroller General of the United States. 1972. *Problems Involving the Effectiveness of Vaccines: Report to the Subcommittee on Executive Reorganization and Government Research, Committee on Government Operations, U.S. Senate* (March 28).

————. 1973. *Problems in Regulating Selected Vaccines: Report to the Subcommittee on Executive Reorganization and Government Research, Committee on Government Operations, U.S. Senate* (February 7).

————. 1980. *Answers to Questions on Selected FDA Bureau of Biologics' Regulation Activities* (June 6).

Department of Commerce. 1980. *1977 Census of Manufactures: Industry Series: Drugs.*

Department of Education. 1984. *Sixth Annual Report to Congress on the Implementation of P.L. 94-142: The Education for all Handicapped Children Act.*

DEPARTMENT OF HEALTH AND HUMAN SERVICES. PUBLIC HEALTH SERVICE
Centers for Disease Control

Diphtheria and tetanus toxoids and pertussis vaccine. *Morbidity and Mortality Weekly Report (MMWR)* 26: 49 (December 9, 1977).

Diphtheria, tetanus, and pertussis: Guidelines for vaccine prophylaxis and other preventive measures. *MMWR* 30: 32 (August 21, 1981).

DPT vaccination and sudden infant deaths—Tennessee. *MMWR* (March 23, 1979).

Pertussis—England and Wales. *MMWR* 31: 47 (December 3, 1982).

Pertussis—Maryland, 1982. *MMWR* 32: 23 (1983). Reprinted in *Journal of the American Medical Association* 250(2): 159–60.

Project grants for preventive health services—Childhood immunization. Availability of funds for fiscal year 1984. *Federal Register* 49: 1 (January 3, 1984).

Report of illness following vaccination and Guidelines for completing the report of illness following vaccination (rev. November 1980).

Sixteenth Immunization Conference Proceedings, May 18–21, 1981, Atlanta, Georgia. USDHHS, PHS, CDC, Atlanta, Georgia (April 1982).

State Immunization Requirements for School Children. Immunization Division, Center for Prevention Services (February, 1981).

Supplementary statement of contraindications to receipt of pertussis vaccine. *MMWR* 33: 13 (April 6, 1984).

Division of Biologics Standards

Legislative History of the Regulation of Biological Products. USDHEW, PHS, DBS. NIH (1971).

Food and Drug Administration

Code of Federal Regulations. Title 21, chap. 1. sec. 601.25 and 601.26, 610.1, 610.53, 620.1–620.7.

Reclassification procedures to determine that licensed biological products are safe, effective, and not misbranded under prescribed, recommended, or suggested conditions of use: Proposed revision. *Federal Register* 46(11): 4634–39 (January 16, 1981).

National Center for Health Services Research

Estimated Economic Costs of Selected Medical Events Known or Suspected to be Related to the Administration of Common Vaccines. USDHHS, PHS, Office of Health Research, Statistics, and Technology (April 9, 1981).

National Institutes of Health

Research Grants Index, 1975–1976, 1976, 1982.

National Institute of Allergy and Infectious Disease

NIAID Awards: Fiscal Year 1982.
NIAID Awards: Fiscal Year 1983.

National Institute of Child Health and Human Development

The NICHHD Cooperative Epidemiologic Study of SIDS Risk Factors. Questionnaire (December 31, 1979).

National Institute of Neurological Disease and Stroke

The Collaborative Study on Cerebral Palsy, Mental Retardation, and other Neurological and Sensory Disorders of Infancy and Childhood. Pt. II-C. Forms: 7—Year and Final (April 1970).

(b) LEGISLATIVE BRANCH

(i) HOUSE OF REPRESENTATIVES

Health Research Extension Act of 1982. *Report of the Committee on Energy and Commerce to Accompany H.R. 6457.* U.S. Congress, House of Representatives, 97th Cong., 2nd sess. Report No. 97–791 (August 23, 1982).

Respecting congressional oversight and agency studies of the appropriateness of continued use of the pertussis vaccine. H. Cong. Res. 313 (April 21, 1982).

(ii) SENATE

Hearings

Consumer Safety Act of 1972. *Hearings Before the Subcommittee on Executive Reorganization and Government Research of the Committee on Government Operations*, U.S. Senate, 92nd Cong., 2nd sess. on Titles I and II of S. 3419 (April 20, 21 and May 3, 4, 1972).

Immunization and Preventive Medicine. *Hearing Before the Subcommittee on Investigations and General Oversight of the Committee on Labor and Human Resources*, U.S. Senate, 97th Cong., 2nd sess., To Examine Adverse Drug Reactions from Immunization, Federal Efforts in Preventive Medicine, and Characteristics of Certain Diseases (May 7, 1982). Testimony by W. H. Foege, R. H. Parrott, V. A. Fulginiti, S. L. Fannin, A. Hinman, and H. Meyer.

Oversight of Immunization Cost. *Hearings Before the Subcommittee on Investigations and General Oversight of the Committee on Labor and Human Resources*, U.S. Senate, 97th Cong. 2nd sess., To Review Federal and State Expenditures for the Purchase of Children's Vaccines (July 22, 1982). Testimony by J. Litvak and A. R. Hinman.

Task Force Report on Pertussis. *Hearing Before the Committee on Labor and Human Resources*, U.S. Senate, 98th Cong., 1st sess., on Examination of the Task Force Report on the Pertussis Vaccine (July 22, 1983). Testimony by W. R. Dowdle, W. S. Jordan, J. C. Petricciani, K. G. Bart, J. H. Schwartz, and G. T. Stewart.

Bills

National Childhood Vaccine-Injury Compensation Act. *Congressional Record*—U.S. Senate (November 17, 1983).

To Require a Study on the Safety and Effectiveness of the Pertussis Vaccine. *Congressional Record*—U.S. Senate (September 23, 1982).

Speeches

Bumpers, Dale. 1981(a). "To Restore Funds for Immunization Programs." *Congressional Record*—*U.S. Senate* (April 2).

————. 1981(b). "Success of Immunization Program." *Congressional Record*—U.S. Senate (June 24).

————. 1982. "Resolution Relating to Preventive Health Programs." *Congressional Record*—U.S. Senate (March 30).

————. 1983. "The DPT Vaccine." *Congressional Record*—U.S. Senate (June 9).

(iii) OFFICE OF TECHNOLOGY ASSESSMENT

Compensation for Vaccine-Related Injuries: A Technical Memorandum (November 1980).

(c) JUDICIARY

Archie Cude et ux., Appellants v. State of Arkansas et al., Appellees. Supreme Court of Arkansas (377 S.W. 2d 816, 1964).

Jacobson v. Massachusetts. U.S. Supreme Court (197 U.S. 11, October term, 1904).

Eric R. Tinnerholm v. Parke, Davis, and Co. U.S. Court of Appeals, 2nd Circuit (411 F. 2d 48, 1950).

UNITED STATES—STATE GOVERNMENTS—HEALTH
DEPARTMENTS

Important Information About Diphtheria, Tetanus, and Pertussis and DTP, DT, and Td Vaccines (rev. 12/1/77, 10/1/80, and 3/1/83).

III. Unpublished Materials

Correspondence

L. J. Baraff, M.D., to H. L. Coulter, Ph.D., 4/1/84.

A. Bernstein, Ph.D., Managing Director, Wyeth Laboratories, to J. Robbins, M.D., Bureau of Biologics, FDA, 6/18/79.

R. Bogash, Ph.D., President, Wyeth Laboratories, to the Honorable P. Hawkins, U.S. Senate, 10/20/83 and 4/30/84.

R. Bogash, Ph.D., President, Wyeth Laboratories, to "Dear Doctor," 6/13/84.

E. N. Brandt, Jr., M.D., Assistant Secretary for Health, USDHHS, PHS to the Honorable D. A. Mica, U.S. House of Representatives, 7/21/82.

J. D. Cherry, M.D., to H. L. Coulter, Ph.D., 1/17/84.

H. L. Coulter, Ph.D., to L. J. Baraff, M.D., 12/19/83 and 1/11/84.

H. L. Coulter, Ph.D., to J. D. Cherry, M.D., 11/4/83.

H. L. Coulter, Ph.D., to W. Falk, M.D., and K. Rosanelli, M.D., 8/19/83, 10/23/83, and 1/11/84.

H. L. Coulter, Ph.D., to A. H. Griffith, M.D., 1/20/84.

H. L. Coulter, Ph.D., to W. C. Torch, M.D., 1/26/84.

W. Falk, M.D., and K. Rosanelli, M.D., to H. L. Coulter, Ph.D., 9/5/83, 12/13/83, and 2/10/84.

J. P. Davis, M.D., State Epidemiologist, State of Wisconsin, to K. C. Geraghty, M.D., 9/29/83.

W. Dowdle, Ph.D., Director, CDC, to J. Schwartz, Esq., 7/20/83 and 8/4/83.

W. Ehrengut, M.D., to B.L. Fisher, 6/14/82 and 9/7/82.

B. L. Fisher to L. J. Baraff, M.D., 7/22/82.

B. L. Fisher to W. Ehrengut, M.D., 5/28/82 and 7/16/82.

B. L. Fisher to A. H. Hayes, Jr., M.D., Commissioner, FDA, 7/30/82.

B. L. Fisher to D. C. Shannon, M.D., 7/19/82.

B. L. Fisher to G. T. Stewart, M.D., 7/16/82 and 6/27/83.

B. L. Fisher to J. Ström, M.D., 5/27/82 and 7/16/82.

A. H. Griffith, M.D., to H. L. Coulter, Ph.D., 1/25/84.

K. C. Geraghty, M.D., to J. W. St. Geme, Jr., M.D., 9/9/83.

K. C. Geraghty, M.D., to E. Ornitz, M.D., 3/17/84.

H. M. Meyer, Jr., M.D., Director, Bureau of Biologics, FDA, to A. Bernstein, Ph.D., Managing Director, Wyeth Laboratories, 7/11/79.

E. M. Ornitz, M.D., to K. C. Geraghty, M.D., 4/19/84.

R. G. Penner, Director, Congressional Budget Office, to the Honorable Orrin Hatch, U.S. Senate, 2/7/84.

J. C. Petricciani, M.D., Director, Office of Biologics, FDA, to B. L. Fisher, 11/17/82.

D. B. Reynolds, Director of Marketing, Connaught Laboratories, to P. A. Brunell, M.D., 8/1/83.

D. B. Reynolds, Director of Marketing, Connaught Laboratories, to K. C. Geraghty, M.D., 9/13/83.

D. C. Shannon, M.D., to B. L. Fisher, 7/27/82.

J. W. St. Geme, Jr., M.D., to K. C. Geraghty, M.D., 9/16/83.

G. T. Stewart, M.D., to B. L. Fisher, 6/11/82, 7/28/82, and 8/7/82.

J. Ström, M.D., to B. L. Fisher, 6/28/82 and 8/18/82.

Interviews

Robert Ancona, M.D., Chairman, Subcommittee on Immunization and Infectious Diseases, Maryland Medical and Chirurgical Faculty, March 15, 1984.

Robert Barrie, M.D., Charing Cross Hospital, London, England, February 19, 1984.

M. Z. Bierly, M.D., Wyeth Laboratories, Radnor, Pennsylvania, February 22, 1984.

George Hardy, M.D., Assistant Administrator, CDC, January 17, 1984.

Charles Manclark, Ph.D., National Center for Drugs and Biologics, FDA, January 6 and 13, 1983.

Daniel Levitt, M.D., Ph.D., Guthrie Research Institute, November 8, 1983.

John Mitchell, M.D., Chief, Bacterial Products Program, Michigan Department of Public Health, February 23, 1984.

J. Anthony Morris, Ph.D., January 12, 1983.

Margaret Pittman, Ph.D., January 19 and February 20, 1984.

John Robbins, M.D., Bureau of Biologics, FDA, December 23, 1982 and January 6, 1983.

News Releases and Talking Papers

American Academy of Pediatrics. "Pediatricians Reaffirm Need for Pertussis Vaccine," April 20, 1982.

Commonwealth of Virginia, Department of Health. "Pertussis Immunization," April 22, 1982.

Dissatisfied Parents Together News. "Statement of Dissatisfied Parents Together (DPT) on Introduction of the National Childhood Vaccine-Injury Compensation Act," November 17, 1983.

State of Maryland, Department of Health and Mental Hygiene. "Maryland

Whooping Cough Epidemic Now Numbers 41 Infants and Youths," August 31, 1982.

—————. "Pertussis Strikes Incompletely Immunized Infants, Study Shows," January 21, 1983.

USDHHS, PHS, CDC. "Pertussis Vaccine Controversy," April 14, 1982.

USDHHS, PHS, FDA. "FDA Talk Paper: Pertussis Vaccine," April 20, 1982.

USDHHS, PHS, FDA. "Comments on DPT Issues Raised on the WRC/NBC TV Program of April 19, 1982." Prepared by a staff member of the Division of Bacterial Products, Office of Biologics, National Center for Drugs and Biologics, FDA.

Transcripts and Memoranda of Meetings, Governmental and Industrial

USDHEW, PHS, CDC. Memorandum from A. David Brandling-Bennett, M.D., Chief, Surveillance and Assessment Branch, to Alan R. Hinman, M.D., Director, Immunization Division, dated May 9, 1979, on "Meeting on DTP Vaccination and Sudden Infant Death Held at the Center for Disease Control on April 28, 1979."

USDHEW, PHS, CDC. Memorandum from William H. Foege, M.D., Assistant Surgeon General, to the Assistant Secretary for Health and Surgeon General, dated June 19, 1979, on "Meeting on DPT Vaccination and Sudden Infant Death, April 26, 1979—INFORMATION MEMORANDUM."

USDHHS, PHS, FDA, NIAID, NIH. New Pertussis Vaccines—Laboratory and Clinical Evaluation, February 11–12, 1982.

USDHHS, PHS, FDA. Open Meeting—Pertussis and Pertussis Vaccines—Interagency Group to Monitor Vaccine Development, Production, and Usage, April 26, 1983.

USDHHS, PHS, Interagency Group to Monitor Vaccine Production, Development, and Usage. Pertussis and Pertussis Vaccines: Executive Summary, Pertussis and Pertussis Vaccines [spring, 1983].

USDHHS, PHS, FDA, National Center for Drugs and Biologics. Office of Biologics Research and Review. Meeting on Pertussis Vaccine: Status of Current Research, November 10, 1983.

USDHHS, PHS, FDA, Bureau of Biologics. Ad Hoc Meeting on Relation Between DPT Vaccines and Sudden Infant Death Syndrome (SIDS), March 19, 1979.

Meetings between officers of DPT (Dissatisfied Parents Together) and FDA officials, February 28 and March 10, 1983.

Meeting between officers of DPT (Dissatisfied Parents Together) and the AAP Red Book Committee, September 13, 1983.

Pharmaceutical Manufacturers Association, Pertussis Vaccine Producers. Meeting at Drake Hotel, Chicago, Illinois, March 5, 1964.

State of Michigan, Department of Public Health. Immunization Bio-Products Cross Program Meetings, October 7 and 21, November 4 and 18, December 2 and 16, 1975; January 27, February 10, September 7, and October 5, 1976.

Television Program Transcripts

DPT: Vaccine Roulette. Broadcast April 19, 1981, WRC-TV, Washington, D.C.

Healthbeat, with Timothy Johnson, M.D. Broadcast December 20, 1982, WTTG-TV, Washington, D.C.

MacNeil-Lehrer Report. July 26, 1983. Transcript no. 2042: "DPT Danger."

Panorama, with Ross Crystal. Broadcast December 21, 1982, WTTG-TV, Washington, D.C.

Testimony Before the U.S. Senate Committee on Labor and Human Resources, May 3, 1984

Richard Bogash, Ph.D., President, Wyeth Laboratories.

Edward N. Brandt, Jr., M.D., Assistant Secretary for Health, PHS, USDHHS.

Connaught Laboratories, Inc.

John E. Lyons, President, Merck Sharp, and Dohme Division of Merck Co., Inc.

Alan R. Nelson, M.D., American Medical Association.

Jeffrey H. Schwartz, Dissatisfied Parents Together (DPT).

Martin H. Smith, M.D., F.A.A.P., American Academy of Pediatrics.

Unpublished Reports and Articles

Association of American Medical Colleges. 1982. *U.S. Medical School Finances* (October).

Christensen, C. N., M.D. 1962. Pertussis vaccine encephalopathy (May).

Ehrengut, W., and Stewart, G. T. 1982. Critique of E. R. Gonzalez, "TV Report on DPT Galvanizes U.S. Pediatricians," *Journal of the American Medical Association* 248(1): 12–23.

Geraghty, K. C. 1983. SIDS, DPT, and the monitoring system for illness following vaccination (MSIFI).

————. 1984. Death events shortly following DPT in Northern California.

Morris, J. A., Ph.D. 1982. Letter to R. Longenecker, Maryland Department of Health, on Maryland whooping cough incidence in 1982 (September 13).

————, and Hoffman, J. C. 1983. *An Analysis of Reported Pertussis Cases in Wisconsin in 1982* (April 26).

Shockley, M. 1982. *Pertussis: A Vaccine's History* (prepared for use by the WRC-TV staff in preparing "DPT: Vaccine Roulette") (spring).

Stetler, H. 1983. Adverse events—Current trends in surveillance. *Eighteenth Immunization Conference*, Atlanta, Georgia (May 17–19).

Torch, W. C. 1982. *Abstract of Presentation made at 34th Annual Meeting of American Academy of Neurology.* April 25–May 1, Washington, D.C.

USDHEW, PHS, FDA. 1979. *Panel on Review of Bacterial Vaccines and Bacterial Toxoids: Report* (April/May).

USDHHS, PHS, FDA, Bureau of Biologics. 1980. *Pertussis Vaccine Project: Rates, Nature and Etiology of Adverse Reactions Associated with DTP Vaccine.* Prepared for the Bureau of Biologics (March 18).

Internal Memoranda and Reports, Government and Industry

Memoranda from the FDA, Connaught Laboratories, and Lederle Laboratories on the Connaught/Lederle "hot lot," March/April 1980.

USDHHS, PHS, FDA, Bureau of Biologics. Twenty-four project reports, October 1, 1980 through September 30, 1981.

————, ————, ————, ————. Instructions, dated May 3 and 12, 1978, on preparation of B. pertussis challenge culture, pertussis vaccine potency assay, mouse weight gain test, and animal randomization.